TELe-Health

Recent advances in technology and medicine are rapidly changing the face of health care. A revolution is occurring in diagnosis and treatment thanks to the implementation of instrumentation and techniques deriving from engineering and research. In addition, a cultural conversion is taking place in which geographical and social boundaries are about to be overcome, resulting in enhanced availability and quality of care. Telemedicine has been considered a possible means of improving health care worldwide that is likely to change the way in which doctors deal with patients and diseases. While various restraints continue to limit the application of telemedicine in different settings and different areas of health, the innovations emerging from eHealth and telecare could stimulate a great leap forward for medicine, provided that some basic rules are taken into consideration and followed. In this series, diverse aspects of tele-health – preventive, promotive, and curative – will be covered by leading experts in the field with the aim of realizing the full potential of the new and exciting technological solutions at our disposal.

Jacopo Demurtas
Editor

Remote Consultation in Primary Care

A Step-by-step Approach to Remote Consultation and Triage

Springer

Editor

Jacopo Demurtas
Family Medicine Department
USL Toscana Sud-Est
Capalbio, Italy

ISSN 2198-6037 ISSN 2198-6045 (electronic)
TELe-Health
ISBN 978-3-031-89660-6 ISBN 978-3-031-89661-3 (eBook)
https://doi.org/10.1007/978-3-031-89661-3

This Springer imprint is published by the registered company Springer Nature Switzerland AG
The registered company address is: Gewerbestrasse 11, 6330 Cham, Switzerland

To Vittoria,

Dad (JD)

Foreword

The demand and service for care are becoming increasingly out of balance. Not only in Europe but everywhere in the world. One of the options for restoring that balance is by developing digital, remote care. Not only to determine the urgency and care for a medical problem but also for follow-up treatment. A necessary but also an enormous challenge.

However, how reliable and safe are these remote ways of consultations? What is the quality of these new digital roads? How should users, doctors and patients, use them? How to respond if you as a user are unsure about a given advice? How do health-insurers deal with these new developments? Who will develop and pay these programs? the government, private companies?

This book discusses these and many other questions about the challenges of providing remote care.

Haaren, Netherlands — Hay Derkx

Preface

If you are holding this book in your hand, or rather scrolling it on some sort of device, you are interested in telemedicine, perhaps involved in remote consultation and/or interested in the peculiar dimension of the doctor-patient relationship that remote consultation implies.

In all cases, you are welcome to this attempt at synthesizing new and older evidence regarding this inexplicably neglected topic.

It still feels like "remote" is just for out of hour physicians. Alas, it is not.

And inevitably, it will involve more and more healthcare professionals in the years to come.

When I give lectures on the topic, I am used to starting by quoting the Depeche Mode and their Personal Jesus: "someone who hears your prayers, someone who cares."

In this era, having someone that is able and competent in dealing with people, delivering a human touch from somewhere remote, adds an enormous value to their skills, as proven by several companies investing in education in this field and experimenting hybrid models of remote care.

After an epidemiological and normative introduction, we will *delve* in the complex *tapestry* of remote communication and relationship, then we will explore several *avenues* and go beyond remote consultation, always considering that technologies are quick to become outdated.

Dive in…This book was deeply and unevenly woven with AI. It took me years before understanding that in research, and notably in this field, the attempt to improve our writing and be more effective was inevitable and forgivable.

I want to whole heartedly thank all the enthusiast, proactive authors of this book.

Guys, we made it.

Now it's up to you, reader. Paraphrasing the Depeche Mode again: Turn the page, I'll make you a believer (hopefully).

Capalbio, Italy — Jacopo Demurtas

Contents

Part I

General Background

1 The Paradigm Shift of Remote Consultation

Jacopo Demurtas, Hans Eguia, Andreas Meer,
and Ana Luísa Neves

1.1 Introduction

Remote consultation is a real medical act, and considering the shortage of healthcare professionals and the burden on healthcare systems, its role will become even more important in the years to come. However, a paradigm shift is needed—a broadened approach in which remote consultation is perceived and recognized as a genuine consultation, comparable to face-to-face encounters with the caring physician [1].

The traditional treatment paradigm is characterized by the dichotomy of outpatient and inpatient care. When COVID-19 struck, doctors and healthcare professionals worldwide were forced to change their care delivery methods. Lockdowns imposed the need for consultations by video or telephone, with severe cases referred to emergency services. Doctors had to develop their skills in remote consultation and triage, even if they had no prior experience in handling calls, and gradually became accustomed to it, at least to manage COVID-19 cases during the lockdowns [2–4].

J. Demurtas
Clinical and Experimental Medicine PhD Program, University of Modena and Reggio Emilia, Modena, Italy

Family Medicine Department, USL Toscana Sud-Est, Capalbio, Italy

H. Eguia
Universitat Oberta de Catalunya, Barcelona, Spain

A. Meer
CEO In4medicine Ltd., Berne, Switzerland

A. L. Neves (✉)
Imperial NIHR Patient Safety Translational Research Centre, Institute of Global Health Innovation, Imperial College London, London, UK
e-mail: ana.luisa.neves14@imperial.ac.uk

J. Demurtas (ed.), *Remote Consultation in Primary Care*, TELe-Health,
https://doi.org/10.1007/978-3-031-89661-3_1

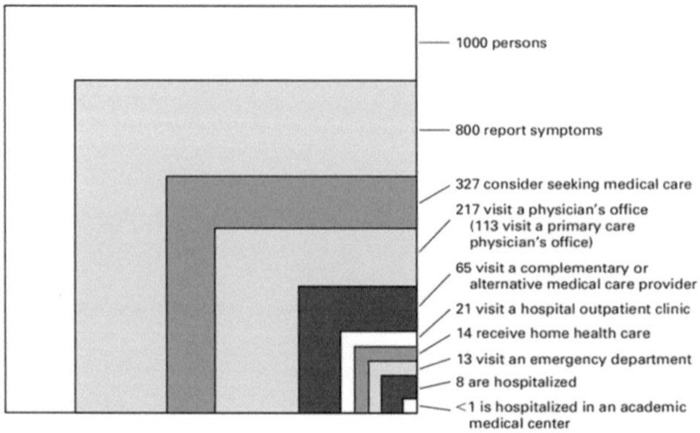

Fig. 1.1 White–Williams–Greenberg diagram [10]

This was a forced change, driven by the pandemic; however, it is widely acknowledged that remote consultation will be a part of the healthcare routine in the future [5]. The need to manage the heavy workload and the shortage of healthcare professionals will necessitate the implementation and scaling up of remote consultation as a standard model of care [6, 7].

After the pandemic, the world has faced a crisis: fewer resources, burned-out healthcare professionals, shortage of healthcare workers, and declining healthcare services [8]. To address this scenario, doctors, notably primary care physicians worldwide, need to embrace the useful tools of remote consultations.

Following the pandemic, a new understanding is gaining ground. Telemedicine is now positioned before outpatient care and has a firm place in follow-up treatment, resulting in a healthcare continuum:

healthy → telemedicine → outpatient → inpatient → outpatient → telemedicine → healthy.

In the digital age, telemedicine must be integrated into the ecology of medical care, including primary care; this is depicted in the White–Williams–Greenberg diagram [9], shown Fig. 1.1, which should be revised accordingly. This evolution of the model is now happening, driven by three major forces: digitalization, the shortage of generalists and specialists in medicine, and a new understanding of communication.

1.2 Models of Remote Care in Primary Care

1.2.1 Remote Consultation

Remote consultation can serve as a relevant alternative to in-person visits, as it allows for prompt and cost-effective healthcare delivery. This modality can be offered via telephone or video, in either a synchronous (real-time interaction between patient and provider) [11] or asynchronous (exchange of information without real-time interaction) manner. Remote consultation holds numerous advantages that make it an appealing option, and it will be the central focus of this book, explored further in the upcoming chapters.

Notably, we will focus on its relevance in triage and correct assessment of patients' conditions and prognosis, by phone or video.

1.2.2 Remote Monitoring

Remote monitoring, also known as remote patient monitoring, uses digital technologies to collect health data from individuals in one location and securely transmit that information to healthcare providers in a different locations for assessment and recommendations [12].

1.2.3 Mobile Health Apps

Mobile health (mHealth) apps, another key component of remote care, leverage smartphone capabilities to provide a range of healthcare services, from appointment scheduling to chronic disease management. These apps can serve as valuable tools for patients to actively engage in their own care and for providers to extend their reach beyond the clinic.

We will further explore their role in symptom checking and remote assessment.

1.2.4 Hybrid Care Models

The future of primary care will likely involve a combination of in-person visits and remote care modalities, creating a hybrid model that capitalizes on the strengths of each approach.

1.3 Importance of the Paradigm Shift, Drivers, and Benefits for Patients

1.3.1 Importance of the Paradigm Shift and Drivers for Transformation

For decades, numerous initiatives have aimed to integrate virtual consultations into healthcare systems—but initiatives have been scattered, with uneven implementation and adoption rates.

In the United States, Kaiser Permanente provides secure email communication and routine telephone and video consultations [13]. In the United Kingdom, telephone consultations have become standard practice. Many other healthcare systems globally have similarly advocated for virtual approaches [14–20]. With the onset of COVID-19, the primary care landscape was radically transformed, with the adoption of digital innovation scaling up globally [21, 22].

The pandemic drove rapid, global acceptance of virtual solutions and spurring services to integrate new technologies, including virtual consultations and remote monitoring, into care delivery [23–25]. In response, many countries issued national guidelines promoting virtual triage and consultation systems, enabling general practitioners (GPs) and patients worldwide to shift from in-person visits to virtual care within just weeks. While previous evidence on virtual care in general practice came from relatively small, localized trials, the pandemic pushed patients, providers, and health systems to rely on virtual consultations as the primary means of accessing care. This unprecedented, global "real-life experiment" provided us with a unique opportunity to understand the key challenges and benefits of virtual primary care, offering insights to help shape its future development.

In a study evaluating the perspectives of general practitioners (GPs) across 20 countries [26], respondents highlighted key drivers for virtual care implementation. They noted that the integration of virtual care during the COVID-19 pandemic has significantly accelerated digital transformation, enhancing awareness and trust, improving digital skills among patients and providers, and expanding technical capabilities. Some participants pointed to the swift rollout of new digital tools, such as e-referrals, e-prescriptions, and electronic fit-to-work certificates. Additional impacts included updates to legal and regulatory frameworks, particularly in terms of the legal context and remuneration for virtual care tasks.

1.3.2 Potential Benefits for Patients

Campbell et al. provided a comprehensive evaluation of GPs' perspectives on the key benefits of virtual consultations [27]. These benefits included reduced COVID-19 exposure risks, improved access, and continuity of care for those with limited access to in-person consultations, as well as the facilitation of remote triage. For patients, virtual consultations enhance convenience, communication, and empowerment. For healthcare providers, they offered greater work flexibility and more control over their schedules. At the health system level, GPs considered that virtual consultations accelerated digital transformation by increasing awareness, trust, adoption, skills, and technical capacity, as well as prompting updates to legal and regulatory frameworks.

While research performed before the pandemic has explored the impact of virtual consultations on care effectiveness and efficiency, often focusing on specific clinical conditions or using broad definitions of remote services, a significant gap remained in the assessment of the effects of virtual consultations on safety, patient-centeredness, timeliness, and equity, with much of the existing literature limited to scoping or rapid evidence reviews. A recent review [27] has systematically assessed the impact of virtual consultations on primary care quality, mapping it, using the Institute of Medicine (IOM) framework to evaluate its impact across six quality domains: efficiency, effectiveness, safety, patient-centeredness, timeliness, and equity [28, 29].

The findings of this systematic review—including a total of 30 studies and encompassing 4,469,333 participants—indicate that virtual consultations can be as effective as, or even more effective than, face-to-face care for managing certain conditions, including mental illness, smoking cessation, and alcohol reduction [27]. Of the five studies examining patient-centeredness, four (80%) reported positive impacts on aspects such as patient engagement, though a negative impact was noted regarding patients' perceived autonomy support—specifically, their sense of authority figures supporting their autonomy. Virtual consultations also appear to reduce waiting times, reduce costs for patients, and decrease follow-up rates in secondary and tertiary care (though they may increase the need for additional GP visits compared to face-to-face consultations) [27].

The adoption of alternative service models during the pandemic will have long-term effects on patient safety; it can equally represent an opportunity for positive change, while maintaining safety as a prerequisite for service transformation [30].

While virtual consultations offer several advantages, they also come with a range of challenges and limitations. In the next section, we will explore these issues in detail, highlighting areas where virtual care may fall short or require further adaptation.

1.4 Challenges, Limitations, and Facilitators

1.4.1 Limitations and Challenges to Remote Consultation Implementation

Remote consultations promise greater accessibility and flexibility in healthcare but face numerous challenges that slow widespread adoption. Technical and infrastructure issues are among the most significant barriers, as effective remote consultations require a reliable internet connection and secure, specialized software to support patient-provider interactions [31]. In many rural and low-resource areas, limited internet bandwidth and insufficient access to technology make remote consultations difficult or even impossible. Integrating telemedicine software with existing electronic health record (EHR) systems further complicates the situation, as compatibility issues and technical complexities hinder seamless data exchange [32–34].

Legal and regulatory obstacles also arise, as remote consultations can span regions with differing rules and requirements. Licensing healthcare providers to practice across state or national boundaries and ensuring access to specific medications are just two of the many regulatory issues that need to be addressed. Without a clear framework, healthcare systems face legal risks and administrative burdens that discourage the adoption of remote consultations.

Privacy and security concerns are also paramount. Remote consultations involve the exchange of sensitive medical information, which makes data protection crucial. Ensuring secure, encrypted connections is necessary to maintain patient trust and comply with privacy laws. Yet, in lower-income regions, healthcare providers may rely on cost-effective platforms that lack adequate security features, putting patient data at risk and further limiting the scope of remote consultations.

Ethical concerns surrounding privacy also need careful consideration. Both patients and providers must feel assured that remote consultations are conducted in private, especially during sensitive discussions. For instance, a patient receiving critical news during a remote consultation in a public or workplace setting may experience distress, raising ethical concerns for the provider. Providers must ensure that remote consultations are conducted in secure, private settings to uphold ethical standards and maintain patient trust.

The financial burden of implementing remote consultation systems also poses a significant challenge. Developing the necessary infrastructure, training staff, and maintaining secure, reliable platforms require substantial investment, often beyond the reach of healthcare providers in underserved regions. In addition, the cost to patients—especially in rural areas where incomes are generally lower—can deter many from using remote consultation services, further restricting the reach of this technology.

Human factors, such as resistance to new technologies and digital literacy challenges, play a major role. Both healthcare providers and patients often show resistance to change, especially when it involves adapting to unfamiliar digital tools. Some healthcare providers express concerns about their ability to build a strong rapport with patients remotely, fearing that remote consultations lack the depth and immediacy of in-person interactions. For patients, particularly older adults, remote consultations can represent a steep learning curve. Although digital literacy improved during the COVID-19 pandemic, many still find the process intimidating or inadequate for addressing their healthcare needs [35].

Concerns about the quality of care in remote consultations contribute to reluctance among both healthcare providers and patients. The lack of face-to-face interaction may lead some to perceive remote consultations as inferior rather than different, and healthcare providers may worry about missing subtle physical cues that could influence diagnosis and treatment. Providers may struggle to incorporate remote consultations into their already full schedules, leading to rushed interactions or inadequate follow-ups [36].

Organizational changes necessary for effective remote consultation also create friction. Adopting telemedicine often requires redefining roles, adjusting workflows, and changing long-standing practices, which can be challenging for healthcare teams accustomed to traditional models. Communication barriers, too, present unique challenges, as remote consultations may be difficult for patients with disabilities or language barriers. During the pandemic, some patients faced considerable difficulties accessing their providers due to hearing or visual impairments or language issues, highlighting the need for more inclusive and supportive solutions [35, 36].

1.4.2 Facilitators

Despite these barriers, several factors can facilitate successful remote consultation systems. Building a strong technological foundation is essential to support reliable connections, secure data transmission, and high-quality video consultations. Proper training for healthcare providers and patients is equally important, helping them adapt to remote consultations with confidence and reducing the frustration that can come with learning to use new digital tools. Support from healthcare leadership and collaboration among providers and technology experts also play a crucial role in making remote consultations effective, ensuring systems are user-friendly and accessible [31].

Remote consultations can offer substantial benefits, especially in underserved and remote areas where travel to healthcare facilities is challenging (costly or impractical). By reducing travel time and costs, they make healthcare more accessible and convenient, particularly for those who face geographic and logistical barriers to in-person care [36, 37]. With thoughtful planning and support, remote consultations can evolve from a promising innovation into a valuable component of the healthcare landscape, making quality care accessible to more people regardless of their location [38–40].

When establishing a telemedicine project, it is essential to have a well-prepared implementation and sustainability plan, with strategies that allow the objectives to be achieved despite any changes that may occur during the project's development. Furthermore, evaluation systems should be in place to obtain feedback on whether the telemedicine project has achieved its goals or if there are areas that need improvement [41]. Finally, it is important to understand the barriers and facilitators in telemedicine, both from the organizational and service facilitator perspectives, to establish an effective and orderly plan that allows the use of technology to help patients and achieve positive results [42]. This will be feasible if the potential problems are identified and strategies to overcome them are developed [43–46].

1.5 Conclusions

Future directions for virtual consultations should focus on a comprehensive evaluation of their impacts, using real-world data and mixed methodologies to assess not only clinical effectiveness but also patterns of use and adoption. A successful implementation will require deliberate efforts to consider the contextual factors, technology infrastructure, awareness and experience, safety and risk management, strategic planning and supporting policies—and continuous monitoring and evaluation [26]. Accompanying policies should aim to minimize digital exclusion, enhance the patient experience, and require rigorous evaluations of virtual primary care both during and beyond the pandemic. These policies should also integrate lessons learned into legal and regulatory frameworks to ensure the long-term, sustainable use of virtual care.

References

1. Johansson AM, Lindberg I, Söderberg S (2014) Patients' experiences with specialist care via video consultation in rural areas. http://downloads.hindawi.com/journals/ijta/2014/143824.pdf
2. Ochal M, Romaszko M, Glińska-Lewczuk K, Gromadziński L, Romaszko J. Assessment of the consultation rate with general practitioners in the initial phase of the COVID-19 pandemic. Int J Environ Res Public Health. 2020;17(21):7710. https://doi.org/10.3390/ijerph17217710.
3. Gabriel C, Mathiot A, Boumediane M, Vernet P, Schwebel M, Figueiredo CD, Gouzou S, Velten M, Liverneaux P, Facca S. Organization of outpatient consultations at a hand surgery department in a French university hospital during the COVID-19 lockdown. Hand Surg Rehabil. 2020, October 29;40(1):17–24. https://doi.org/10.1016/j.hansur.2020.10.006.
4. Murphy M, Scott LJ, Salisbury C, Turner A, Scott A, Denholm R, Lewis R, Iyer G, Macleod J, Horwood J. Implementation of remote consulting in UK primary care following the COVID-19 pandemic: a mixed-methods longitudinal study. Br J Gen Pract. 2021;71(704):e166–77. https://doi.org/10.3399/bjgp.2020.0948.
5. Iyengar KP, Jain VK, Vaishya R. Pitfalls in telemedicine consultations in the era of COVID 19 and how to avoid them. Diabetes Metab Syndr. 2020;14(5):797–9. https://doi.org/10.1016/j.dsx.2020.06.007.
6. Ramos PM, Lamela AV, González-Juanatey JR. Reorganización de la actividad asistencial ambulatoria en la era de la COVID-19. La hora de la e-consulta. Revista Española de Cardiología. 2020;20:21–6. https://doi.org/10.1016/s1131-3587(20)30031-5.
7. Roberts L, Osborn-Jenkins L. Delivering remote consultations: talking the talk. Musculoskelet Sci Pract. 2021;52:102275. https://doi.org/10.1016/j.msksp.2020.102275.
8. Singh V, Sarbadhikari SN, Jacob AG, John O. Challenges in delivering primary care via telemedicine during COVID-19 pandemic in India: a review synthesis using systems approach. J Family Med Prim Care. 2022;11(6):2581. https://doi.org/10.4103/jfmpc.jfmpc_1559_21.
9. DeFriese GH. The visualization of primary care: the White-Williams-Greenberg diagram. N C Med J. 2002;63(4):186–8.
10. White et al. Monthly Prevalence Estimates of Illness in the Community and the Roles of Physicians, Hospitals, and University Medical Centers in the Provision of Medical Care. Data are for persons 16 years of age and older. Reprinted from the 1961. The New-England Medical Review and Journal. 344(26):2021–5. https://doi.org/10.1056/NEJM200106283442611.
11. Fry MW, Saidi S, Musa A, Kithyoma V, Kumar P. "Even though I am alone, I feel that we are many" – an appreciative inquiry study of asynchronous, provider-to-provider teleconsultations in Turkana, Kenya. PLoS One. 2020;15(9):e0238806. https://doi.org/10.1371/journal.pone.0238806.
12. Patel H, Hassell A, Cyriacks B, Fisher B, Tonelli W, Davis C. Building a real-time remote patient monitoring patient safety program for COVID-19 patients. Am J Med Qual. 2022;37(4):342–7. https://doi.org/10.1097/jmq.0000000000000046.
13. Pearl R. Kaiser Permanente Northern California: current experiences with internet, mobile, and video technologies. Health Aff (Millwood). 2017;33:251–7. PMID: 24493768
14. McGrail KM, Ahuja MA, Leaver CA. Virtual visits and patient-centered care: results of a patient survey and observational study. J Med Internet Res. 2017:19, e177. PMID: 28550006
15. Fatehi F, Menon A, Bird D. Diabetes care in the digital era: a synoptic overview. Curr Diab Rep. 2018;18:38. PMID: 29748905
16. Greenhalgh T, Vijayaraghavan S, Wherton J, Shaw S, Byrne E, Campbell-Richards D, et al. Virtual online consultations: advantages and limitations (VOCAL) study. BMJ Open. 2016;6:e009388. PMID: 26826147
17. NHS England and British Medical Association. Investment and evolution: a five-year framework for GP contract reform to implement the NHS long term plan. 2019.

18. Digital Health and Care Scotland. Scotland's Digital Health and Care Strategy: enabling, connecting and empowering. 2018; 20. Available: https://www.gov.scot/publications/scotlands-digital-health-care-strategy-enabling-connecting-empowering/
19. US Department of Veterans Affairs. Department of Veterans Affairs FY 2018–2024 Strategic Plan. Available: https://www.va.gov/oei/docs/VA2018-2024strategicPlan.pdf
20. National Digital Health Strategy and Framework for Action | Australian Digital Health Agency. [cited 13 Jul 2021]. Available: https://www.digitalhealth.gov.au/about-us/national-digital-health-strategy-and-framework-for-action
21. Majeed A, Maile EJ, Bindman AB. The primary care response to COVID-19 in England's National Health Service. J R Soc Med. 2020:208–10. PMID: 32521196
22. Tsopra R, Frappe P, Streit S, Neves AL, Honkoop PJ, Espinosa-Gonzalez AB, et al. Reorganisation of GP surgeries during the COVID-19 outbreak: analysis of guidelines from 15 countries. BMC Fam Pract. 2021;22:1–16. PMID: 33388038
23. Neves AL, et al. Use and impact of virtual primary care on quality and safety: the public's perspectives during the COVID-19 pandemic. J Telemed Telecare. 2024;30(2):393–401.
24. Neves AL, Li E, Gupta PP, Fontana G, Darzi A. Virtual primary care in high-income countries during the COVID-19 pandemic: policy responses and lessons for the future. Eur J Gen Pract. 2021;27(1):241–7. https://doi.org/10.1080/13814788.2021.1965120.
25. Clarke J, Flott K, Crespo RF, Ashrafian H, Fontana G, Benger J, et al. Assessing the safety of home oximetry for COVID-19: a multisite retrospective observational study. BMJ Open. 2021;11(9):e049235.
26. Li E, Tsopra R, Jimenez G, Serafini A, Gusso G, Lingner H, et al. General practitioners' perceptions of using virtual primary care during the COVID-19 pandemic: an international cross-sectional survey study. PLOS Digit Health. 2022;1(5):e0000029.
27. Campbell K, Greenfield G, Li E, O'Brien N, Hayhoe B, Beaney T, et al. The impact of virtual consultations on the quality of primary care: systematic review. J Med Internet Res. 2023;25:e48920.
28. Leape L, Berwick D, Clancy C, Conway J, Gluck P, Guest J, et al. Transforming healthcare: a safety imperative. BMJ Qual Saf. 2009;18(6):424–8.
29. IOM (Institute of Medicine). Telemedicine: a guide to assessing telecommunications for health care. Washington, DC: National Academy Press; 1996.
30. Demaerschalk BM, Hollander JE, Krupinski E, Scott J, Albert D, Bobokalonova Z, et al. Quality frameworks for virtual care: expert panel recommendations. Mayo Clin Proc Innov Qual Outcomes. 2023;7(1):31–44.
31. Eguia H, Vinciarelli F, Villoslada Muñiz RL, Sanz García FJ. Remote consultation: information for Primary Care physicians [Internet]. Vol. 46, Semergen. Ediciones Doyma, S.L.; 2020 [cited 2021 Jun 30]. p. 560–5. Available from: https://doi.org/10.1016/j.semerg.2020.08.005.
32. Kruse CS, Krowski N, Rodriguez B, Tran L, Vela J, Brooks M. Telehealth and patient satisfaction: a systematic review and narrative analysis. BMJ Open. 2018;7(8):e016242.
33. Wade VA, Karnon J, Elshaug AG, Hiller JE. A systematic review of economic analyses of telehealth services using real-time video communication. BMC Health Serv Res. 2010;10(1):233.
34. Kvedar J, Coye MJ, Everett W. Connected health: a review of technologies and strategies to improve patient care with telemedicine and telehealth. Health Aff. 2014;33(2):194–9.
35. Kruse CS, Karem P, Shifflett K, Vegi L, Ravi K, Brooks M. Evaluating barriers to adopting telemedicine worldwide: a systematic review. J Telemed Telecare. 2017;24(1):4–12.
36. Mair F, May C, O'Donnell C, Finch T, Sullivan F, Murray E. Factors that promote or inhibit the implementation of e-health systems: an explanatory systematic review. Bull World Health Organ. 2012;90(5):357–64.
37. Dinesen B, Nonnecke B, Lindeman D, Toft E, Kidholm K, Jethwani K, et al. Personalized telehealth in the future: a global research agenda. J Med Internet Res. 2016;18(3):e53.
38. Ekeland AG, Bowes A, Flottorp S. Effectiveness of telemedicine: a systematic review of reviews. Int J Med Inform. 2010;79(11):736–71.

39. Bashshur RL, Howell JD, Krupinski EA, Harms KM, Bashshur N, Doarn CR. The empirical foundations of telemedicine interventions in primary care. Telemed J E Health. 2016;22(5):342–75.
40. McKethan A, Brammer C, Fatemi P, Kim M, Kirtane J, Kunzman J, McClellan M. An early status report on the Beacon communities' plans for transformation via health information technology. Health Aff. 2009;30(4):782–8.
41. Porter ME, Teisberg EO. Redefining health care: creating value-based competition on results. Harvard Business Press; 2006.
42. Dorsey ER, Topol EJ. State of telehealth. N Engl J Med. 2016;375(2):154–61.
43. Acheampong F, Vimarlund V. Business models for telemedicine services: a literature review. Health Syst. 2014;4(3):189–203. https://doi.org/10.1057/hs.2014.20.
44. Bashshur, R L. (1995). Telemedicine effects: cost, quality, and access. J Med Syst, 19(2), 81–91. https://doi.org/10.1007/bf02257059
45. Hassibian MR, Hassibian S. Telemedicine acceptance and implementation in developing countries: benefits, categories, and barriers. Razavi Int J Med. 2016;4(3) https://doi.org/10.17795/rijm38332.
46. Vitacca M, Scalvini S, Spanevello A, Balbi B. Telemedicine and home care: controversies and opportunities. Breathe. 2006;3(2):148–58. https://doi.org/10.1183/18106838.0302.148.

Epidemiology of Telephone and Remote Consultation

2

Lee Smith, Sanjiv Ahluwalia, Ulrik Bak Kirk, and Jacopo Demurtas

2.1 Introduction

Historically, the first exempla of telemedicine were health-seeking attempts using the telephone, dating back to 1876 and 1879. Indeed, the first words said on the receiver of a telephone were from one of the inventors, Alexander Graham Bell. He said, "Mr. Watson, come here, I want you.' It has been reported that the very first telephone call was the very first telemedicine act, a call for medical assistance, as Bell had just upset the wet battery powering the transmitter, spilling sulphuric acid on his clothes [1].

The second was reported in the *Lancet* on November 1879 and cited the case of an anxious mother who made her baby's grandmother call a physician to seek help and request a home visit, as they were convinced that the baby had croup. The doctor said, 'Lift the child to the telephone and let me hear it cough.' In this way, he could hear that the cough was indeed not croup.

L. Smith (✉)
Centre for Health Performance and Wellbeing, Anglia Ruskin University, Cambridge, UK
e-mail: lee.smith@aru.ac.uk

S. Ahluwalia
Faculty of Health, Medicine and Social Care, School of Medicine, Anglia Ruskin University, Chelmsford, UK
e-mail: sanjiv.ahluwalia@aru.ac.uk

U. B. Kirk
Faculty Fellow, Department of Public Health, Aarhus University, Aarhus, Denmark

Digital Health, Research Unit for General Practice, Aarhus, Denmark
e-mail: ubk@ph.au.dk

J. Demurtas
Clinical and Experimental Medicine PhD Program, University of Modena and Reggio Emilia, Modena, Italy

Family Medicine Department, USL Toscana Sud-Est, Capalbio, Italy

J. Demurtas (ed.), *Remote Consultation in Primary Care*, TELe-Health,
https://doi.org/10.1007/978-3-031-89661-3_2

Nevertheless, for centuries, the telephone did not get an important place in medical practice, notwithstanding several important studies on its utility [2–5]; however, its use spread, along with that of other means of remote consultation, particularly after the outbreak of the COVID-19 pandemic.

The pandemic has indeed shifted healthcare consultations from traditional face-to-face methods to remote consultations that are broadly defined as any situation in which the patient and clinician are not in the same room. Specifically, these are generally consultations conducted by telephone, video or through asynchronous text-based GP–patient communication via email or an online portal (e-consultation or telehealth).

To decline and prevent the spread of SARS-CoV-2, face-to-face contact was minimized [6], and several social distancing and isolation measures were implemented [7]. Such preventive strategies resulted in a drive towards more remote consultations, as well as telemedicine, and accelerated the adoption of online and video consultations with healthcare practitioners. This will be revisited later in this chapter.

2.2 Prevalence of Telephone and Remote Consultations Prior to the COVID-19 Pandemic

Prior to the COVID-19 pandemic, telephone and remote consultations were relatively rare and few countries had implemented telephone and remote consultation procedures and systems. Indeed, prior to the COVID-19 pandemic, nine countries (Estonia, Hungary, Iceland, Ireland, Korea, Luxembourg, Mexico, Turkey and the United States) allowed medical consultations to be performed. While it was possible to use telemedicine services in other countries, many governments had requirements specific to telemedicine that effectively disincentivized its use. Although the number of services was growing, in countries such as Australia, Canada and Portugal, teleconsultations were only between 0.1% and 0.2% of all appointments.

Denmark is one country with an early adoption of remote consultation. On 1 January 1992, Denmark implemented a systems reform: locally negotiated rota systems were replaced with county-based services. Each county had a coordination centre, where all patients' calls were received by a team of doctors. The doctors could give a telephone consultation, advise the patient to attend one of the emergency clinics strategically placed around the county, or arrange for a home visit. Doctors on home visiting duty were located at bases throughout the county and kept in touch with the coordination centre with mobile telephones [8].

One study carried out an evaluation of the reform five years after its implementation and concluded that the organization of the out-of-hours service, with a fully trained general practitioner (GP) in a telephone triage function, is working satisfactorily. Many calls that previously would have required home visits were dealt with by telephone. The out-of-hours workload for general practitioners decreased considerably [9].

In 2009, a collective agreement made it mandatory for all Danish GPs to offer email consultations. A 2015 study found that Denmark had the highest number of doctor–patient emails sent/received in Europe [10] making it a forerunner in the adoption of email consultations. By 2019, the number of email consultations in Denmark had risen from 1.3 million in 2008 to 7.2 million per year, corresponding to just under 21% of all GP consultations.

A media-theoretical qualitative study found that from the patients' perspective, email consultations provided more convenient contact with their GP. From the GPs' perspective, email consultations facilitated contact with patients whom they otherwise rarely saw, but also resulted in overuse and inappropriate use. Patients and GPs considered email consultations as inviting new interactions and also facilitating communication about emotional and sensitive issues. Both patients and GPs experienced email consultations as a way in which patients could achieve easier access to face-to-face consultations (access to access) [11].

In 2008, Kaiser Permanente Northern California (KPNC) implemented an inpatient and ambulatory care electronic health record system for its 3.4 million members and developed a suite of patient-friendly internet, mobile and video tools. Indeed, the number of virtual 'visits' grew from 4.1 million in 2008 to an estimated 10.5 million in 2013 [12].

In another study using 2005–2017 data from OptumLabs Data Warehouse—a de-identified claims database for privately insured and Medicare Advantage enrollees in a large private US health plan –observed that annual telemedicine visits among all members increased from 206 in 2005 (0.020 per 1000 [95% CI, 0.018–0.021]) to 202,374 in 2017 (6.57 per 1000 [95% CI, 6.54–6.60]), at an average annual compound growth rate of 52% (95% CI, 45–61%) (43% [95% CI, 37–49%] from 2005 to 2014 and 261% [95% CI, 206–331%] from 2015 to 2017).

Moreover, most telemedicine visits were either telemental health (53%) or primary care telemedicine (39%). Primary care telemedicine visits grew 36% annually before 2016 and then increased sharply to 136,366 visits in 2017, while telemental health grew 56% annually to 57,095 visits in 2017. By 2017, primary care telemedicine was the most frequently used form of telemedicine [13]. While another US study found that only 15% of physicians in the United States worked in health practices that used telehealth services in 2016 [14].

In the United Kingdom, prior to the COVID-19 pandemic, remote consultations were rare and take-up was low although it was increasing. For example, in a recent UK study including 350,966 registered patients in 21 practices, it was observed that, in April 2019 (pre-COVID-19 pandemic), there were 218 GP consultations per 1000 registered patients; 31% were by telephone, and no video consultations were recorded [15].

In the United Kingdom, in 2014, a pilot study of an online consultation system in primary care was carried out in 36 general practices covering 396,828 patients. Just 7472 patients went on to complete an 'e-consultation' (indicating 200 online consultations per 1000 patients per month). E-consultations were mainly performed on weekdays and during normal working hours. Patient records (n = 485) were abstracted for eight practices and showed that women were more likely to use e-consultations than men (64.7% vs. 35.3%) and users had a median age of 39 years (IQR 30–50).

The most common reason for an e-consultation was an administrative request (e.g. test results, letters and repeat prescriptions [22.5%]) followed by infections/immunological issues (14.4%). The majority of patients (65.2%) received a response within two days. The most common outcome was a face-to-face (38%) or telephone consultation (32%). The former was more often needed for patients consulting about new conditions (OR 1.56, 95% CI 1.05 to 2.27, $p = 0.049$). The study concluded that use of e-consultations is significantly low, particularly at weekends. Unless this can be improved, any impact on staff workload and patient waiting times is likely to be negligible [16].

There are few other studies on the prevalence of telephone and remote consultations prior to the COVID-19 pandemic highlighting the rarity of this approach prior to 2020. Moreover, data from low-and middle-income countries is scarce and the prevalence in such settings is likely to be lower than in high-income countries, owing to financial and technological limitations.

2.3 Change in Prevalence of Remote Consultations Owing to the COVID-19 Pandemic

As we mentioned in the opening statements, telephone and remote consultations have grown significantly in developed countries since the beginning of the COVID-19 pandemic and will likely remain an integral part of medical care hereon. However, the maintenance of telephone and remote consultation will be heavily influenced by policy. Indeed in some countries, such as the United Kingdom, policy change is attempting to drive an increase in face-to-face provision within general practices, a discussion of which is beyond the scope of this chapter.

Although the number of face-to-face appointments (hospital and GP surgeries) in England decreased from 8,758,600 in February 2020 to 2,783,535 in April 2020 (COVID-19 pandemic phase), they have since increased by 89% (5,248,932 in August 2021). Simultaneously, telephone consultations almost trebled during this period (from 2,203,203 in February 2020 to 6,221,869 in August 2021) [17].

Moreover, in a UK study including 350,966 registered patients in 21 general practices, it was found that in April 2019 (pre-COVID-19 pandemic), there were 218 GP consultations per 1000 registered patients; 31% were by telephone, and no video consultations were recorded. In April 2020 (COVID-19 pandemic period), this had reduced to 180 GP consultations per 1000 registered patients, 89% by telephone and 1% coded as video, increasing to 3% for patients aged >85 years [15].

In another study including 27 European countries and Israel, almost one in three [33%, 95% CI (31.2, 34.8)] older adults aged 50 and over have had remote medical consultations over the phone, computer or any other electronic means, with or without video since the start of the COVID-19 outbreak [18].

In a study in Denmark, it was observed that the number of face-to-face in-clinic consultations declined during the lockdown in March 2020. A subsequent increase in the number of clinic consultations occurred, rising to a level above that of the pre-pandemic period; this increase resulted mainly from the introduction of telehealth consultations (that is, video and extended telephone, taking longer than regular telephone consultations). The number of daytime email consultations increased, whereas the number of daytime home visits decreased. Likewise, the number of out-of-hours telephone consultations increased, whereas the number of out-of-hours home visits and clinic consultations decreased. Consultation rates of patients who are vulnerable, that is, those with low education, old age and comorbidity, were most adversely affected by the pandemic. The most adverse impact in out-of-hours clinic consultations was seen for children aged 0 to 9 years [19].

Moreover, in a register-based study of all consultations in daytime general practice in Denmark from 1 January 2019 to 30 November 2021, it was observed that video consultations were used mostly during the early-stage pandemic period (March to mid-June 2020), declining to about 2% of all clinic consultations in the late-stage period (mid-June 2020 to 30 November 2021). Patients having more video consultations were young, had a higher level of education, were employed and living in big cities, while older patients and retired patients had lower odds [20].

In a study in the United States, it was observed that in April 2020 (pandemic period), overall telehealth utilization for office visits and outpatient care was 78 times higher than in February 2020 (pre-pandemic), although the prevalence somewhat declined after this period in February 2021 it was still 38 times higher than February 2020 [21].

In another study, it was found that since COVID-19, Langone Health Centre in New York City in the United States reported an increase in telemedicine visits from 102.4 to 801.6 per day between March and April 2020, implying a 683% increase in visits in less than a month [22].

A further study from the United States included insurance claims data from the OptumLabs Data Warehouse to capture all outpatient visits over a 24-week period from 1 January to 16 June 2020. The study found that among 16,740,365 enrollees, the weekly rate of telemedicine visits increased during the pandemic period, peaking in the week of 15 April 2020, before declining by the week of 10 June 2020. From the weeks of 1 January to 10 June, the rates for telemedicine visits increased from 0.8 to 17.8 visits per 1000 enrollees (increase of 17.0 or 2013% change); in-person visits dropped from 102.7 to 76.3 (decrease of 26.4 or −30.0% change); total visits (telemedicine and in-person visits combined) decreased from 103.5 to 94.1 (−9.1% change). By the last 4 weeks of the study period, 20 May through 16 June 2020, there was wide geographic variation in per cent of total visits delivered by telemedicine (ranging from 8.4% in South Dakota to 47.6% in Massachusetts) and the per cent change from baseline in total visit rates (ranging from −73.2% in Hawaii to −16.0% in Alaska). Some states, especially in the South, had a small decline in total visits and lower rates of telemedicine use (i.e. Tennessee: −23.6% change in total visits with 10.4% of all visits as telemedicine; Alabama: −21.5% and 13.4%, respectively) [23].

Some literature on telephone and remote consultation uptake in specific healthcare settings exist. Researchers analysed electronic health records between 7 January 2019 (pre COVID-19) and 20 September 2020 (COVID-19 pandemic) for all people receiving mental healthcare from South London and Maudsley NHS Foundation Trust in the United Kingdom. The Trust provides clinical services to around 37,500 patients each week within its catchment area, a region diverse in terms of area-level deprivation, ethnic composition and education. It was found that prior to the COVID-19 pandemic, video calls accounted for less than 1% of remote consultations. Since July 2020, they have accounted for around 30% indicating a rapid uptake in the use of video call software to conduct mental healthcare assessments [24]. Moreover, the change was less pronounced in older adults, who experienced a 105% increase in remote consultations between the weeks of 9 March and 8 June 2020, compared with a 262% and 298% increase for those aged under 18 and 18 to 65 years respectively.

One study focused on the uptake of telehealth among people living with HIV in the United States. It was observed that at the beginning of the COVID-19 pandemic there was an initial increase in video visits to 30%, the proportion then subsequently declined and plateaued at ~10%. A substantial proportion of face-to-face visits were replaced by phone visits (~50% of all visits were by phone early in the pandemic, now stable at 10–20%). Logistic regression demonstrated that older age (>50 or > 65 years old compared with 18–35 years old), Black, Asian or Pacific Islander race (compared with White race) and Medicaid insurance (compared with private insurance) were significantly associated with never completing a video visit, whereas history of patient portal login was significantly associated with completing a video visit [25].

Other specialities have also observed increases including, paediatric diabetes management [26], cancer care [27], physiotherapy [28] and urology [29].

2.4 Telephone and Remote Consultations in Low- and Middle-Income Countries

It should be noted that data on the prevalence and trends in relation to telephone and remote consultations has predominantly come from developed countries. Not much is known about corresponding figures for low- and middle-income countries. However, it has been reported that the global growth in telephone and remote consultations has been steady and much slower in low- and middle-income countries due to the lack of sustainable models, limited financial resources, health policy priority of the country, poor knowledge and limited access to telehealth technologies [30].

2.5 Evidence from Systematic Review

To conclude, several systematic reviews showed [31–33], regardless of the COVID-19 pandemic, that a remote approach, by video or telephone consultation, may be acceptable as an alternative to face-to-face consultation in several settings. Byambasuren et al. provided a direct comparison of telephone and video telehealth consultations for ongoing care of patients with established diagnoses, finding no significant differences in clinical effectiveness, patient satisfaction and healthcare use (cost-effectiveness) [31]. Chair et al. found in their review on RCTs comparing telephone consultation to face-to-face consultation that telephone consultations may improve call resolution and reduce face-to-face contacts with doctors on the day of first management for regular day service with some evidence that nurse-led telephone consultation may provide better effects than that by doctors for out-of-hours service [33].

2.6 Summary

Prior to the COVID-19 pandemic telephone and remote consultations were rarely implemented although there were increasing trends in their use in developed countries. The need to reduce face-to-face contact during the COVID-19 pandemic subsequently resulted in a dramatic increase in the use of telephone and remote consultations, which has seemed to have declined and plateaued since the start of the pandemic but remains considerably higher than the pre-COVID-19 period. However, it should be noted that there seems to be some variation in the direction of trends between within-country locations. Importantly, there is a scarcity of data on the prevalence and trends of telephone and remote consultations in low- and middle-income countries. While most of the prevalence and trend data is from developed countries, this data is still collected infrequently and no robust monitoring system is in place; such systems with frequent data collection would facilitate a better understanding regarding the epidemiology of telephone and remote consultations. Moreover, future epidemiological work is required in low- and middle-income countries in relation to telephone and remote consultations to inform policy and practice.

References

1. Aronson SH. The Lancet on the telephone 1876–1975. Med Hist. 1977;21(1):69–87.
2. Bunn F, Byrne G, Kendall S. Telephone consultation and triage: effects on health care use and patient satisfaction. Cochrane Database Syst Rev. 2004;3:CD004180.
3. Newbould J, Abel G, Ball S, Corbett J, Elliott M, Exley J, et al. Evaluation of telephone first approach to demand management in English general practice: observational study. BMJ. 2017;358:j4197.

4. Campbell JL, Fletcher E, Britten N, Green C, Holt T, Lattimer V, et al. ESTEEM trial: pilot study report. The clinical effectiveness and cost-effectiveness of telephone triage for managing same-day consultation requests in general practice: a cluster randomised controlled trial comparing general practitioner-led and nurse-led management systems with usual care (the ESTEEM trial). Health Technol Assess. 2015;19:1.
5. Lattimer V, George S, Thompson F, Thomas E, Mullee M, Turnbull J, et al. Safety and effectiveness of nurse telephone consultation in out of hours primary care: randomised controlled trial. BMJ. 1998;317(7165):1054–9.
6. Greenhalgh T, Koh GCH, Car J. Covid-19: a remote assessment in primary care. BMJ. 2020;368:m1182.
7. Ohannessian R, Duong TA, Odone A. Global telemedicine implementation and integration within health systems to fight the COVID-19 pandemic: a call to action. JMIR Public Health Surveill. 2020;6(2):e18810.
8. Olesen F, Jolleys JV. Out of hours service: the Danish solution examined. BMJ. 1994;309(6969):1624–6.
9. Christensen MB, Olesen F. Out of hours service in Denmark: evaluation five years after reform. BMJ. 1998;316(7143):1502.
10. Newhouse N, Lupiáñez-Villanueva F, Codagnone C, Atherton H. Patient use of email for health care communication purposes across 14 European countries: an analysis of users according to demographic and health-related factors. J Med Internet Res. 2015;17(3):e58.
11. Grønning A, Hvidt EA, Brøgger MN, Fage-Butler A. How do patients and general practitioners in Denmark perceive the communicative advantages and disadvantages of access via email consultations? A media-theoretical qualitative study. BMJ Open. 2020;10(10):e039442.
12. Pearl R. Kaiser Permanente Northern California: current experiences with internet, mobile, and video technologies. Health Aff. 2014;33(2):251–7.
13. Barnett ML, Ray KN, Souza J, Mehrotra A. Trends in telemedicine use in a large commercially insured population, 2005–2017. JAMA. 2018;320(20):2147–9.
14. Kane CK, Gillis K. The use of telemedicine by physicians: still the exception rather than the rule. Health Aff. 2018;37(12):1923–30.
15. Murphy M, Scott LJ, Salisbury C, Turner A, Scott A, Denholm R, et al. Implementation of remote consulting in UK primary care following the COVID-19 pandemic: a mixed-methods longitudinal study. Br J Gen Pract. 2021;71(704):e166–e77.
16. Edwards HB, Marques E, Hollingworth W, Horwood J, Farr M, Bernard E, et al. Use of a primary care online consultation system, by whom, when and why: evaluation of a pilot observational study in 36 general practices in South West England. BMJ Open. 2017;7(11):e016901.
17. Green MA, McKee M, Katikireddi SV. Remote general practitioner consultations during COVID-19. Lancet Digit Health. 2022;4(1):e7.
18. Monaghesh E, Hajizadeh A. The role of telehealth during COVID-19 outbreak: a systematic review based on current evidence. BMC Public Health. 2020;20:1–9.
19. Huibers L, Bech BH, Kirk UB, Kallestrup P, Vestergaard CH, Christensen MB. Contacts in general practice during the COVID-19 pandemic: a register-based study. Br J Gen Pract. 2022;72(724):e799–808.
20. Kirk UB, Høstrup Vestergaard C, Hammer Bech B, Bondo Christensen M, Kallestrup P, Huibers L. Video consultation in general practice during COVID-19: a register-based study in Denmark. BJGP Open. 2024;8(2):BJGPO.2023.0208.
21. Bestsennyy O, Gilbert G, Harris A, Rost J. Telehealth: a quarter-trillion-dollar post-COVID-19 reality. McKinsey & Company; 2021. p. 9.
22. Mann DM, Chen J, Chunara R, Testa PA, Nov O. COVID-19 transforms health care through telemedicine: evidence from the field. J Am Med Inform Assoc. 2020;27(7):1132–5.
23. Patel SY, Mehrotra A, Huskamp HA, Uscher-Pines L, Ganguli I, Barnett ML. Trends in outpatient care delivery and telemedicine during the COVID-19 pandemic in the US. JAMA Intern Med. 2021;181(3):388–91.

24. Appleton R, Williams J, Vera San Juan N, Needle JJ, Schlief M, Jordan H, et al. Implementation, adoption, and perceptions of telemental health during the COVID-19 pandemic: systematic review. J Med Internet Res. 2021;23(12):e31746.
25. Wood BR, Lan KF, Tao Y, Mose EY, Aas E, Budak JZ, et al. Visit trends and factors associated with telemedicine uptake among persons with HIV during the COVID-19 pandemic. Open forum infectious diseases. Oxford University Press US; 2021. p. ofab480.
26. Tornese G, Schiaffini R, Mozzillo E, Franceschi R, Frongia AP, Scaramuzza A. The effect of the COVID-19 pandemic on telemedicine in pediatric diabetes centers in Italy: Results from a longitudinal survey. Diabetes Res Clin Pract. 2021;179:109030.
27. Burbury K, Wong ZW, Yip D, Thomas H, Brooks P, Gilham L, et al. Telehealth in cancer care: during and beyond the COVID-19 pandemic. Intern Med J. 2021;51(1):125–33.
28. Barton C, Caneiro J, Haines T, Malliaras P, Merolli M, Williams C. 'It's not hands-on therapy, so it's very limited': Telehealth use and views among allied health clinicians during the coronavirus pandemic. J Sci Med Sport. 2021;24:S43.
29. Naik N, Nandyal SR, Nayak SG, Shah M, Ibrahim S, Hameed B, et al. Telemedicine and Telehealth in Urology: uptake, impact and barriers to clinical adoption. Front Surg. 2022;9:911206.
30. Tiwari BB, Kulkarni A, Zhang H, Khan MM, Zhang DS. Utilization of telehealth services in low-and middle-income countries amid the COVID-19 pandemic: a narrative summary. Glob Health Action. 2023;16(1):2179163.
31. Byambasuren O, Greenwood H, Bakhit M, Atkins T, Clark J, Scott AM, Glasziou P. Comparison of telephone and video telehealth consultations: systematic review. J Med Internet Res. 2023;25:e49942.
32. Downes MJ, Mervin MC, Byrnes JM, Scuffham PA. Telephone consultations for general practice: a systematic review. Syst Rev. 2017;6(1):1–6.
33. Chair SY, Chien WT, Kendall S, Zang Y, Liu T, Choi KC. Effects of telephone consultation on safety, service use, patient satisfaction, and workload: systematic review and meta-analysis of randomized trials. Telemed J E Health. 2024;30(2):364–80.

Remote Healthcare Around the World

3

Vanja Lazic, Jumana Antoun, Adel Fouad Yasky, Vildan Mevsim, Meena Nathan Cherian, Hans A. Eguia, Oğulcan Çöme, Yasemin Özkaya, and Almas Fatma

3.1 Introduction

Leveraging the power of technology, remote healthcare has transcended geographical barriers, enabling healthcare providers to reach more patients, particularly in high-income countries, which have seen a revolution in primary care delivery. This

V. Lazic (✉)
Association of Teachers in General Practice/Family Medicine, Zagreb, Croatia

J. Antoun
Department of Family Medicine, American University of Beirut, Beirut, Lebanon
e-mail: ja46@aub.edu.lb

A. F. Yasky
Family Medicine Department, King Abdulaziz Medical City, Riyadh, Saudi Arabia

V. Mevsim
Department of Family Medicine, Faculty of Medicine, University of Dokuz Eylul, Izmir, Turkey

M. N. Cherian
Global Health New Challenges: Online Courses, Geneva, Foundation for Medical Education & Research (GFMER), Geneva, Switzerland

H. A. Eguia
Lægehuset Engdraget, Rudkøbing, Denmark

eHealth – WONCA, Rudkøbing, Denmark

Digital Health Working Group of the Spanish Society of Family Medicine (SEMERGEN), Barcelona, Spain

Danish Society of Primary Care (DSAM), Copenhagen, Denmark

Universitat Oberta de Catalunya, Barcelona, Spain
e-mail: heguia@uoc.edu

J. Demurtas (ed.), *Remote Consultation in Primary Care*, TELe-Health,
https://doi.org/10.1007/978-3-031-89661-3_3

chapter delves into the multifaceted realm of remote healthcare, exploring its definitions, trends, perspectives, success stories and the pivotal roles played by governments and the private sector in countries with different features in technological and financial resources, by international standards.

3.2 Remote Consultation in High-Income Countries

High-income countries are characterised by robust economies and advanced healthcare infrastructures. These nations typically prioritise public health and invest significantly in healthcare systems to ensure the well-being of their citizens. Despite their shared goal of delivering quality care, high-income countries exhibit diverse healthcare systems, including single-payer systems, insurance-based systems or a combination of both [1]. Examples of high-income countries with varying healthcare systems include the United States, Canada, Germany, Australia, Saudi Arabia and Japan.

In recent years, remote primary care has gained momentum in high-income countries, catalysing healthcare accessibility and improving patient outcomes. Through telehealth platforms and digital communication tools, the internet positively affected several areas, including electronic scheduling appointments (29% improvement in specialty care), improved referral and booking and identifying and addressing medication adverse events [2].

A study conducted in the United States found that telehealth services for primary care increased by 53% from 2016 to 2017, demonstrating the growing trend of remote healthcare in high-income countries [2].

Moreover, the COVID-19 pandemic further accelerated the adoption of remote primary care, with telehealth visits skyrocketing in various countries, such as Canada, the United Kingdom and Australia [3].

Several high-income countries have successfully implemented remote consultation programmes, setting examples for effective healthcare delivery. For instance, the National Health Service (NHS) 111 online service, which provides remote healthcare consultations, enables patients to access medical advice and assistance remotely, and Australia's 'Health Direct Video Call' service has facilitated virtual consultations with healthcare professionals, notably affecting rural areas.

Remote medical services arrangements have shown promising outcomes in overseeing ongoing sicknesses. For example, the Constant Consideration Model, which was carried out through remote conferences, has further developed results for patients with conditions like diabetes and hypertension. These projects concentrate more on remote observation, patient instruction and customary virtual discussions to improve self-administration and diminish medical clinic visit requirements [4].

O. Çöme
Faculty of Medicine, Family Medicine Department, Dokuz Eylul University, Izmir, Turkey

Y. Özkaya
Izmir Tepecik Training and Research Hospital, İzmir, Turkey

A. Fatma
Family Physician & Certified Digital Health Professional at Alcura Family Clinic, Navi Mumbai, India

High-income countries require collaboration between governments and the private sector to implement remote consultation.

Governments may play a crucial role in establishing policies, regulations and reimbursement frameworks to support integrating remote healthcare solutions into existing healthcare systems. A firm policy can enhance the potential boost of remote healthcare consultancy. For instance, the United Kingdom's National Health Service (NHS) implemented policies to promote the use of telehealth and provide guidance for healthcare providers [5].

On the other hand, the private sector, including healthcare technology companies and telecommunication providers, contributes by developing innovative platforms, secure communication tools and interoperable systems. Many healthcare technology providers have developed so far innovative platforms with interoperable systems to support remote consultations with secure communication tools which have produced more effectiveness in remote healthcare systems [6].

High-income countries, by improving healthcare accessibility, notably for poor people, removing geographical barriers and lowering travel costs may benefit from remote tools with quick accessibility and even improve their wealth by lowering the costs of healthcare delivery without impairing the quality of services.

According to Canadian research, remote consultations reduced emergency department visits, hospital admissions and healthcare expenses [7]. Remote consultations also encourage and promote continuity of care. Patients can easily connect with their primary care providers, specialists and other healthcare professionals, fostering a coordinated and integrated approach to healthcare delivery.

Remote consultations also empower patients, providing them with tools and resources for self-management, education and active participation in their healthcare decisions. Patients can indeed track their vital signs through remote monitoring devices and telehealth platforms, receive educational materials, and engage in shared decision-making with healthcare providers [8].

In conclusion, remote healthcare solutions can transform healthcare delivery in high-income countries.

It offers a wealth of benefits, encompassing improved accessibility, reduced costs, enhanced patient satisfaction and effective management of chronic diseases. Successful examples from various countries demonstrate the positive impact of remote consultation programmes on patient outcomes and healthcare systems. However, collaboration between governments, healthcare providers and the private sector is crucial to unlocking the full potential of remote consultations.

3.3 Remote Consultation in Low- and Middle-Income Countries

LMIC countries share several common characteristics, including low national incomes, a high rural population density, weak infrastructure, insufficient healthcare services, education deficiencies, political instability, high birth rates and environmental issues. These factors can create significant challenges for citizens living in LMIC countries, including poverty, limited access to basic amenities, inadequate healthcare and educational opportunities and environmental hazards [9]. Moreover, in LMIC countries, many people lack access to basic healthcare services, including preventive care, routine check-ups and immunisations, leading to increased rates of infectious diseases, maternal and child mortality and other preventable health issues [10].

In addition to challenges with access to healthcare, many LMIC countries struggle with a high burden of non-communicable diseases (NCDs), such as diabetes, cancer and heart disease. Various factors, including poor diet, lack of exercise and tobacco and alcohol use, can cause NCDs. Addressing NCDs requires a comprehensive approach that includes improving healthcare infrastructure and access and addressing underlying social and economic factors that contribute to poor health outcomes [11].

Improving health outcomes in LMIC countries is a complex challenge that requires coordinated efforts from multiple stakeholders, including governments, international organisations and civil society.

The current state of communication infrastructure in LMIC countries varies widely depending on the specific country and region. While some countries have made significant progress in developing communication infrastructure, others face significant challenges.

In some LMIC countries, limited regulatory oversight and weak governance can also contribute to challenges in developing adequate communication infrastructure. For example, corruption and political instability can hinder progress in infrastructure development, leading to inadequate or poorly functioning communication networks.

The current state of communication infrastructure in LMIC countries is rapidly evolving due to ongoing technological advancements and increased investment in infrastructure development. While challenges remain, many LMIC countries are making significant progress in expanding access to communication technologies and improving the reliability and affordability of communication networks.

The expansion of mobile networks and internet access drives progress in LMIC countries. By investing in infrastructure development, such as the deployment of 3G and 4G networks, low-cost mobile devices, mobile money and other mobile-based services, many LMIC countries have significantly increased their mobile network and internet access in recent years.

In addition to improving access to mobile networks and the internet, many LMIC countries invest in developing fixed-line broadband networks to provide faster and more reliable internet access to businesses and households.

However, significant disparities in access to communication technologies persist, particularly between urban and rural areas and across income groups. In addition, limited regulatory oversight and weak governance remain significant challenges in some LMICs, hindering progress in infrastructure development.

The increasing population in LMICs has led to a rise in demand for affordable and quality healthcare. However, access to healthcare remains a significant challenge, particularly for the poor and vulnerable populations. Quality of care and appropriate healthcare assessment have also been neglected in LMICs, focusing more on technical aspects than interpersonal components. The cost of healthcare in LMICs is also a significant issue, with out-of-pocket expenditure on healthcare increasing significantly and posing a threat to household finances.

Geographical access, availability, affordability and acceptability are all barriers to accessing healthcare in LMICs, particularly for women, children, the elderly and the physically handicapped. The rapid developments in information and communication technologies, particularly web-based technologies, offer new possibilities for providing better healthcare to populations. Telemedicine is gradually emerging as a viable policy option for governments in LMICs.

The current state of remote consultation in LMICs is rapidly evolving due to ongoing technological advancements and the COVID-19 pandemic. Remote consultation involves using digital technologies to provide healthcare services and consultations remotely, including video conferencing, telephone consultations and mobile health applications.

The COVID-19 pandemic has accelerated the adoption of remote consultation in many LMIC countries as governments and healthcare providers seek to reduce the risk of virus transmission in healthcare facilities and ensure continuity of care for patients. Many LMIC countries have rapidly implemented policies and infrastructure to support remote consultation, including developing telemedicine platforms and expanding internet and mobile network coverage [12, 13].

Despite these developments, significant challenges remain in adopting and using remote consultation in LMIC countries. Limited access to digital technologies, including smartphones and high-speed internet, remains a significant barrier to adoption for many people in LMIC countries, particularly those living in rural areas. In addition, regulatory frameworks and policies around telemedicine are still evolving in many LMIC countries, which can create uncertainty for healthcare providers and patients alike [14].

The history of telemedicine in low- and middle-income countries (LMICs) is marked by innovative initiatives and projects that have aimed to address various healthcare challenges in these regions. In LMICs, telemedicine has been used as a strategy to increase access to healthcare services and improve health outcomes.

In 2017, only 33–49% (between one-third and half) of the global population was covered by essential health services. Middle-income (both (upper and lower) countries had the largest number (1.9 to 2 billion) of people lacking coverage of essential health services. With the rising population by 2030, the essential health service coverage to meet Sustainable Development Goals (SDG) Targets could be slow. We need to accelerate the implementation of innovative digital health technologies to maximise the capacities of health workers and the utilisation of quality healthcare facilities [15].

The World Health Organization (WHO) estimates that '18 million more health workers are needed to achieve UHC by 2030' [16].

With the current shortage of surgical health workforce, the use of smartphone apps (other health technologies) in LMIC would allow not only timely surgical interventions and referrals but also postoperative home follow-up. Scheduling for a telephone call follow-up will depend on the availability of time, whereas a smartphone enables close monitoring and a quick review for any complications, a review of photos and closer contact with patients, particularly in remote rural settings. It reduces costs and time (long travels, waiting periods at the outpatient clinic, early hospital discharge, burden of the family carer) for the patients.

Médecins Sans Frontières (MSF, Doctors Without Borders), a medical humanitarian organisation, have evaluated the quality of 7 years of field experience in telemedicine. The study shows that despite the increasing patient load, the quality of MSF telemedicine service is maintained, thus providing improved clinical management in low-resource settings for patients and long-term education by specialists for field physicians [17].

Today, we are globally connected through digital technologies far better than decades ago, and nearly half the population globally has access to the internet. In LMIC, 8 in 10 people own a mobile phone. These technologies are more equitably distributed across the world than income [18].

Telehealth has the potential to reach the vulnerable and marginalised population living in remote, rural and conflict-affected areas to meet SDG Targets 3.8 (SDG indicator 3.8.1 on the coverage of essential health services and SDG indicator 3.8.2 on catastrophic health spending) on UHC [19].

It is essential to include investments for the training of the health workforce in the implementation plan for telemedicine programmes in LMIC. Otherwise, the quality and sustainability become questionable.

A study in a rural district in Tanzania reported the feasibility and acceptability of online training of the health workforce for remote consultation in PHC. It successfully initiated behaviour change in healthcare workers, cascading teaching and learning skills to remotely consult the health system to bill patients for remote consulting. The online MoodleApp was used for training, including education resources and WhatsApp for remote patient consultations [20].

With the experience of remote consultation during the COVID-19 pandemic and considering the current gaps in the healthcare systems, including the shortage of health workers, it is crucial to invest in sustainable Telehealth technologies to ensure equitable access to quality healthcare services in LMIC.

Remote consultation in low- and middle-income countries (LMIC) is an effective solution to overcome barriers to access to healthcare. In many of these areas, people live in poverty, remote locations and slums with high incidences of mortality and morbidity, making it challenging to access health services. Remote consultation can overcome those barriers by allowing patients to consult with healthcare providers from the comfort of their homes, reducing the need for travel and saving time and money. A retrospective cross-sectional study of 25,182 teleconsultation visits has shown a cumulative patient savings of USD 9,175,132, and 1,876,146 h, or 213.1 years compared with hypothetical in-person consultations due primarily to eliminating travel costs and time, including accommodation and round trips to the nearest health facility [21].

The implementation of remote consultation faces several challenges in LMICs. The infrastructure and technological barriers, including the availability and reliability of the internet and electricity supply, are the most common challenges. The lack of digital literacy and shortage of personnel trained in virtual healthcare also hinder the implementation of mobile consultation in primary care. The need for electronic solutions in healthcare is another challenge. Therefore, using technology in remote consultations may highlight vulnerabilities and inequities for people living in slums, older patients and those without access to smartphones or digital devices, as well as for digital illiteracy.

Common barriers were weak infrastructure and regulatory mechanisms. Some of the highlighted challenges included the need to develop awareness and education for patients and health workers to accept remote consulting. Health workers need to be supported through training skills and education in ethics, transparency and local culture to gain patients' confidence [13].

3.4 Remote Consultation in Rural Settings

Although the rural population has grown slowly since 1950, it is thought that it has now peaked and will continue to decline gradually. The rural population is estimated to be around 3.4 billion globally and will decrease to 3.1 billion people by 2050 [22]. The most significant rural population is in Africa and Asia, with almost 50% living in rural settings. India has the largest number, around 893 million people, and China has 578 million.

This means that despite the gradual decline, the number of people in these areas is still relatively high, and due to their location, they have fewer resources at hand than in urban areas, such as means of transportation and access to adequate health systems.

To help with this problem, we can count on telemedicine to enhance health access in rural areas, allowing geographical and distance barriers to be overcome and, simultaneously, allowing patients to access health services without the need to make trips or long journeys.

Telemedicine can overcome geographical barriers by bringing medical attention to people in rural areas with no access to medical specialities. This way, patients can receive diagnostic or follow-up medical consultations from their homes, avoiding unnecessary travel and sparing resources. It must be considered that well-implemented telemedicine can affect the quality, access and equality of rural primary healthcare [23]. Moreover, by allowing more patients to have access to healthcare services, as well as better and more frequent monitoring of chronic patients, it allows for a reduction in hospital admissions and patient mortality, improving the overall social and healthcare results of a certain healthcare area.

3.5 Potential Future Development of Remote Healthcare Solutions

The future of remote healthcare solutions holds immense promise as technological advances and societal needs evolve. Integrating emerging technologies like artificial intelligence, wearable devices and virtual reality can revolutionise healthcare delivery. Artificial intelligence (AI) algorithms can analyse patient data, aiding accurate diagnoses and personalised treatments. Wearable devices enable remote monitoring, proactive management of chronic conditions and early intervention. Virtual reality creates immersive environments for virtual consultations and therapy, overcoming geographical barriers. Integrating remote healthcare with data analytics can provide insights into public health trends and enable early interventions. Collaboration among stakeholders is crucial in establishing standards, policies and ethical guidelines. Investments in infrastructure and digital literacy are needed for equitable access.

References

1. Smith PC, Anell A, Busse R, et al. Leadership and governance in seven developed health systems. Health Policy. 2012;106(1):37–49. https://doi.org/10.1016/j.healthpol.2011.12.009.
2. Bashshur RL, Howell JD, Krupinski EA, Harms KM, Bashshur N, Doarn CR. The empirical foundations of telemedicine interventions in primary care. Telemed J E Health. 2016;22(5):342–75. https://doi.org/10.1089/tmj.2016.0045.
3. Sodhi A, van Winkle C, Goudreau M, Poliquin K, Almonte V. The rise of telemedicine during the COVID-19 pandemic. J Am Coll Radiol. 2021;18(7):1074–82.
4. Gagnon MP, Duplantie J, Fortin JP, Landry R. Implementing telehealth to support medical practice in rural/remote regions: what are the conditions for success? Implement Sci. 2012;7:18. https://doi.org/10.1186/1748-5908-7-18.
5. Greenhalgh T, Shaw S, Wherton J, Hughes G, Lynch J, A'Court C, Hinder S, Fahy N. SCALS: a fourth-generation study of telehealth in the home. University of Southampton; 2018.
6. Ekeland AG, Bowes A, Flottorp S. Effectiveness of telemedicine: a systematic review of reviews. Int J Med Inform. 2010;79(11):736–71. https://doi.org/10.1016/j.ijmedinf.2010.08.006.
7. Gupta A, Anjomshoa M, Kainth N, Goyal M, Patel N, Ranasinghe T, et al. Impact of telehealth remote patient monitoring on hospital admissions and 30-day readmissions in heart failure patients. Telemed e-Health. 2018 Nov;24(11):883–9.
8. Hailey D, Roine R, Ohinmaa A. The effectiveness of telemental health applications: a review. Can J Psychiatry. 2017 Jan;62(1):14–24.
9. UNDP (United Nations Development Programme), OPHI (Oxford Poverty and Human Development Initiative). 2022 global multidimensional poverty index (MPI): unpacking deprivation bundles to reduce multidimensional poverty. New York; 2022.
10. Laurie Marczak PD, Kevin O'Rourke MFA, Dawn Shepard BA, et al. Mortality in children and adolescents, 1990–2013. JAMA. 2016;315(19):2055. https://doi.org/10.1001/jama.2016.5891.
11. WHO. Non-communicable diseases. 2022. Retrieved from https://www.who.int/news-room/fact-sheets/detail/noncommunicable-diseases
12. Babu Tiwari B, Kulkarni A, Zhang H, Khan MK, Zhang DZ. Utilisation of telehealth services in low- and middle-income countries amid the COVID-19 pandemic: a narrative summary. Glob Health Action. 2023;16:1. https://doi.org/10.1080/16549716.2023.2179163.

13. Mahmoud K, Jaramillo C, Barteit S. Telemedicine in low- and middle-income countries during the COVID-19 pandemic: a scoping review. Front Public Health. 2022 June 22;10:914423. https://doi.org/10.3389/fpubh.2022.914423. PMID: 35812479; PMCID: PMC9257012.
14. Mohamad SI, Defi RI. Telerehabilitation in low- and middle-income countries [internet]. Biomedical Engineering IntechOpen; 2023. Available from: https://doi.org/10.5772/intechopen.107449.
15. WHO. Primary Health Care on the Road to Universal Health Coverage 2019 GLOBAL MONITORING REPORT. https://www.who.int/publications/i/item/9789240004276
16. WHO. Health workforce. Available from: www.who.int/data/gho/data/themes/health-workforce. Accessed on 25 May 2023.
17. Delaigue S, Bonnardot L, Steichen O, Garcia DM, Venugopal R, Saint-Sauveur J-F, Wootton R. Seven years of telemedicine in Médecins Sans Frontières demonstrate that offering direct specialist expertise in the frontline brings clinical and educational value. JOGH. 2018;8(2):0204142023. https://doi.org/10.7189/jogh.08.020414.
18. Anderson M, Albala SA, Patel N, Lloyd J, Mossialos E, At the London School of Economics. Building the economic case for primary healthcare: a scoping review, technical series on primary healthcare. WHO; 2018.
19. WHO. Service coverage. Available from: https://www.who.int/data/gho/data/themes/topics/service-coverage. Accessed on 25 May 2023.
20. Downie A, Mashanya T, Chipwaza B, Griffiths F, Harris B, Kalolo A, Ndegese S, Sturt J, De Valliere N, Pemba S. Remote consulting in primary health care in LMIC: feasibility study of an online training program to support care delivery during the COVID-19 pandemic. JMIR Form Res. 2022;6(6):e32964.
21. Sayani S, Muzammil M, Saleh K, Muqeet A, Zaidi F, Shaikh T. Addressing cost and time barriers in chronic disease management through telemedicine: an exploratory research in select low- and middle-income countries. Ther Adv Chronic Dis. 2019;10:2040622319891587.
22. UN. World population. Available from: https://www.un.org/en/desa/68-world-population-projected-live-urban-areas-2050-says-un. [cited 2023 Apr 7].
23. Lindberg J, Bhatt R, Ferm A. Older people and rural eHealth: perceptions of caring relations and their effects on engagement in digital primary health care. Scand J Caring Sci [Internet]. 2021 Dec 1 [cited 2023 Apr 15];35(4):1322–1331.

Remote Consultation Appropriateness: Legal Issues and Ethical Concerns

4

Erika Céspedes Suzuki

4.1 Introduction

4.1.1 Definition and Scope

Telemedicine, from the Greek *τελε* meaning 'distance' and the Latin *medicum* derived from *mederi* meaning 'heal, cure', refers to the practice of medicine at a distance facilitated by telecommunications. In the words of the WHO: 'The delivery of health care services, where distance is a critical factor, by all health care professionals using information and communication technologies for the exchange of valid information for diagnosis, treatment and prevention of disease and injuries, research and evaluation, and for the continuing education of health care providers, all in the interests of advancing the health of individuals and their communities' [1].

Telemedicine encompasses a wide variety of services, as mentioned by the European Commission Communication COM/2008/689 on telemedicine for the benefit of patients, healthcare system and society [2], namely 'teleradiology, telepathology, teledermatology, teleconsultation, telemonitoring, 'telesurgery and teleophthalmology. Other potential services include call centres/online information centres for patients, remote consultation/e-visits, or videoconferences between health professionals'.

Telemedicine uses information and communication technologies (ICTs) to overcome geographical barriers and increase access to healthcare services. Thus, among its advantages, we find accessibility, agility, ubiquity, sustainability and cost-effectiveness [3].

E. C. Suzuki (✉)
Accident and Emergency consultant physician, Basque Country, Spain

Family physician, Basque Country, Spain

Law Degree, Basque Country, Spain

J. Demurtas (ed.), *Remote Consultation in Primary Care*, TELe-Health,
https://doi.org/10.1007/978-3-031-89661-3_4

Four elements characterize telemedicine [4]:

1. Its aim is to provide clinical support.
2. Its purpose is to overcome geographical barriers, connecting users who are not in the same physical location.
3. It involves the use of various types of ICT.
4. Its goal is to improve health outcomes.

Notice that remote consultation (RC) does not exclude the need for personal contact and does not intend to substitute face-to-face medicine. Both practices are complementary, so prior triage plays a very important role, in knowing when each of them is indicated. A consultation can begin digitally and continue in person or the other way around, according to the needs of each case [3].

4.1.2 Importance of Ethical and Legal Considerations

We must remember that medical practice must continue to be based on the same ethical principles, quality conditions, safety and warmth of an in-person doctor–patient relationship. The fact that the patient is not physically in front of the physician cannot shift the responsibility onto a communication system [5]. Furthermore, healthcare professionals must act more cautiously because, on the one hand, the lack of physical presence increases the risk of errors during service delivery, and on the other hand, technical problems such as transmission errors, security incidents or data storage issues are likely to occur. In other words, the use of ICTs increases the precautions that professionals must take since they not only rely on their scientific knowledge but also on a means of communication, such as telephony or optical fibre [5]. It is evident that ICTs themselves do not pose ethical dilemmas; rather, it is their use that can create ethical conflicts.

Therefore, an appropriate and up-to-date legal framework is necessary to guarantee respect for patient rights and to maintain the essence of the doctor–patient relationship in any form of care delivery.

4.2 Regulatory Framework

4.2.1 National Regulations

Most countries of the European Union (EU) do not have specific legal regulations on telemedicine, and only some of them have adopted national regulations or professional and ethical guidelines regarding the provision of health telemedicine services [6]. In Europe, countries such as France, Sweden, Germany and Switzerland have specific regulations applicable to telemedicine. In other countries such as Belgium or Italy, there is no law that incorporates the requirements of telemedicine; however, in Belgium, several institutions have published good practices recommendations and, in Italy, National Guidelines for the development of telemedicine was enacted [6].

In the United States, there is no specific regulation at the federal level, but there is one in each state. The United States has a federal legal system with 50 independent states that traditionally controlled healthcare within the borders of each state. That is why US doctors face many legal and technical barriers to providing efficient telemedicine care to patients in other states [7]. As a US physician, you must know your state's regulations (distant site) and the rules relative to the state where your patients reside (originating site) [8].

In Latin America, despite the deficiency of resources in health systems, some countries have made significant progress in implementing specific regulations regarding telehealth, while others are still in the early stages of legislative development. About 90% have regulations at the national level, most of them since before 2019. However, references to confidentiality and professional secrecy in telemedicine are scarce [9].

On the Asian continent, China's telemedicine policies have significantly evolved, contributing to improved healthcare accessibility, especially in remote areas. The implementation of telemedicine policies has grown rapidly since the medical reform of 2009 and the 'Opinions on Promoting Telemedicine Services in Medical Institutions' policy in 2014. Similarly, the 'Healthy China 2030' plan has been an important driving force for the expansion of telemedicine, with more than 900 virtual hospitals and 24,000 medical institutions offering telemedicine services. There are mandatory (most of them), voluntary, economic and informational instruments. These address issues of compliance, supervision, inspection, permission regulation, legal liability, reimbursement security and data privacy [10].

The situation in Africa is different. In the Sub-Saharan African region, the panorama is characterized by the lack of policies and regulatory frameworks to support the use of ICT in health. Likewise, there are concerns about the security and confidentiality of medical data, which generates mistrust in both patients and clinicians. In member states (MS) of the Sahel-Sahara Community, there is low acceptance of telemedicine due to the government's lack of understanding of its benefits [11].

In many Middle Eastern countries, there is a lack of specific e-health policies and legal frameworks, inadequate governmental support and a slow pace of policy formulation. The organizational structure and the existing healthcare regulations in many Eastern countries do not support the implementation of telemedicine. Furthermore, in countries like Saudi Arabia, consultations between different sexes are a sensitive topic, influenced by cultural and religious beliefs, which may affect the acceptance of telemedicine [12].

4.2.2 International Standards

Although today RC is more accessible than ever before, many works show that the legislation on telemedicine activity is lacking in many cases [13]. Thus, the regulatory uncertainty entails further difficulty that adds to the curative activity of telemedicine itself [13] and constitutes another obstacle to the spread of its use. In this chapter, we will focus on the EU framework and match it to that of the United States.

The legal regulation of telemedicine in Europe varies considerably from country to country and presents specific challenges due to differences in healthcare systems, medical practices and data protection laws. However, there are some common trends in telemedicine regulation across the region.

According to the European Commission, 'Telemedicine is the provision of healthcare services, through the use of ICT, in situations where the health professional and the patient (or two health professionals) are not in the same location' [2]. The quoted definition must be interpreted in conjunction with Articles 56 and 57 of the Treaty on the Functioning of the EU [14] and the definition of 'health professionals' of Article 3/f of Directive 2011/24/EU [15, 16]: '"health professional" means a doctor of medicine, a nurse responsible for general care, a dental practitioner, a midwife or a pharmacist within the meaning of Directive 2005/36/EC [17], or another professional exercising activities in the healthcare sector which are restricted to a regulated profession as defined in Article 3(1)(a) of Directive 2005/36/EC, or a person considered to be a health professional according to the legislation of the Member State of treatment.' In other words, remote consultation, as a type of practice of health professions, is based on the free movement of services.

In the European legal framework, RC is both a health service and an information society service [2]; thus, both regulations should be applied [15]. Respecting health services, we must consider the Directive 2011/24/EU [18], on the application of patients' rights in cross-border healthcare and the Directive 2005/36/EC, on the recognition of professional qualifications [17]. Regarding ICT, we must refer to the following regulations: Directive 95/46/EU [19], the Data Protection Directive and the General Data Protection Regulation (GDPR) [20]; Directive 98/34/EC, the Directive on Services of the Information Society [21]; Directive 2000/31/EC, the Electronic Commerce Directive [22] and Directive 2002/58/EC, the Directive on Privacy and Electronic Communications or e-Privacy Directive [15, 23].

Besides, the EU developed several initiatives to increase the use of telemedicine such as the eHealth Action Plan 2012–2020, 'Innovative Healthcare' for the twenty-first century [24]. It proposed a set of actions to boost the deployment of eHealth and the use of interoperable eHealth services within and between national healthcare systems, with the goal of turning telemedicine into a standard medical service and accessible to every European patient.

4.2.3 Licensing Requirements

RC introduces the need to determine which national legal jurisdiction defines the qualification and licensing requirements, as it often involves doctors providing services in a location different from the patient's home country. The EU's Directive 2005/36/EC on recognition of professional qualifications [17] does not directly apply to telemedicine as it pertains to temporary movement to another EU member state (MS). Consequently, only the qualifications mandated by the provider's home country apply. Each national entity regulating medical practice must oversee the qualifications and other aspects of healthcare providers, including those involved in cross-border telemedicine. Moreover, no additional requirements can be imposed by the receiving country's legal system, and doctors are not obligated to obtain authorization or licensing there. An EU healthcare professional offering telemedicine services only needs to be licensed in the country where they are physically located without regard to the location where the services are received, as defined by the E-Commerce Directive [22] and the Cross-Border Healthcare Directive [18]. Nonetheless, some propose the idea of a specific licence for telemedicine, focusing on expertise in handling the new related technologies [15].

On the contrary, most US states require a medical licence for both the state where the patient resides and the state where the physician is practicing. Federal legislation has led to the creation of the Interstate Medical Licensure Compact (IMLC) by the Federation of State Medical Boards, aiming to ease interstate licensing restrictions for physicians. Currently, 32 states [25], participate in the IMLC. To participate, physicians must meet specific qualifications, including maintaining unrestricted licensure in their primary state, maintaining board certification in their specialty and having a clean disciplinary record [8].

4.3 Informed Consent in Remote Consultation

4.3.1 Definition of Informed Consent (IC)

IC embodies a communication process between a patient and a healthcare provider, often culminating in the patient's agreement or authorization for medical care, treatment, services or investigation. This involves a comprehensive understanding of the associated risks, benefits, consequences or potential complications.

IC entails the explicit endorsement of a competent individual in participating in decisions regarding their health. IC constitutes a legal obligation for healthcare professionals, integral to the *lex artis*. It represents an ethical mandate that upholds the patient's right to self-determination, aiming not solely at obtaining a signed document but rather ensuring the supply of pertinent information, a fundamental patient entitlement [26].

Four components [27] are fundamental to make the consent valid: adequate and clear information, comprehension of information, capacity to consent and voluntariness.

4.3.2 Consent Requirements in Teleconsultation

The physician must provide all the necessary information to the patients so that they are able to make their own decisions especially regarding treatment options. However, IC in telemedicine is somewhat more complex, and that is why it is important to inform about the limits of remote medical evaluation. Before participating in a teleconsultation, patients should receive clear, complete and understandable information about the risks, benefits and alternatives to telemedicine. Further, according to the Directive 2011/24/EU [18], patients are entitled to be informed about the quality and safety standards and guidelines in the MS where the treatment is administered or, where the physician is located [15]. Likewise, the health professional should be available to resolve any questions that may arise.

IC in RC entails informing patients about their rights under data protection laws, potential system errors, teleconsultation protocols, prescription guidelines, and coordination with other healthcare professionals [28]. In addition, patients should be aware that despite safety measures, their data are not entirely secure. Finally, caregivers must ensure that patients understand instructions, provide consent and possess the means and skills to use the ICTs effectively.

According to Article 7 of GDPR, the burden of proof regarding the existence of the consent falls on the controller. For this reason, it is advisable that consent be given in writing or by digital signature.

4.4 Malpractice and Liability

Regarding professional liability, it is important to emphasize that telemedicine services should be treated similarly to any other diagnostic and therapeutic health service. Nonetheless, there is a lack of uniformity regarding medical liability since the EU does not have common regulations regarding tort and criminal liability [15].

The rules vary significantly among European MSs, particularly between continental law systems and common law systems. Moreover, within the same legal framework, regulations concerning medical liability may differ depending on the context of the medical procedure, such as whether it is performed within the national health service (where tort law is applied) or in the private sector (where contract law is applicable) [15]. Also, the competent court in the event of a malpractice claim is yet to be determined.

It is essential to regulate RC at a level comparable to face-to-face medical services. This ensures that professionals are not exempt from accountability for their actions or performance conducted remotely.

However, teleconsultation not only involves different countries and regulations but also covers a series of different domains (medicine, ICT, privacy, social security), making it more complex to define and the most adequate entity to regulate and control it [15].

Consequently, legal doctrine aligns in recognizing three distinct categories regarding liability: the telemedicine service provider or the company that produces and distributes the device and the ICT support; the healthcare facility offering the teleconsultation service; and the individual caregiver [29].

Health practitioners also bear direct liability for ensuring their own training is sufficient for their roles and for the tasks they perform [30].

In brief, each MS is responsible for regulating this matter; they determine the qualifications and prerequisites for practicing medicine and, consequently, telemedicine [15]. Enhancing adherence to current regulations and clearly outlining the liability responsibilities of all relevant parties can mitigate defensive medical practices and facilitate wider adoption of telemedicine [30].

4.5 Confidentiality and Clinical Records

4.5.1 Data Privacy and Confidentiality

The concept of safeguarding medical information has always been present, but the GDPR [20], applicable in the EU, has enhanced this by specifying and categorizing data points for better comprehension and management of personal data.

Personal data can be simplified as 'any information related to an identified or identifiable natural person' (Article 4(1) of GDPR). Certain data is deemed particularly sensitive as it reveals intimate details about individuals, such as health-related or sexual information (Article 9(1) of GDPR).

Moreover, ensuring maximum protection is essential when transmitting data concerning minors and entire groups of subjects, such as families [13].

Patient information includes detailing the purpose behind data collection (diagnosis, treatment), disclosing any intended sharing of data with third parties and informing patients if their data will be transferred outside the EU territory. In addition, patients must understand that despite implementing safety measures, their data cannot be guaranteed to be completely secure [15].

Nevertheless, there are various exceptions to this general principle. Personal data may be processed: with explicit consent from the data owner, when necessary for fulfilling employment and social security obligations, or if justified by reasons of public interest. Furthermore, there may be exceptions for archiving, scientific research or statistical purposes of public interest [31].

Patients must provide consent for the handling of their data, but several other requirements must be met: the data collection should adhere to the principle of proportionality (meaning caregivers should only collect necessary data for effective medical care); the collected data must be used exclusively for this purpose and not for any other purpose; and the data must be processed by a healthcare professional who is obligated by professional secrecy [15].

Otherwise, patients must be ensured access to a copy of all data concerning themselves, including their health records, whether in paper or electronic format. In addition, patients have the right to request oblivion—also known as the 'right to be forgotten'—and the deletion of their data [13].

4.5.2 Privacy Regarding Teleconsultation

Cross-border data sharing faces stringent requirements under the GDPR, especially for non-EU countries. Specific contracts or guidelines may be needed for data movement, particularly involving the United States. On the other hand, challenges arise with cloud databases used in telemedicine, complicating compliance. In addition, involving ICT staff accessing health data may conflict with confidentiality requirements, suggesting a need for more flexible regulations requiring this staff to sign confidentiality agreements [15].

Despite the implementation of a uniform legal framework across all MSs, variations exist in how each national legislature has transposed it and in how it is interpreted by national entities responsible. Consequently, while there is a common core, certain practices may be deemed acceptable in one MS but not in another, potentially leading to legal complexities, especially in the context of cross-border telemedicine [15].

In the United States, compliance with the Health Insurance Portability and Accountability Act (HIPAA) regulations is mandatory, alongside adherence to any state, local or organizational standards. It is crucial to note that personal health information extends beyond medical reports to encompass patients' email addresses, phone numbers, street addresses and other related data, all of which require protection [25].

4.5.3 Regulations Compliance

The current EU regulations prioritize the protection of collected data by imposing severe penalties for unauthorized disclosure, loss or destruction and privacy breaches. Data handlers—companies, hospitals or caregivers—are obligated to implement appropriate measures to ensure data security, such as reliable encryption techniques and robust firewalls. Vulnerabilities within hospitals often stem from issues like inadequate encryption, insufficient separation of internal and external networks, lack of device inventories, weaknesses in user authentication, and difficulty identifying unauthorized devices on wireless networks [15].

While current guarantees for patient data are significant, ensuring maximum protection for patient data in the future is imperative. This responsibility lies not only with device suppliers but also with all healthcare professionals involved in the process [13]. That is why it would be advisable to educate telemedicine professionals on best practices for protecting health data.

4.6 Ethical Aspects

4.6.1 Ethical Principles

The World Medical Association Statement on the Ethics of Telemedicine adopted in Copenhagen in 2007 [32] asserts that face-to-face consultation between physician and patient remains the gold standard of clinical care. In this vein, it is understood that the four mandatory principles of medical ethics also apply to the practice of RC.

These principles are as follows:

- `Autonomy: patients' right to make decisions regarding their medical assistance and their health information. Also, the patient's freedom to access (or not) their information and thereby, to accept or decline, initiate or discontinue remote care.
- Beneficence: the provider's obligation to act in the patient's best interest under all circumstances. That is why the physician must prioritize their training and ensure the quality and proper condition of the ICTs they utilize.
- Nonmaleficence: the provider's duty not to intentionally harm the patient or society while caring for that patient. The health professional's opinion should not be influenced by their own benefit or their institution's.
- Justice: refers to equity and impartiality in the distribution of medical resources and the time dedicated to each patient. Physicians must treat all patients equally, without discriminating based on gender, race, etc.

4.6.2 Doctor–Patient Relation in Telemedicine [33]

RC has revolutionized doctor–patient interactions, emphasizing the importance of trust in the absence of physical cues. Some psychiatric studies show that video consultations are as effective as in-person visits, fostering open dialogue. Email communication allows for remote updates and adjustments to treatment plans. Patients may initially feel uneasy with camera-based interactions, but reassurance of privacy and quality care can mitigate concerns. In some cases, a third party may aid communication.

Ensuring a successful outcome involves recognizing that the core of medical practice lies in the doctor–patient relationship, built on trust and the acknowledgement of the patient's dignity. In the future, this will be facilitated as people become familiar with new ICTs.

When RCs prioritize measures to establish a strong, professional and empathetic therapeutic connection, it can achieve the same level of humanity and intimacy as in-person interactions.

4.6.3 Addressing Equity and Access Issues [34]

The development of telemedicine occurs within a specific socio-political and economic environment, which influences how and who can access it, sometimes resulting in an unfair paradox. On the one hand, more than a third of the world's population, 2.9 billion people, lacks internet access, with nearly all excluded individuals (96%) living in poor countries. However, many of the raw materials used in technology production come from these same countries.

The United Nations also notes a global gender digital gap—pronounced in Africa—and a breach between urban and rural areas globally, with urban residents being twice as likely to use the internet. Lastly, there is an evident generational gap worldwide, with an average of 71% of the global population aged 15 to 24 using the internet, compared to 57% of other age groups.

Furthermore, the implementation of telemedicine is a complement to healthcare systems, but undoubtedly not the most critical, considering that many countries still lack strong public healthcare systems equipped with sufficient resources.

Therefore, for an equitable implementation of RC, it will be essential to continue strengthening universal access to primary healthcare systems and overcoming digital divides, ensuring not to leave anyone behind and not to represent a new face of inequality but rather a tool to improve access to health.

4.7 Conclusions

- RC—utilizing ICTs to provide healthcare remotely—requires adherence to ethical and legal standards to ensure patient rights, safety and the integrity of the doctor–patient relationship, recognizing that it supplements rather than replaces traditional in-person consultation.
- The evolution of telemedicine poses a series of legal problems ranging from licensing, liability and special IC, to the protection of patient's personal data.
- Data privacy and confidentiality are decisive. Challenges include cross-border data sharing, compliance with varying national interpretations of laws, and ensuring robust security measures to safeguard patient data from unauthorized disclosure or breaches.
- RC faces regulatory uncertainty and lacks consistent legislation across the world. An effective regulatory framework is required to safeguard patients and provide direction for healthcare professionals. Laws should promote collaboration between doctors and patients, as well as among various stakeholders in the healthcare system.
- While regulating RC and, particularly concerning medical liability, it is advisable to consider the rules of the country from which the services are being provided.

- It is the duty of the physician to uphold the essence of the doctor–patient relationship and apply the ethical principles. For this purpose, continuous training is essential, not only in medical science but also in ethics, law, social sciences, digital skills and communication with the patient in virtual environments.

References

1. WHO. A health telematics policy in support of WHO's health-for-all strategy for global health development: report of the WHO group consultation on health telematics, 11–16 December 1997. Geneva, World Health Organization, 1998.
2. Communication from the Commission to the European Parliament, the Council, the European Economic and Social Committee and the Committee of the Regions on telemedicine for the benefit of patients, healthcare systems and society. /COM/2008/0689 final/. Available from: http://eurlex.europa.eu/legal-content/EN/TXT/?uri=COM:2008:0689:FIN.
3. Barbagallo G. La telemedicina en tiempos de COVID-19 [Internet]. Archive.consejo.org.ar [cited 2024 Apr 16]. Available from: https://archivo.consejo.org.ar/consejodigital/RC60/barbagallo.html
4. WHO Global Observatory for eHealth. Telemedicine: opportunities and developments in Member States: report on the second global survey on eHealth. World Health Organization; 2010. Available from: https://iris.who.int/handle/10665/44497
5. El Hospital. Telemedicina: la mala aplicación del término [Internet]. El Hospital [cited 2024 Apr 18] Available from: https://www.elhospital.com/es/blog/telemedicina-la-mala-aplicacion-del-termino
6. Esade Creapolis. Estudio sobre la consulta de salud virtual y sus beneficios para el sistema sanitario [Internet]. Esadeedu, 2020. [cited 2024 Apr 26]. Available from: https://itemsweb.esade.edu/wi/Prensa/EsadeCreapolis_BHH_Estudio-Salud.pdf
7. Chang SL, Pines JM, Thorpe JH. How the European Union is embracing cross-border telemedicine and what the U.S. State Medical Boards can learn from it. [Internet] 2018. [cited 2024 Apr 26]. Available from: https://hsrc.himmelfarb.gwu.edu/gw_research_days/2018/SMHS/5/
8. Fields BG. Regulatory, legal, and ethical considerations of telemedicine. Sleep Med Clin. [Internet] 2020 [cited 2024 Apr 26];15(3):409–416. Available from: https://doi.org/10.1016/j.jsmc.2020.06.004.
9. Alegre V, Álvarez MY, Bianchini A, et al. Salud digital en América Latina: legislación actual y aspectos éticos. Rev Panam Salud Publica. [Internet] 2024 [cited 2024 May 31];48:e40. Available from: https://www.ncbi.nlm.nih.gov/pmc/articles/PMC11069326/
10. Zhang W, He D, Wang G, Zhu C, Evans R. Analyzing national telemedicine policies in China from the perspective of policy instrument (1997–2020). Int J Med Inform [Internet] 2022 [cited 2024 May 31], 166, 104854. Available from: https://www.sciencedirect.com/science/article/pii/S138650562200168X?via%3Dihub4
11. Dodoo JE, Al-Samarraie H, Alzahrani AI. Telemedicine use in Sub-Saharan Africa: barriers and policy recommendations for Covid-19 and beyond. Int J Med Inform [Internet] 2021 [cited 2024 May 31]; *151*, 104467. Available from: https://www.ncbi.nlm.nih.gov/pmc/articles/PMC9761083/
12. Al-Samarraie H, Ghazal S, Alzahrani AI, Moody L. Telemedicine in middle eastern countries: progress, barriers, and policy recommendations. Int J Med Inform [Internet] 2020 [cited 2024 May 31]; 141, 104232. Available from: https://www.sciencedirect.com/science/article/abs/pii/S1386505620303579?via%3Dihub

13. Nittari G, Khuman R, Baldoni S, Pallotta G, Battineni G, Sirignano A, Amenta F, Ricci G. Telemedicine practice: Review of the current ethical and legal challenges. Telemed J E-Health [Internet] 2020 [cited 2024 Apr 18] 26(12), 1427–1437. Available from: https://www.ncbi.nlm.nih.gov/pmc/articles/PMC7757597/
14. European Union. Consolidated version of the Treaty on the Functioning of the European Union. Official J Eur Union C 326, 26 October 2012. Available from: https://eur-lex.europa.eu/legal-content/EN/TXT/?uri=celex%3A12012E%2FTXT.
15. Raposo VL. GMS | GMS Health Innovation and Technologies | Telemedicine: The legal framework (or the lack of it) in Europe. [cited 2024 Apr 18]; Available from: https://www.egms.de/static/en/journals/hta/2016-12/hta000126.shtml
16. EU Parliament and the Council. Directive 2011/24/EU of 9 March 2011 on the application of patients' rights in cross-border healthcare. OJ L 88 of 4 April 2011.
17. Directive 2005/36/EC of the European Parliament and of the Council of 7 September 2005 on the recognition of professional qualifications. OJ L 255 of 30 September 2005. Available from: https://eur-lex.europa.eu/eli/dir/2005/36/oj
18. Directive 2011/24/EU of the European Parliament and of the Council of 9 March 2011 on the application of patients' rights in cross-border healthcare. Off J. 2011;L 88:45–65. Available from: http://data.europa.eu/eli/dir/2011/24/oj
19. Directive 95/46/EC of the European Parliament and of the Council of 24 October 1995 on the protection of individuals with regard to the processing of personal data and on the free movement of such data. Off J 1995; L 281:31–50. Available from: http://data.europa.eu/eli/dir/1995/46/oj
20. Regulation (EU) 2016/679 of the European Parliament and of the Council of 27 April 2016 on the protection of natural persons with regard to the processing of personal data and on the free movement of such data, and repealing Directive 95/46/EC (General Data Protection Regulation) (Text with EEA relevance) OJ L 119 of 4 May 2016. Available from: http://data.europa.eu/eli/reg/2016/679/oj
21. Directive 98/34/EC of the European Parliament and of the Council of 22 June 1998 laying down a procedure for the provision of information in the field of technical standards and regulations. Off J. 1998;L 204:37–48. Available from: http://data.europa.eu/eli/dir/1998/34/oj
22. Directive 2000/31/EC of the European Parliament and of the Council of 8 June 2000 on certain legal aspects of information society services, in particular electronic commerce, in the Internal Market ('Directive on electronic commerce'). Off J. 2000; L 178:1–L 116. Available from: http://data.europa.eu/eli/dir/2000/31/oj
23. Directive 2002/58/EC of the European Parliament and of the Council of 12 July 2002 concerning the processing of personal data and the protection of privacy in the electronic communications sector (Directive on privacy and electronic communications). Off J 2002; L 201:37–47. Available from: http://data.europa.eu/eli/dir/2002/58/oj
24. Communication from the Commission to the European Parliament, the Council, the European Economic and Social Committee and the Committee of the Regions on eHealth Action Plan 2012–2020—Innovative healthcare for the 21st century /COM/2012/0736 final/. Available from: http://eurlex.europa.eu/legal-content/EN/ALL/?uri=CELEX:52012DC0736
25. Interstate Medical Licensure Compact. US state participation in the compact. [Internet]. 2016 [cited 2024 Apr 28]. Available from: https://www.imlcc.org/
26. Pantoja Zarza L. El consentimiento informado: ¿sólo un requisito legal? Rev Esp Reumatol [Internet]. 2004 [cited 2024 Apr 29];31(8):475–478. Available from: https://www.elsevier.es/es-revista-revista-espanola-reumatologia-29-articulo-el-consentimiento-informado-solo-un-13067152
27. Mondragón-Barrios L. Consentimiento informado: una praxis dialógica para la investigación [Informed consent: a dialogic praxis for the research]. Rev Investig Clin. 2009;61(1):73–82.
28. Gil Membrado C, Barrios V, Cosín-Sales J, Gámez JM. Telemedicina, ética y derecho en tiempos de COVID-19. Una mirada hacia el futuro [Telemedicine, ethics, and law in times of COVID-19. A look towards the future]. Rev Clin Esp. [Internet]. 2021 [cited 2024 Apr 29];221(7):408–410. Available from: https://doi.org/10.1016/j.rce.2021.03.002

29. Ferorelli D, Nardelli L, Spagnolo L, Corradi S, Silvestre M, Misceo F, et al. Medical legal aspects of telemedicine in Italy: Application fields, professional liability and focus on care services during the COVID-19 health emergency. J Prim Care Community Health [Internet]. 2020 [cited 2024 Apr 29];11. Available from: https://journals.sagepub.com/doi/10.1177/2150132720985055
30. Parimbelli E, Bottalico B, Losiouk E, et al. Trusting telemedicine: a discussion on risks, safety, legal implications, and liability of involved stakeholders. Int J Med Inform. [Internet]. 2018 [cited 2024 Apr 29]; 112:90-98. Available from: https://doi.org/10.1016/j.ijmedinf.2018.01.012
31. Botrugno C. Telemedicine in daily practice: addressing legal challenges while waiting for an EU regulatory framework. Health Policy Technol. [Internet] 2018 [Cited 2024 Apr 29];7(2):90–98 Available from: https://doi.org/10.1016/j.hlpt.2018.04.003.
32. The World Medical Association (WMA) statement on the ethics of telemedicine [Internet]. wma.net. [cited 2024 May 6]. Available from: https://www.wma.net/policies-post/wma-statement-on-the-ethics-of-telemedicine/
33. Macarena M, Iván PH. El acto médico en la era de la telemedicina. Rev méd Chile [Internet] 2020 [cited 2024 May 6]; 148(6): 852–857. Available from: http://www.scielo.cl/scielo.php?script=sci_arttext&pid=S0034-98872020000600852&lng=es. https://doi.org/10.4067/S0034-98872020000600852.
34. Jiménez M. Telemedicina y Equidad. OSEKI Osasun eskubidearen aldeko ekimena-Iniciativa por el derecho a la salud. [Internet] 2022 [cited 2024 May 6]. Available from: https://oseki.eus/articulos/telemedicina-y-equidad/

Part II

Remote Consultation

Clinical Reasoning in the Remote Consultation

5

Giuseppe Parisi, Cristina Vito, and Jacopo Demurtas

5.1 Clinical Reasoning: An Overview of the Literature

5.1.1 Three Approaches to Clinical Reasoning

The first approach that we consider is the analytical one: it is based on critical, logically grounded thinking and the exhaustive collection of all data prior to the deductive phase and also employing the help of Bayesian probability calculation.

The second approach that we consider is the non-analytical one, based on the intuitive recognition of diseases that are recalled in memory by means of 'scripts', or the recognition of patterns or overall 'gestalt' configurations, and applying inductive logic. It involves the use of heuristic strategies.

A heuristic is a strategy that is based on two rules: the exploration of the most promising conclusion by ignoring some of the information and the stop rule, i.e. moving on to a decision when the information is considered sufficient [1] or, in other words, 'satisfying' [2]. Especially in situations of high uncertainty, complexity or emergencies, the use of these strategies has proved to be fruitful [1,

G. Parisi (✉)
Postgraduate School of Specific Training in General Practice, (Scuola di Formazione Specifica in Medicina Generale), Trento, Italy

Italian Society of Medical Education (SIPeM), Torino, Italy

Interdepartmental Center for Medical Sciences, University of Trento, Trento, Italy

C. Vito
Family Physician Consultant, Hair Disorders Specialist, AraMedica, Lecce, Italy

J. Demurtas
Clinical and Experimental Medicine PhD Program, University of Modena and Reggio Emilia, Modena, Italy

Family Medicine Department, USL Toscana Sud-Est, Capalbio, Italy

J. Demurtas (ed.), *Remote Consultation in Primary Care*, TELe-Health,
https://doi.org/10.1007/978-3-031-89661-3_5

2]. Their benefits include timeliness and pliability, but they also risk methodological errors of early closure of diagnostic reasoning or other cognitive biases, although there is no agreement on this [3]. This is why they must always be accompanied by control cognitive routines (see below) or they must be in interaction with a recursive comparison with the results obtained from other approaches [4].

Recently, a third approach has also been described using gut feelings [5].

Gut feelings have been studied since the 1980s, mainly in nursing [6], and since the 2000s in medical literature. Stolper [7, 8] operationalized the concept in uncertain clinical situations in general practice. The full inclusion of gut feelings in the core curriculum of general practice has recently been advocated [9, 10] as a distinctive feature of general practice.

The debate is still open as to which approach is best, but it is certain that there is no universal approach to the problems that doctors encounter in their practice. Doctors have to use different tools for different situations or different stages of the reasoning process, so they have to carry a toolbox, not just a single tool [4, 11, 12].

5.1.2 The First Section of the Clinical Reasoning: From Symptoms to Diagnosis

Reasoning from a base of signs and symptoms to reach a formulated diagnosis is well described by Elstein and Schwartz, who refer to the deductive hypothetical model, a combination of the first and second approach described above:

> Solutions to difficult diagnostic problems were found by generating a limited number of hypotheses early in the diagnostic process and using them to guide subsequent collection of data. Each hypothesis can be used to predict what additional findings ought to be present if it were true, and the diagnostic process is a guided search for these findings [13].

The simple formulation of the process identifies two phases: an inductive phase of hypothesis generation and a subsequent phase of hypothesis verification. This second phase is performed through verbal and objective examination during the consultation itself, or through requests for further examinations, thereby extending the phase beyond the consultation.

5.1.3 The Second Section of the Clinical Reasoning: From Diagnosis to Action

Clinical reasoning does not stop there. The diagnosis is only the first step towards the final decision; it is a means to an end.

This section of clinical reasoning is based on the first evaluative step followed by the second step of designing and choosing a course of action, the so-called plan and choose phase.

The *evaluative step* consists of a set of cognitive routines aimed at diagnosing the degree and nature of uncertainty [14] and analysing the reliability of the process through meta-reflection [15] [[16]: 129]. The objective is not merely diagnosis, but an overall clinical judgement, defined as:

> … the awareness of the doctor of the whole situation of the patient, which is the effect of the burden of multi-morbidity on the prognosis in terms of physical and mental functioning, quality of life and life expectancy, but also in terms of the capacity of patients of coping with it [[17]: 68].

In the *plan and choose* step, the physician must identify the options, share them with the patient if necessary or requested, choose the course of action and reach a shared decision with the patient [18–22].

At this point in the process the consultation stops, but the care continues as the patient will be followed up and reviewed through surveillance strategies.

In this step, doctors may use all three approaches, depending on the clinical situation and the grade of uncertainty.

5.1.4 Clinical Reasoning in Primary Care: Four Peculiar Features

In primary care, the process of clinical reasoning is different and more complex, although the 'building blocks' are always the same.

We found four peculiar features.

First of all, in primary care *the prevalence of illnesses is low*. Faced with this epidemiological assumption, the physician must exclude serious illnesses, rather than make a certain diagnosis. This situation of rarely achieving 'diagnostic satiation' [23] is difficult to sustain: as a matter of fact it is more difficult to diagnose 'what is not' than 'what is', or to 'manage' instead of 'diagnose', to resist the temptation to be exhaustive [24].

In addition to the epidemiological peculiarities of 'real' diseases, the doctor in primary care works with *uncertainty (second feature).* They encounter borderline situations, which are characterized by high uncertainty: boundaries between health and illness, between perception of illness, illness characterized by anatomical-pathological changes and experience of illness [25], and between psychological and physical problems, e.g., 'medically unexplained symptoms' [26]. There is often uncertainty even in the assessment of initial and non-specific symptoms [27].

Moreover, as it is well known, uncertainty is also present in the case of chronic diseases, patients with multi-morbidity and complex patients.

Therefore, in the epidemiological framework of general practice, hypothesis generation uses probability [28] *followed closely by a series of tests with a high predictive power of exclusion* [16, 23].

It follows that we can hardly ever speak of a diagnosis, but of a working diagnosis, i.e. *a diagnosis detailed enough to make a decision* [29], *often negotiated with the patient* [16].

Table 5.1 Clinical and non-clinical problems

Classical clinical problems:
Physical symptoms (i.e. sore throat).
Beside diagnoses (i.e. thyroid node in neck scan).
Laboratory test results (i.e. anaemia).
Functional problems (i.e. elderly with walking difficulties).
Risk behaviour (i.e. alcohol intake).
Psychological problems (i.e. anxiety).
Non-clinical problems:
Family problems (i.e. marital tension).
Coping problems (i.e. after her father's illness she feels depressed).
Social problems (i.e. elderly alone).
Existential problems (feelings and moods that cannot be medicalized as psychological problems or sub-threshold psychological problems).
Administrative problems (certificate).

The *third aspect* is that in primary care *more attention is required to the context*, preferences, and values of the patient and all the problems they bring, following the indications of the biopsychosocial model [30] even if not directly related to the clinical problem that is the primary reason for the encounter. The general practitioner is a specialist of the individual embedded in the community and not of a specific part of an individual's body; therefore, they must take into account the context in which the patient lives, and not only selected factors of the environment [31, 32].

The concept of problem is central to the method of general practice. A problem is defined as:

> anything that requires action on the part of the doctor or the patient himself/herself anything that the doctor and/or patient perceives as a deviation from the normal state of health or that threatens, has threatened or will threaten the patient's functional capacity [33]

We distinguish between 'clinical' problems and 'non-clinical' problems [34], which are not directly related to the physician's current disciplinary knowledge (Table 5.1) The problems are classified by the international coding system for problems in general practice [35].

> *Therefore, identifying the causes and considering the effects of problems on both the medical aspects and the patient's life* [36] *should be a process that runs alongside the medical disciplinary process for achieving working diagnoses.*

The *fourth feature*, the most important and peculiar in primary care, is the *longitudinal relationship* with patients, so that information gathering and clinical decision-making occur over several encounters [37]: after the present remote consultation the same doctor or someone of their team will meet the patient another time, for the same problem or another episode of illness, and the present remote consultation becomes the previous step in taking care of them.

Therefore, the timeframe of clinical reasoning in primary care does not comprise of merely the one consultation, but a set of consultations which are 'transit stations' [[16]: 262] *of a care strategy. Hence, we have a reasoning strategy inside the remote consultations and a managing strategy including the next appointment with the patient.*

5.1.5 Clinical Reasoning in Remote Consultation

The processes and components of clinical reasoning in a remote consultation are largely the same as those of a face-to-face consultation. However, one of the major limitations and potential source of errors is the difficulty of performing an adequate physical examination. In the following sections, we will highlight ways to prevent this from happening.

5.1.6 Conclusion

In the case of experienced practitioners, the aforementioned reasoning processes and cognitive routines usually play out in a parallel, and often subtle, way. However, for expositive and didactic convenience we can identify an ideal process, which, when respected by the novice practitioner, can be useful to connect what doctors elaborate with what and how they communicate. The analysis of the steps of this process allows us to reflect and to evaluate it.

5.2 Clinical Reasoning on the Run

5.2.1 Step 1

Gather information to generate clinical hypotheses and gather non-clinical information focusing on:

Reason for the call
Symptoms and problems
Ideas, concerns and expectations
Personal situation
Implicit questions
Your emotional reactions

The first step in any decision-making process—and thus also in medical decision-making—is the gathering of information.

The information in a remote consultation is first provided by the caller, who expresses a series of symptoms, problems, requests, observations, reflections or fears in a narrative form.

Of these, some lead to the automatic generation of a series of clinical hypotheses (the so-called clinical information) through 'forward reasoning' [38], the first step of clinical reasoning. Other narratives help the doctor to understand the preferences of the patient and to decide the course of action that is useful and appreciated by the individual patient (the so-called non-clinical information). To focus on the reason for the call, the ideas, concerns, and expectations the caller has is a strong determinant of a satisfying consultation [39].

More difficult is to understand the implicit questions of the caller: the most effective way to train yourself to be aware of them is to observe the sensitivity to your own emotional reaction.

Remember that you do not have to make a detailed diagnosis but to decide the best course of action for that individual patient.

5.2.1.1 Notes on This Step in Remote Consultation

This step is quite different in remote consultation from the face-to-face one, because communicative elements that come to us from the paraverbal are less evident in remote than in face-to-face consultations. For this reason, it is essential to be attentive and sensitive to words, silence and tone of voice.

Remember that also in a remote consultation it is possible to understand the patients' subjectivity, their discomfort, their preferences, and allow them to express themselves freely.

Empathic listening is correlated to satisfaction and enablement of the patient [40]. Moreover, encouraging patients to freely express themselves allows the doctor to collect *more* pieces of information, whereas asking questions narrows the area of research and allows the doctor to collect more *detailed* pieces of information.

In other words, the doctor's aim is to open an unrestricted area—as stated in RICE—in an empathetic, silent and passive but attentive manner, and wait to ask for details in the second step of the reasoning process, which will start as soon as the spontaneous flow of information from the patient is exhausted.

Check List Step 1

Did you generate early diagnostic hypotheses?
Did you gather non-clinical information?

5.2.2 Step 2

Select and test the clinical hypotheses, in order to reach the working diagnoses and to rule out severe pathologies
Focus on problems
Start collecting and investigating problems and other determinants

This second step of the clinical reasoning process is the 'backward reasoning' [38], the deductive cognitive routine. This step corresponds to the second phase of the RICE process: collecting specific information on medical problems.

It consists of actively gathering additional information to test the generated hypotheses—through closed questions with high predictive power—rule out severe conditions, investigate 'red flags', and to detail the nature of the non-clinical problems, including their causes, and their effects, on the patient's life and on clinical problems.

The communication style of the doctor changes from conversational to interviewing style, from open (ended) question, or brief repetition of the patient's words, to the more traditional doctor-centred history taking.

The goal is to reach working diagnoses based on the testing of previously generated clinical hypotheses, and to investigate other determinants of the life and health of the patient.

5.2.2.1 Notes on This Step in Remote Consultation

In a remote consultation, the doctor has less information due to the physical absence of the patient, and enough data must be collected to rule out acute, life-threatening diseases. A list of closed-ended questions could be of good support.

Once life-threatening, severe problems are ruled out, the doctor can gain time by applying a premature diagnostic closure, or 'freezing', that prevents any search for new information ('stopping rule'). The working diagnosis can also be a simple, broad evaluation of severity [37].

The stopping rule involves three criteria: the ruling out of high risk conditions requiring the referral to the emergency department, the agreement with the patient on the management of the problem, and the reliable safety netting (see below) [37].

Check List Step 2

1. Have you investigated all the physical, psychological, family and social factors involved?
2. Did you focus on the symptoms in order to understand their significance?
3. Did you select and test the hypotheses generated?
4. Have you used appropriate questions in the verbal examination that are sufficiently sensitive and specific, avoiding redundancy?
5. Have high-risk conditions and severe illness that require urgent hospital attention been excluded?
6. Have you responded directly to the patient's needs?
7. Is there a reliable safety netting in place?

5.2.3 Step 3

In order to reach an overall clinical judgement:

Contextualize the working diagnoses:
Reframe and prioritize problems.
Describe interactions (not excluding the doctor him/herself).
Evaluate grade and type of uncertainty.
Activate forced cognitive strategies to avoid errors, the so-called safety routines.

The consultation can be divided into two sections: (first) information gathering and (second) projecting, planning and choosing a course of action. In between these two, we recommend the evaluation step.

Evaluation is the most important step in clinical reasoning, in which all the elements collected must be integrated to reach the outcome: an overall clinical judgement.

We have called this process of information integration 'contextualization of working diagnoses'.

The other tasks are the evaluation of the uncertainty and the scrutiny of the overall reasoning process to avoid methodological errors.

We describe the tasks one by one, even though in practice they may be indistinguishable from each other and occur in any order. Moreover, the evaluation step itself can be invisible, because it may be an instantaneous process or a parallel cognitive routine during the previous steps.

5.2.3.1 Contextualize the Working Diagnoses

Reframe and prioritize problems.
Describe interactions (not excluding the doctor him/herself).

In general practice—but also in every discipline of medicine—the diagnosis is not the end point of clinical reasoning, rather a concept useful to justify a course of action that must be decided. The course of action is directed to a patient with ideas, concerns and expectations, often with a previous illness, living in the community with a caregiver and/or a family. These aspects influence the course of action. So, the working diagnosis must be contextualized and connected with these problems or other aspects of the patient's life (Table 5.2).

For example, if the caregiver of a complex, elderly person (multi-morbid and non-autonomous) is unreliable and the social network is poor, in the case of an acute event the decision to hospitalize may depend almost exclusively on the unreliability of the caregiver, regardless of the working diagnosis.

Table 5.2 Problems and aspects of patient's life that need to be related to the working diagnosis

Psychological
Psychosocial
Social
Familiar
Administrative
Economic status
Patient's care situation
Nature of the social network
Reliability of the patient and caregivers
Commitment of the relatives
Organizational and contextual opportunities

Here you see that the working diagnoses can be contextualized if the doctor knows the nature of the problems identified, their relevance, their causes and effects on each other and on the clinical problems presented. In other words, this can happen if the doctor understands the system formed by the patient, his family, professionals and other caregivers, up to the community.

Knowing *the nature* of the problems helps to reframe them: in fact, a problem does not exist in the world, but is a creation of our thinking. The problem is the consequence of the failure to achieve a goal that is not immediately attainable, finding an obstacle that prevents one from reaching it. Therefore, it can be presented in a different way. It can, in other words, be manipulated by the subject or their advisor, in this case the doctor. Specifically, the problem can be broken down into subproblems and then solved more easily, but can also be considered from another point of view, that of the physician, and presented back to the patient [41].

In addition, you have to define *the relevance* of problems for both the patient and the physician, both clinical and social, in order to prioritize the necessary actions.

Finally, you have to take into account *the effects* of the problems in relation to each other in order to understand the system. If the system is complex, a simple list of problems is not enough, you have to draw a problem map or an 'influence diagram'. This can highlight the complex interaction between problems, best highlighted by several arrows [42]. In this map, you describe the interactions by also considering yourself as a determining factor.

Another way to approach this step of clinical reasoning is to analyse scenarios. A scenario is defined as the description or portrayal of a situation. The attention is focused on its uncertain aspects and forecast how they would evolve or emerge.

The scenario allows for manipulations and mental experiments, thus aiding in the envisioning of its evolution. It is useful to generate multiple scenarios, including at least a best-case scenario and a worst-case scenario.

In addition, the scenario is a useful tool for self-observation because it also includes the doctor, who is not just a spectator but an actor in that scenario. This means the doctor is in relationships with other actors.

It is methodologically robust because it is not just an analysis tool for the evolution of disease patterns but for any uncertain evolutionary aspect (psychological, social and so on) [23, 43].

The scenario contains working diagnoses, the patient's relationships, their requests and their internal world. It is generated automatically by the physician and has immediate effects on clinical reasoning.

5.2.3.2 Evaluate Source and Grade of Uncertainty

Uncertainty has been defined as an inability to decide because of the subjective perception of ignorance [44], which occurs in the face of an unknown risk. This is different from the situation of known risk, in which doctors possess probabilistic knowledge of the occurrence of an event, where logic and statistical tools are invaluable in making a decision [[45]: 29, 39, 320].

First of all, to have more control over behaviour facing uncertainty, it is useful to reflect on emotions connected with it (Table 5.3).

Investigate the Source of Uncertainty

The doctor should not ignore uncertainty because of unpleasant feelings, but instead investigate its source (Table 5.4) and assess its grade [44].

Each type of uncertainty demands a different strategy: for instance, if uncertainty is due to ambiguity of information of a probabilistic nature, doctors have to find further evidence-based information, while if uncertainty is due to unreliability of patients, doctors have to build a trusting relationship with them.

Table 5.3 Checklist to control behaviour in facing uncertainty [14]

Recall an instance where you were uncertain.
How did you feel?
What emotions arose?
What thoughts came to mind?

Table 5.4 Source of uncertainty

The Source of uncertainty may lie in:
A) *Information of a probabilistic nature, if it is ambiguous.*
Imprecise: when the probability is expressed by a wide range of values.
Unreliable:
When the estimation of probabilities is derived from unreliable methods or instruments.
If there are multiple causal factors, states of events, outcomes or possible interpretations.
When the boundaries between events are vague or are difficult to describe (situations of complexity).
B) *Practical-organizational uncertainty*, because any diagnostic and therapeutic intervention cannot disregard the quality of the health care system in which it is embedded.
C) *Information disclosed by the patient* about themselves and their care network can be uncertain. This is particularly relevant in primary care, where almost all interventions start from the patient's subjectivity, and is even more relevant in remote consultation.

It should be remembered, however, that the indeterminacy of future events is not eliminable, because it still remains a probabilistic, and not a deterministic, prediction [[45]: 40].

> Identifying, articulating and prioritizing of 'unnecessary uncertainties' are the first step and a specific strategy for a better management of clinical uncertainty.

Investigate the Grade of Uncertainty
Clinical situations can be represented as consisting of a core of known risk, determined by probabilistic knowledge, shrouded in a cloud of uncertainty [10] (Fig. 5.1). We also know that the cloud of uncertainty can be thick or thin, leading to very different situations from the clinical and practical point of view [10], which we discuss further in this chapter.

It is believed that the physician's duty is always primarily to explore the known risk, using expert systems or clinical prediction rules, and to assess what can be considered "certain" (even if it is probabilistic and therefore 'not certain' for the individual patient). However, we should not stop there, but instead further explore the cloud of uncertainty, either to reduce it through additional information, or to tolerate it, and help the patient tolerate it, with the stark awareness that uncertainty is constitutive of the real world.

5.2.3.3 Strategies to Avoid Errors

Safety cognitive routines are the last part of clinical reasoning and are used to confirm the assessment before entering the plan-and-choose section of the consultation [15].

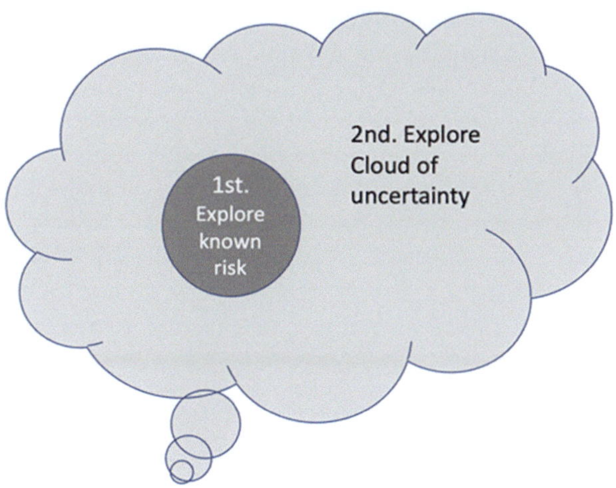

Fig. 5.1 Representation of clinical situations: a core of known risk and a cloud of uncertainty

Table 5.5 Activation of safety cognitive routines [14]

Are there alternative diagnoses that would greatly change the assessment?
For example:
Are there more likely diagnoses (to avoid the availability bias)?
Are there more convincing diagnoses than the one I generated from the beginning (to avoid anchoring bias)?
Is there information disconfirming the diagnosis I generated from the outset (to avoid confirmation bias)?
Could it be an atypical presentation of an alternative diagnosis (to avoid representativeness bias)?
Did I stop at the right moment? Do I need to achieve more certainty? Am I too certain of the generated diagnosis?

In the telephone consultation, which is a setting in which errors are more likely to occur, doctors can use cognitive routines that 'forcibly' check the process carried out in order to identify any errors, and avoid premature closure of the diagnostic process, with respect to the desired degree of certainty or detail.

You have to stop the reasoning process and, before moving on to the project/decision phase, force yourself to answer a set of questions (Table 5.5), much like the 'cash machine' forces you to withdraw the card before taking the cash.

5.2.3.4 Notes on This Step in Remote Consultation

Complex situations could be a contraindication to remote consultation in principle, but we state that is possible to face these complex situations with an accurate evaluation.

Check List Step 3

1. Have you analysed the context?
2. Have you reframed the problems?
3. Have you prioritized the problems?
4. Did you take into account the interactions among the problems?
5. Did you investigate the sources and the grade of uncertainty?
6. Did you check the reasoning process to identify any errors?
7. Did you consider prognosis, quality of life of the patient, degree of medicalization and intensity of care in your clinical judgement?

5.2.4 Step 4

Generate multiple evolution scenarios and design future course of actions.
Choose a course of action:

Identify the options, share them with the patient if necessary or if requested by them, choose the course of action and reach a shared decision with the patient.

Use strategies to manage uncertainty if uncertainty is high: *The higher the uncertainty, the higher the involvement of the patient in the process. Build the safety net.*

5.2.4.1 Generate Multiple Evolution Scenarios and Design Future Course of Actions

After assessing the present situation, the physician generates possible scenarios and course of actions which are never black or white, but rather always shrouded in some cloud of uncertainty: these are the so-called multi-attribute options. Hence, at the end of this process, the doctor will have a list of options at hand.

Be prepared for the flexibility to choose alternative routes if proposals are rejected when shared with the patient. In other words, remember the importance of 'plan B'.

Check List Step 4
Designing and Planning in Primary Care

1. Have you planned appropriate tests or referrals in the appropriate sequence in a satisfactory manner, in appropriate timing, taking into account the characteristics of the service you are sending the patient to?
2. Did you design the care pathway making sure to give an answer to each problem, physical, psychological, social and existential?
3. If you planned to do nothing, did you ask yourself why, and did you find a good reason for this choice?
4. For the design of the treatment:

Who is the patient?
Who should or can be the care giver?
How often do I contact the patient and for how long?
How do I communicate with the patient or the caregiver?

5.2.4.2 Choose a Course of Actions

Definition of "Decision"
Goal-driven behaviour that occurs in the presence of options on the basis of a cognitive process in which a series of related actions are selected in order to achieve a satisfactory resolution.

During a consultation you make a lot of decisions, and often you are not aware of it.

Decisions are not only about therapy or diagnostic pathway, but also are related to taking care of the patient (Table 5.6) [45].

Moreover, medical decisions are challenging because they are not a mere administrative job of enforcing rules, but rather a more complex reasoning process that considers the meaning of medical action in the relationship to the patient, and considers the uniqueness of the situation [[16]: 174]. Therefore, the entire process of decision-making must be shared with the patient: the patient has to co-built the process.

As we have stated above, options in medicine are multi-attribute, and therefore, the doctor relies on weighing up the pros and cons in order to choose an option based on the best existing evidence, according to the EBM method.

The second step is *fine tuning* to the specific patient, which is neither simple nor automatic [46]. We use, as an example, the ideal process of prescribing a drug, which is the most frequent medical act and not without risk for the patient's safety (Table 5.7). The logic of reasoning also applies to other therapeutic or diagnostic acts.

In fact, the efficacy and safety of a drug is tested on patient populations that do not necessarily have the characteristics of the real patient. Delvecchio and Vettore [17] state:

> The outcome of therapy is a statistical result for the generality of similar cases, but is casual for the individual case.

Table 5.6 Decision types

Decision types.
Gathering additional information
Evaluating test results
Defining problem
Drug related decisions
Therapeutic procedure related decisions
Legal and insurance related decisions
Organizational decisions (i.e. how to manage social network of the family, or the referrals)
Giving advice and precaution
Treatment goal
Referral

Table 5.7 Drugs prescription

Have you designed the drug therapy by identifying a set of useful drugs?
Have you analysed this set of drugs by asking yourself the therapeutic objective (cure, heal, chronicize or simply remove the symptom? Therapy: background, collateral, adjuvant)?
Have you checked the safety profile of the drugs?
What do you expect when the drug is administered? (therapeutic threshold, dose side effects, interactions).
What reliability in administration and compliance?

Table 5.8 Goals and values in decision-making

Goals	Underlying values
I am not a mere prescriber of what the patient wants	Professional dignity
I am very attentive to the needs of the elderly	Improving quality of life is as important as prolonging it
I am very strict with patients who want antibiotics to avoid stock piling at home	Avoid overtreatment Avoid side effects from non-indicated drugs Avoid wastage

For this reason, consider the safety of the drug by weighing up the pros and cons in relation to the seriousness of the situation. The more risky the drug, the clearer and more justified the goals must be.

A drug must be a helpful means to reach a health objective: to treat the illness, to prolong life, or to alleviate pain or troublesome symptoms, always in accordance with the patient's preferences, values and requirements. The objective is the patient as a whole person.

In patients being treated with a range of drugs, special attention must be paid to interactions.

Finally, the third and last step is the shared choice with the patient: if you shared the entire process, you know the patient's values and preferences, and if you informed them honestly, preferences become 'informed preferences' [22].

Furthermore, the doctors have to be aware of their own underlying values. As doctors become aware of their values and their patient's values and informed preferences, they can make better, and more balanced, shared decisions. If a conflict with the patient arises, the doctor might wonder if they hold different values (Table 5.8).

5.2.4.3 Use Strategies to Manage Uncertainty if It Is High

We suggest two effective strategies to manage the high uncertainty of a chosen medical action.

Within the Consultation: Shared Decision-Making

The strategy is to share with the patient both the steps of decision-making and the final choice: the higher the uncertainty, the higher the involvement. Shared decision-making should be implemented to a greater extent if the uncertainty is higher [47], reaching greater agreement between physician and patient [48].

Remote Solution: Safety Net (Call Back, New Contact)

The second strategy is to use time as a test with strong confirmatory or exclusion power [49]. Time may bring an increase (or decrease) in the severity of symptoms, or number of symptoms, thus crossing into the area of low decision uncertainty (Figs. 5.2 and Fig. 5.3).

The test of time should be used in all clinical situations whose worsening or recovery directs us towards a more precise diagnosis or allows us to rule out more serious diagnoses, once severe conditions have been excluded. In addition, the test of time must be embedded in a framework –the so-called safety net [50] (Fig. Fig. 5.3) organized by the physician, characterized by:

1. the use of precise communication tools (instructing the patient on what to do depending on the evolution of the clinical situation);
2. a solid relationship between physician and patient/person; and,
3. an effective call reception system that ensures immediate feedback [51].

Test of time is recommended as a tool to close the decision-making process [37] although little research is reported on its effectiveness [51].

If the uncertainty is greater and the patient is unreliable, or if there is something that does not fit with the clinical situation, the doctor should call back, following gut feelings, because the clinical reasoning is based not only on cognitive routines, but also on instinctive feelings [5], often within fast and frugal heuristic strategies [45]

Fig. 5.2 Threshold of decision uncertainty

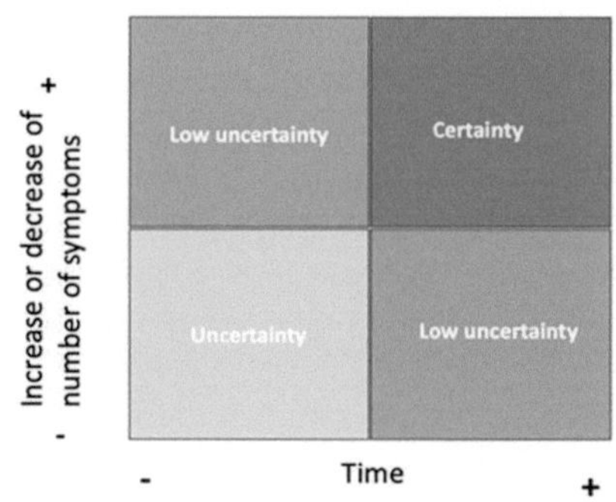

SAFETY NETTING
Inform the patient:
That there is uncertainty
What exactly to look out for
How exactly to seek further help
What to expect about time course
Safety-net advice should be documented in the medical notes
Written format rather than verbally

Fig. 5.3 Safety-netting process

(see above). These two simple questions: ‘Is something wrong here?’ and ‘Does everything fit?’ can help the doctor to decide if the chosen course of action is ‘good enough’ [5, 7, 8].

5.2.4.4 Notes on This Step in Remote Consultation

Doctors in remote consultation can design the same pathways as they would design in person, but they can also refer the patient to a face-to-face visit, in order to have the opportunity to do a physical examination or to gather more information, enhancing diagnostic accuracy (Table 5.9).

Moreover, sharing with the patient in the remote consultation is a duty, and reaching an agreement is always necessary. Information provided to the patient on all aspects of the treatment must be complete and honest.

Safety net and call-back are necessary tools and must always be used, because to consider a second thought is always a wise choice.

Check List Step 4
Decision-Making in Primary Care/Uncertainty Management

1. Have you followed evidence-based guidelines?
2. Have you adapted it to your patient?
3. Have you explored the pros and cons of each option and shared them with the patient if necessary or requested by them?
4. Have you made explicit to yourself the values against which you will decide and compared them with those of the patient?
5. Have you reached a shared decision with the patient?
6. Have you involved the patient if uncertainty is high?
7. Have you built the safety netting?
8. Have you used intuition: ‘Is there something that does not add up?’ or ‘Does everything add up?’

Table 5.9 Paths in remote consultation

Emergency/Hospital Visit
Home/surgery face-to-face visit
Advice and/or drugs
Diagnostic route

References

1. Marewski JN, Gigerenzer G. Heuristic decision making in medicine. Dialogues Clin Neurosci. 2012;14(1):77–89.
2. Gigerenzer G. Risk savvy: how to make good decisions. Penguin; 2015. p. 336.
3. McLaughlin K, Eva KW, Norman GR. Reexamining our bias against heuristics. Adv Health Sci Educ. 2014;19(3):457–64.
4. Croskerry P. A universal model of diagnostic reasoning. Acad Med. 2009;84(8):1022–8.
5. Stolper E, Van de Wiel M, Van Royen P, Van Bokhoven M, Van der Weijden T, Dinant GJ. Gut feelings as a third track in general practitioners' diagnostic reasoning. J Gen Intern Med. 2011;26(2):197–203.
6. Kozlowski D, Hutchinson M, Hurley J, Rowley J, Sutherland J. The role of emotion in clinical decision making: an integrative literature review. BMC Med Educ. 2017;17(1):255.
7. Stolper E, Van Royen P, Van de Wiel M, Van Bokhoven M, Houben P, Van der Weijden T, et al. Consensus on gut feelings in general practice. BMC Fam Pract. 2009;10:66.
8. Stolper E, van Bokhoven M, Houben P, Van Royen P, van de Wiel M, van der Weijden T, et al. The diagnostic role of gut feelings in general practice. A focus group study of the concept and its determinants. BMC Fam Pract. 2009;10:17.
9. van Weel C. The extraordinary diagnostic sensitivity of family physicians. Fam Pract. 2020;37(4):431–3.
10. Parisi G, Kurotschka PK. From evidence-based medicine to shared decision making: how to manage uncertainty in clinical practice. Recenti Prog Med. 2022;113(5):305–16.
11. Pelaccia T, Tardif J, Triby E, Charlin B. An analysis of clinical reasoning through a recent and comprehensive approach: the dual-process theory. Med Educ Online. 2011;16
12. Balla JI, Heneghan C, Glasziou P, Thompson M, Balla ME. A model for reflection for good clinical practice: model for reflection on practice. J Eval Clin Pract. 2009;15(6):964–9.
13. Elstein AS, Schwartz A. Clinical problem solving and diagnostic decision making: selective review of the cognitive literature. BMJ. 2002;324(7339):729–32.
14. Gheihman G, Johnson M, Simpkin AL. Twelve tips for thriving in the face of clinical uncertainty. Med Teach. 2020;42(5):493–9.
15. Croskerry P. Cognitive forcing strategies in clinical decisionmaking. Ann Emerg Med. 2003;41(1):110–20.
16. Parisi G, Pasolli L. Clinica, relazione, decisione. La consultazione medica nelle cure primarie. 1° edizione. Franco Angeli; 2016. 358.
17. Delvecchio G, Vettore L. Decidere in terapia. Dialogo sul metodo nella cura. Liberodiscrivere, curatore. Vol. 13, Liberodiscrivere. Genova; 2013.
18. Charles C, Gafni A, Whelan T. Shared decision-making in the medical encounter: what does it mean? (or it takes at least two to tango). Soc Sci Med. 1997;44(5):681–92.
19. Stiggelbout AM, Pieterse AH, De Haes JCJM. Shared decision making: concepts, evidence, and practice. Patient Educ Couns. 2015;98(10):1172–9.
20. Kon AA. The shared decision-making continuum. JAMA J Am Med Assoc. 2010;304(8):903.
21. Whitney SN, McGuire AL, McCullough LB. A typology of shared decision making, informed consent, and simple consent. Ann Intern Med. 2004;140(1):54–9.
22. Elwyn G, Edwards A Thompson R (a cura di). Shared decision making in health care. Achieving evidence-based patient choice. Oxford: Oxford University Press; 2016.
23. Delvecchio G. Logica e diagnosi. Principi di metodologia medica. Rubbettino; 2020. 186.
24. Dixon AS. «There's a lot of it about»: clinical strategies in family practice. J R Coll Gen Pract. 1986;36(291):468–71.
25. Marshall M. Redefining quality: valuing the role of the GP in managing uncertainty. Br J Gen Pract. 2016;66(643):e146–8.
26. Jadhakhan F, Romeu D, Lindner O, Blakemore A, Guthrie E. Prevalence of medically unexplained symptoms in adults who are high users of healthcare services and magnitude of associated costs: a systematic review. BMJ Open. 2022;12(10):e059971.

27. Malterud K, Guassora AD, Reventlow S, Jutel A. Embracing uncertainty to advance diagnosis in general practice. Br J Gen Pract. 2017;67(659):244–5.
28. Doust J. Using probabilistic reasoning. BMJ. 2009;339:b3823.
29. Ilgen JS, Eva KW, Regehr G. What's in a label? Is diagnosis the start or the end of clinical reasoning? J Gen Intern Med. 2016;31(4):435–7.
30. Engel GL. The need for a new medical model: a challenge for biomedicine. Science. 1977;196(4286):129–36.
31. McWhinney IR. Why we need a new clinical method. Scand J Prim Health Care. 1993;11(1):3–7.
32. Watsjold BK, Ilgen JS, Regehr G. An ecological account of clinical reasoning. Acad Med. 2022;97(11S):S80–6.
33. Gervas J. Los problemas de salud en atencion primaria y su clasificacion. Aten Primaria. 1987;4:429–31.
34. Procter S, Stewart K, Reeves D, Bowen L, Purdy S, Ridd M, et al. Complex consultations in primary care: a tool for assessing the range of health problems and issues addressed in general practice consultations. BMC Fam Pract. 2014;15(1):105.
35. Classification Committee of the World Organization of family doctors. In: ICPC-2: international classification of primary care. Oxford University Press; 1992.
36. Pendleton D. The consultation: an approach to learning and teaching. Oxford: University Press; 1984. (Oxford general practice series)
37. Balla J, Heneghan C, Thompson M, Balla M. Clinical decision making in a high-risk primary care environment: a qualitative study in the UK. BMJ Open. 2012;2(1):e000414.
38. Groen GJ, Patel VL. Medical problem-solving: some questionable assumptions. Med Educ. 1985;19(2):95–100.
39. Ruiz-Moral R, Pérula de Torres LÁ, Jaramillo-Martin I. The effect of patients' met expectations on consultation outcomes. A study with family medicine residents. J Gen Intern Med. 2007;22(1):86–91.
40. Mercer SW, Jani BD, Maxwell M, Wong SY, Watt GC. Patient enablement requires physician empathy: a cross-sectional study of general practice consultations in areas of high and low socioeconomic deprivation in Scotland. BMC Fam Pract. 2012;13(1):6.
41. Newell A, Shaw JC, Simon HA. Elements of a theory of human problem solving. Psychol Rev. 1958;65(3):151–66.
42. Sturmberg JP. Systems and complexity thinking in general practice: part 1 – clinical application. Aust Fam Physician. 2007;36(3):170–3.
43. Delvecchio G. Metodo e diagnosi. Società editrice Universo; 2011.
44. Han PKJ, Klein WMP, Arora NK. Varieties of uncertainty in health care: a conceptual taxonomy. Med Decis Mak. 2011;31(6):828–38.
45. Ofstad EH, Frich JC, Schei E, Frankel RM, Gulbrandsen P. What is a medical decision? A taxonomy based on physician statements in hospital encounters: a qualitative study. BMJ Open. 2016;6(2):e010098.
46. Bissessur SW, Geijteman ECT, Al-Dulaimy M, Teunissen PW, Richir MC, Arnold AER, et al. Therapeutic reasoning: from hiatus to hypothetical model: therapeutic reasoning. J Eval Clin Pract. 2009;15(6):985–9.
47. O'Riordan M, Dahinden A, Aktürk Z, Ortiz JMB, Dağdeviren N, Elwyn G, et al. Dealing with uncertainty in general practice: an essential skill for the general practitioner. Qual Prim Care. 2011;19(3):175–81.
48. Innes AD, Campion PD, Griffiths FE. Complex consultations and the 'edge of chaos'. Br J Gen Pract. 2005;55(510):47–52.
49. Almond SC, Summerton N. Test of time. BMJ. 2009;338(jun15 1):b1878.
50. Almond S, Mant D, Thompson M. Diagnostic safety-netting. Br J Gen Pract. 2009;59(568):872–4.
51. Jones D, Dunn L, Watt I, Macleod U. Safety netting for primary care: evidence from a literature review. Br J Gen Pract. 2019;69(678):e70–9.

Communication Setting and Skills on the Telephone

6

Cristina Vito, Giuseppe Parisi, Jacopo Demurtas, Adel Yasky, and Almas Fatma

6.1 Introduction

6.1.1 Telephone Consultation in General Practice Over the Years

Although it is a common opinion that telephone consultation is a recent phenomenon, it is worth remembering that the first telephone consultation reported in scientific literature dates back to 1879 [1]. Since then, and notably in the last 20 years, telephone medical consultations in general practice have progressively increased, as they offer a quick and straightforward way to access medical care, allowing general practitioners to improve time and resource management.

C. Vito (✉)
Family Physician Consultant, Hair Disorders Specialist, AraMedica, Lecce, Italy

G. Parisi
Postgraduate School of Specific Training in General Practice, (Scuola di Formazione Specifica in Medicina Generale), Trento, Italy

Italian Society of Medical Education (SIPeM), Torino, Italy

Interdepartmental Center for Medical Sciences, University of Trento, Trento, Italy

J. Demurtas
Clinical and Experimental Medicine PhD Program, University of Modena and Reggio Emilia, Modena, Italy

Family Medicine Department USL Toscana Sud-Est, Capalbio, Italy

A. Yasky
Family Medicine Department King Abdulaziz Medical City, Riyadh, Saudi Arabia

Ministry of National Guard Health Affairs, Riyadh, Saudi Arabia

A. Fatma
Family Physician & Certified Digital Health Professional at Alcura Family Clinic, Navi Mumbai, India

J. Demurtas (ed.), *Remote Consultation in Primary Care*, TELe-Health,
https://doi.org/10.1007/978-3-031-89661-3_6

Furthermore, in the context of our service, most initial contacts take place by telephone. Teleconsultation also allows for interaction with the general practitioner even where this may not be possible or may be challenging, and can help limit the spread of contagious infectious diseases, as recently emerged in the context of the COVID-19 pandemic in 2020 [2].

As is well known, the pandemic has played a decisive role in implementing the use of telemedicine, and, in particular [3]:

- In Europe, teleconsultations became the preferred mode of primary care delivery, where physicians were recommended to triage patients remotely, and face-to-face consultations were discouraged unless considered necessary by the attending doctor [4–6].
- In Italy, 20% of the teleconsultations carried out during the pandemic were telephone-based, 38% were conducted through web-based systems, 29% on specific platforms, and 13% via apps [7].
- Telephone consultations in US outpatient centers, by April 2020, accounted for 65.4% of primary care consultations and 71.6% of behavioral health visits [8].

6.1.2 Telephone Consultation: Main Purpose and Basic Requirements

Telephone contacts are increasingly used as an extension of, or a substitute for, traditional face-to-face contacts with a range of primary and secondary healthcare professionals. Telephone services now include delivery of routine and emergency care, facilitating health promotion interventions, prompt communication of laboratory investigations, and repeated medical prescriptions [9, 10]. In primary care, telephone consultation is increasingly used to replace an in-person visit, when this is required and possible. It is clear that telephone consultation, by its nature, cannot have the same structure and content as face-to-face medical consultations in an outpatient or home setting; in the same way, remote video consultations are distinguished. In medical teleconsultation, the patient is provided with an answer to a clinical problem in the absence of visualization of the patient and in the absence of clinical data available through the visit; clearly, the output of the consultation may also be the need for an in-person visit or hospital admission. Therefore, given the importance of teleconsultation, it is unthinkable that this is limited to a chaotic and disorganized exchange of information. Thus, it is essential to understand the scope of teleconsultation (i.e., what is permissible and appropriate to do remotely), especially in a field where available evidence in the literature is limited and developments are ongoing.

In primary care, telephone consultations can act as:

- *Replacements* for in-person visits, when feasible
- *Triage tools,* to determine the need for further action, including referral for in-person consultations or hospital admissions
- *The outcome of a telephone consultation may fall under one of the following categories:*

Consultation outcome	Description
Telephone consultation	Simple cases that can be resolved through advice or prescription
Video consultation needed	Issues requiring visual confirmation or additional patient interaction
In-person visit required	Situations where physical examination or further diagnostics are necessary
Urgency/Emergency referral	Cases requiring immediate referral to emergency services

In summary, the GP must keep in mind that the purpose of a teleconsultation is not to formulate a remote diagnosis, but rather to carry out a selection (see Table 6.1), a telephone triage.

Furthermore, we must not forget that teleconsultation (especially in general medicine) can also be an opportunity for prevention and health promotion, rather than being exclusively aimed at addressing an active clinical problem, as shown in Table 6.2.

Table 6.1 Triage categories in telephone consultations

Triage category	Description	Possible actions	Examples
Manageable by telephone	Situations that can be resolved entirely over the phone	Provide telephone advice Issue a drug prescription	Mild seasonal allergies, prescription refills
Manageable by video consultation	Cases where visual assessment or more interaction is needed	Switch to video consultation Provide advice or prescription	Skin rash, follow-up for chronic conditions
Requires face-to-face consultation	Cases where physical examination is essential	Arrange an outpatient or home visit	Abdominal pain, suspected fractures
Urgency/Emergency referral	Critical conditions that demand immediate medical intervention	Direct referral to emergency services	Chest pain, severe breathlessness

Greenhalgh, T., Koh, G. C. H., & Car, J. (2020). COVID-19: A remote assessment in primary care. BMJ, 368, m1182. https://doi.org/10.1136/bmj.m1182

Table 6.2 Key opportunities in telephone consultations

Opportunity	Description	Examples
Prevention	Use the opportunity to promote healthy behaviors	Advise on smoking cessation Encourage regular exercise
Health promotion	Educate patients on wellness and preventive care	Discuss vaccination schedules Promote screening programs
Building rapport	Strengthen the doctor–patient relationship by offering accessible care	Follow up on previous visits Acknowledge patients' concerns with empathy

World Health Organization. (2020). Telemedicine: Opportunities and developments in member states (second ed.). WHO Global Observatory for eHealth. https://www.who.int/goe/publications/telemedicine

Table 6.3 Requirements for a safe and effective telephone consultation

Requirement	Details	Examples of best practices
Safety	Ensure clinical safety through accurate history-taking and decision-making	Confirm allergies before prescribing medications
Respect for privacy	Conduct calls in private spaces to protect patient confidentiality	Avoid public areas for consultations
Preserving doctor–patient relationship	Maintain professional communication to build trust and empathy	Use reassuring language and listen actively
Distraction-free environment	Ensure both doctor and patient are in settings free from audio-visual interference	Avoid background noise (e.g., TV, children) Ask patients to move to a quieter place if needed

Bunn, F., Byrne, G., & Kendall, S. (2005). Telephone consultation and triage: Effects on healthcare use and patient satisfaction. The Cochrane Database of Systematic Reviews, (4), CD004180. https://doi.org/10.1002/14651858.CD004180.pub2

Medical telephone consultation must ensure some basic requirements, such as safety, respect for privacy, and the protection and respect of the general practitioner-patient relationship. It is also essential that teleconsultation takes place in an environment undisturbed by audio-visual interferences (e.g., noise from children playing, TV on in the background). Both the general practitioner and the individual must be in a suitable location without external interferences that could hinder effective communication (Table 6.3).

6.2 Peculiar Aspects of Telephone Consultation in General Practice

6.2.1 Safety, Advantages, and Disadvantages of Telephone Consultation

Telephone consultations can be a safe and appropriate means of care, provided that physicians understand their limitations and boundaries (Greenhalgh et al., 2020). The British Medical Association states that properly conducted telephone consultations offer a safe and acceptable way of managing patient care (BMA, 2020) [9, 11]. Evidence shows that telephone consultations in primary care can be comparable in quality to in-person visits (Bunn et al., 2005) [12].

The main advantages and disadvantages of telephone consultation are summarized in Table 6.4.

Table 6.4 Advantages and disadvantages of telephone consultation

Advantages of telephone consultation	Disadvantages of telephone consultation
Quicker access to care More choice in the way healthcare is received Improve the doctor–patient relationship Increase patient and doctor satisfaction Reducing transmission of infectious agents Monitoring for chronic diseases and therapy adjustment Possibility of guiding self-examinations Improve outcomes Improve adherence to chronic therapies Prevent inappropriate access to the emergency department Allow the patient to communicate from a more comfortable environment Promotes early diagnosis Lead home care management Reduce lost working days Avoids cancellation of appointments and therefore reduces waiting time Eco-sustainability and economic sustainability (reduce access cost)	Absence of clinical visual cues[a] Absence of visual signals inherent to communication/relationship[a] (e.g., nonverbal cues) Absence of physical examination[a] Impossibility of guiding self-examinations Impossibility of evaluating some types of patients firsthand (e.g., children, elderly people, patients with cognitive impairment), for which it is necessary to speak with a third person Environmental interference (e.g., background noises) Environmental distractions for both patients and doctors. Possibility of technical problems (e.g., call drops, poor audio quality) Limited suitability for patients with low health literacy May result in missed red flags or signs Privacy concerns in shared spaces

[a]Absence of visual clues, facial expressions, and postures that often provide vital signs regarding an individual's true thoughts and state of mind are either not available or less obvious during telephone consultation [13] (Bunn et al., 2005)

NB: Despite the obvious differences between video consultations and telephone consultations listed in the table, we note that a recent systematic review on the comparison between telephone and video consultations concludes that "Based on a small set of different studies, we found no notable differences between consultations telephone and video services for the management of patients with confirmed diagnoses. There is also a significant lack of research on telemedicine in primary care settings, despite its high diffusion" [14].

6.2.2 Recognizing Limitations and Minimizing Potential Risks of Telephone Consultations

Telephone consultations cannot always fully address a patient's concerns. They may not be suitable for the following:

- Complex patients (e.g., those with cognitive impairment or language barriers).
- Situations that require clinical examination or diagnostic testing.
- Conditions where in-person or video consultation is necessary (Bunn et al., 2005) [13].

Risks related to the protection of patient privacy must also be taken into consideration and will be discussed elsewhere. Some strategies to minimize risks deriving from telephone consultations are summarized in Table 6.5.

Table 6.5 Strategies to minimize risks in telephone consultations

Strategies to minimize the risks of telephone consultation
Use of detailed protocols for the organization of a telephone service [9]
Structured evaluation of the urgency of calls [9]
Establishing clinical facts, including relevant history, management plans, and good practice points [13]
Ask the patient to repeat their understanding of what has been discussed and agreed, making sure he/she clearly understands the medication instructions and potential side effects [13]
A dedicated and protected telephone consultation setup with no interruptions is recommended to focus on the appointment and allow good time management [13]
Enhanced documentation to compensate for the lack of physical examination will clarify agreed treatment plans for follow-up care [13]
Know the issues related to confidentiality and protect patient data and yourself from medical–legal problems [9]
Use specific strategies aimed at reducing clinical risk of teleconsultation that hesitate with remote advice (discussed in detail in the chapter …), such as:
The "Safety-net" or the "safety net" → It involves providing detailed information to the person about what to do in case of worsening/nonimprovement of symptoms or where particular events occur conditions (e.g., a new alarm symptom appears). Simply put, the person, at the end of the teleconsultation, must have understood under what circumstances, with what timing and methods carry out a specific action (e.g., contact the GP again, contact emergency services, go to the emergency department)
"Call back" = Scheduled telephone check → the doctor calls the person back at an agreed time
"New contact" → the person calls the doctor back at an agreed time

Table 6.6 Matching patients' needs to consultation formats

Consultation format	Suitable patient groups	Examples
Telephone consultation	Patients with chronic conditions, those requiring follow-ups, or those with travel difficulties [3]	Hypertension monitoring Postdischarge follow-up
Video consultation	Patients requiring visual assessments or those with high anxiety levels [3, 15]	Skin rashes Patients with mental health needs
Face-to-face consultation	Patients with complex conditions or those requiring physical exams [3, 16]	Acute abdominal pain Neurological assessment
Inappropriate for telephone consultation	Patients with low health literacy, cognitive impairment, or language barriers	Dementia patients Young children

6.2.3 Matching Patients with the Most Suitable Consultation Format

Certain patient groups are better suited for telephone consultations, while others may benefit more from video or in-person consultations based on their needs and abilities (Table 6.6).

Reversing Diagnostic Assumptions: From Likely to Worst-Case Scenarios

In traditional practice, clinicians often base their diagnostic hypothesis on the most probable and common conditions rather than rare but severe cases. However, this strategy needs to be adapted for teleconsultations. The absence of a clinical examination requires a more cautious approach to avoid missing urgent or emergent situations. The goal of gathering information through telephone consultations should be to *exclude any possibility of an emergency or serious condition*.

If the GP *cannot confidently rule out* an urgent or emergency scenario, the case should be redirected to:

- *In-person consultation* for further evaluation, or.
- *Emergency services* if immediate care is required.

This cautious approach ensures patient safety by prioritizing early detection of potentially severe conditions. GPs must avoid confirmation bias, where they focus too heavily on details supporting their initial hypothesis, rather than thoroughly evaluating for red flags.

And What if It Was Not an Appropriate Call?

Sometimes, a consultation may initially seem unnecessary or unrelated to medical care. However, the GP must remain alert to the possibility that the *patient may not be expressing their true concerns*. Embarrassment, fear, or anxiety can prevent individuals from openly discussing sensitive issues (e.g., mental health struggles, domestic abuse).

It is essential to probe beyond the surface and ensure the patient feels safe and comfortable to talk. Key strategies include:

1. *Check for barriers to communication.*
   - "Are you comfortable talking right now?"
   - "Is there anything stopping you from sharing your concerns freely?"
2. *Explore hidden concerns.*
   - "Is there anything else on your mind that you haven't mentioned yet?"
   - "Are you worried about something different from what we've discussed so far?"
3. *Assess potential danger or harm.*
   - "Are you currently safe?"
   - "Do you feel threatened or in danger from anyone?"

Such questions can reveal critical information that may not be apparent initially and guide the GP in providing appropriate care or referrals (e.g., mental health services, social support) (Table 6.7).

Pitfalls in Telephone Consultation

Telephone consultations can be effective, but they require specific caution and awareness to avoid diagnostic errors or mismanagement. Unlike in-person visits, the lack of visual and physical examination means that the clinician must rely solely on verbal communication, patient-reported symptoms, and epidemiological reasoning. However, this poses certain risks that general practitioners (GPs) must mitigate through structured approaches.

Table 6.7 Summary of key pitfalls and solutions in telephone consultations

Pitfalls	Description	Solutions
Confirmation bias	Focusing too early on the most likely diagnosis and missing severe conditions	Systematically exclude emergencies before confirming any hypothesis
Overreliance on patient reports	Sole reliance on patient-provided information may miss critical signs	Ask detailed, open-ended questions to probe for red flags
Hidden patient concerns	Patients may not express their true problems due to embarrassment or fear	Use probing questions to explore unexpressed concerns
Missed urgency/emergency	Some emergency conditions may not be obvious through phone consultation	Redirect to in-person care or emergency services if in doubt
Environmental distractions	Background noise or interruptions may affect communication	Ensure both the patient and clinician are in a quiet, private environment
Communication barriers	Language difficulties or cognitive impairments can hinder effective communication	Consider video or in-person consultation if communication is insufficient

Key Takeaways for Safe Telephone Consultation

- *Err on the side of caution:* Always prioritize ruling out emergencies before focusing on likely diagnoses.
- *Remain vigilant for unexpressed concerns:* Seemingly inappropriate calls may mask deeper or more sensitive issues.
- *Use open-ended and probing questions:* Encourage patients to share any additional information or concerns they might hesitate to express.
- *Transition to in-person care when needed:* If there is any doubt about the diagnosis or urgency, switch to face-to-face consultation.

A successful telephone consultation requires balancing diagnostic efficiency with patient safety. By focusing on ruling out emergencies first and using sensitive communication strategies, GPs can mitigate the risks inherent to remote consultations and ensure optimal patient care.

6.2.4 Telephone Consultation Techniques

Conducting an organized telephone consultation is essential for general practitioners (GPs) to effectively meet the needs of callers while ensuring no critical elements are overlooked. Although there are no standardized guidelines for telephone consultations, this manual provides theoretical and practical elements to guide GPs in their clinical actions. For example, we will explore the telephone consultation framework based on the RICE model developed by Hay Derkx. Iyengar and El-Nahas offer a concise guide to telephone medical consultations, summarizing vital steps for effective interactions, which we present here in an adapted format.

6.2.4.1 Vital Steps for a Successful Phone Consultation (Adapted from Iyengar and El-Nahas)

Stage	Step	Details
Before the consultation	Preparation of patient records	Open the electronic patient record application on your computer screen Familiarize yourself with the patient's history, including previous consultations, medications, and surgical procedures. This foundational knowledge is crucial for informed decision-making during the call
	Documentation setup	Populate necessary fields for the patient consultation Ensure easy access to relevant information during the call, streamlining the conversation and enhancing the quality of care provided
During the consultation	Time management	Set a time limit for the consultation (e.g., 10–15 mins) to maintain focus and efficiency Inform the patient of this time frame at the beginning of the call to manage expectations and encourage concise communication
	Case discussion	Engage in a thorough discussion of the patient's case and specific problems they are experiencing Actively listen to their concerns, asking clarifying questions to gain a comprehensive understanding of their situation.
	Confirmation of management plans	Clearly outline and confirm the management plans with the patient Ensure they understand the proposed approach, including any medications, referrals, or lifestyle modifications, which is essential for patient adherence and satisfaction
	Follow-up appointment	Establish an appropriate follow-up appointment, specifying the timeline for the next contact This practice fosters continuity of care and reassures the patient that their health is a priority
After the consultation	Documentation of the consultation	Dictate a detailed letter summarizing the consultation and documenting all pertinent information using an electronic dictation system This step is crucial for maintaining accurate medical records and providing continuity of care in future interactions

(continued)

Stage	Step	Details
	Face-to-face consultation arrangements	If a comprehensive plan cannot be established during the telephone consultation, prioritize scheduling an in-person appointment as soon as possible This approach ensures that patients with complex needs receive the appropriate level of care
Integrating additional telemedicine techniques	Sending multimedia	Encourage patients to send photos or videos relevant to their condition This visual information can provide valuable context that aids in diagnosis and treatment planning
	Sharing specialist reports and laboratory results	Patients can share diagnostic reports and lab results electronically during the consultation This real-time access to critical information allows for more informed discussions and decision-making
	Use of diagnostic equipment	Patients equipped with diagnostic tools, such as blood pressure monitors or pulse oximeters, can provide real-time readings during the call This data can significantly enhance clinical assessment
	Guided self-evaluation	GPs may instruct patients on performing guided self-evaluations to assess their symptoms This approach empowers patients to take an active role in their healthcare while providing the practitioner with additional data for clinical decision-making

Effective telephone consultation techniques are essential for GPs to deliver high-quality care in a remote setting. By adhering to structured steps before, during, and after the consultation, and by integrating additional telemedicine methods, practitioners can enhance their communication and diagnostic capabilities. These techniques ultimately contribute to improved patient outcomes and satisfaction in the evolving landscape of healthcare delivery.

6.3 Communication Skills and Settings for Telephone Consultations in General Practice

6.3.1 Communication Skills for Telephone Consultations

Telephone consultations require refined communication skills to bridge the gap caused by the absence of visual cues and body language. Effective communication helps build trust, ensure patient safety, and foster adherence to treatment plans. Moreover, research suggests that empathy in medical consultations improves patient satisfaction, quality of life, and pain outcomes (Neumann et al., 2007; Mercer & Reynolds, 2002) [17–22]. Therefore, general practitioners (GPs) must adopt a deliberate approach to ensure that patient interactions remain professional, empathetic, and efficient over the phone.

6.3.1.1 Communication Skills for Telephone Consultations

Table 6.8 lists the essential communication strategies to optimize telephone consultations:

Table 6.8 Communication skills for telephone consultations

Skill/Strategy	Description and techniques	Example phrases
Clear introduction	Start with a formal introduction to establish rapport and set the agenda for the call. State who you are, your role, and the purpose of the call.	"Good morning, I am Dr. Green from the general medicine clinic. I'm calling to check on your blood pressure since your medication was adjusted."
Clarifying the purpose of the call	Ask open questions to identify the patient's concerns or reasons for calling. This promotes transparency and ensures that both parties understand the purpose.	"How can I assist you today?" or "What specific issue would you like to discuss?"
Speaking clearly and slowly	Speak more slowly and clearly than you would in person to avoid misunderstandings. Clear articulation ensures that patients follow instructions correctly, especially over poor audio connections.	N/A
Avoiding medical jargon	Use simple language and provide instructions in an accessible way. Repeat key concepts to reinforce understanding.	"Take this medicine twice a day: once in the morning and once at night. Can you repeat that back to me?"
Asking effective questions	Use a combination of open-ended questions (to encourage detailed responses) and closed-ended questions (for specific information). Open-ended questions elicit broader information, while closed questions confirm details.	Open-ended: "Can you describe your symptoms in more detail?" Closed-ended: "Are you currently taking your medication?"
Agreeing on a management plan	Discuss the treatment options or next steps with the patient, encouraging them to ask questions. Involve them in decision-making to promote adherence and satisfaction.	"We have a couple of options: we could either try a new medication or monitor your condition for a few more days. Which one are you comfortable with?"
Checking for understanding	Periodically confirm the patient's understanding by asking them to repeat the instructions. This ensures clarity and reduces the risk of errors.	"Can you explain to me how you'll take the new medication, just to make sure I was clear?"
Active listening	Use verbal cues to demonstrate attentiveness. Pay attention to pauses, voice tone, and hesitations, which may indicate underlying concerns.	Brief affirmations such as: "I see," "Tell me more"

(continued)

Table 6.8 (continued)

Skill/Strategy	Description and techniques	Example phrases
Demonstrating empathy	Convey warmth and understanding through voice modulation. Use a calm and reassuring tone to make the patient feel supported, especially during stressful situations.	"I understand this situation is worrying for you, but I'll help you through it step by step."
Engaging in small talk	Small conversational touches (such as commenting on the weather or the patient's daily routine) help create a connection and humanize the interaction. This strengthens the doctor–patient relationship.	"It sounds like you've had a busy day. Have you been able to get some rest?"

6.3.1.2 Key Considerations for Effective Telephone Communication

In addition to communication techniques, several environmental and contextual factors affect the success of telephone consultations.

Factor	Details	Recommendations
Privacy and confidentiality	Both the GP and the patient must be in private spaces to ensure the confidentiality of the conversation.	Confirm with the patient: "Are you in a private place where we can talk freely?" Use encrypted communication lines if available
Minimizing interruptions	Environmental distractions (such as children, TV noise, or pets) can hinder effective communication.	Advise both parties to be in a quiet room Schedule calls at times with minimal external interference
Overcoming technical limitations	Poor audio quality or dropped calls can disrupt conversations, leading to frustration and miscommunication.	Ensure a good phone connection before starting the call Confirm backup contact details in case of disconnection
Handling language or cognitive barriers	Patients with cognitive impairments, hearing difficulties, or limited language proficiency may struggle with phone consultations.	Use simple language and repeat key concepts If necessary, involve a caregiver or family member to assist
Cultural sensitivity	Cultural differences may influence how patients communicate and interpret health advice.	Be mindful of cultural norms and preferences during interactions Adapt your communication style as needed to suit the patient's background

Telephone consultations require deliberate communication strategies to compensate for the absence of visual cues. GPs must be empathetic, clear, and proactive in seeking the patient's input to ensure effective information exchange and collaborative decision-making. Paying attention to environmental factors, privacy, and potential barriers helps create a professional and patient-centered experience. When executed with care, telephone consultations can maintain the same quality of care as in-person visits and foster lasting relationships between doctors and patients.

How Do Patients Perceive Empathy Telephone Consultation in General Practice [17]?

Empathy is a cornerstone of effective medical practice, directly influencing patient satisfaction, adherence to treatment, and clinical outcomes (Mercer & Reynolds, 2002). However, delivering empathy through telephone consultations—without the benefit of nonverbal cues—presents unique challenges. A recent mixed-methods study examined how patients perceive empathy during telephone consultations in primary care. The study found that although patients generally reported satisfactory levels of empathy, specific factors can either enhance or hinder its expression. Patients also valued the comfort and convenience of receiving care from their homes, which contributed positively to their overall experience (Rich et al., 2023).

Factors That Influence the Perception of Empathy in Telephone Consultations

Facilitators of empathy	Barriers to empathy
Comfortable environment: Patients appreciated the ability to consult with doctors from home, which fostered relaxation and openness. *Focused verbal communication:* When doctors used active listening techniques and clear verbal cues, patients felt acknowledged and understood. *Personalized communication:* Asking follow-up questions or engaging in small talk made patients feel connected and cared for.	*Lack of visual cues:* Without facial expressions, gestures, and body language, it is harder for patients to sense empathy, which can impair emotional connection. *Professional detachment:* A distant or overly formal tone may reduce warmth and human connection. *Interruptions:* Environmental distractions or call quality issues can disrupt the flow of conversation, undermining empathic engagement.

The Role of Professional Training in Enhancing Empathy

The study emphasizes the importance of specific training for healthcare professionals to enhance empathy during telephone consultations. Unlike in-person care, where nonverbal cues play a crucial role, telephone consultations rely entirely on verbal communication to convey understanding and compassion. Training programs could focus on several key areas:

- *Verbal empathy techniques*: Doctors could use phrases that reflect active listening, such as, “It sounds like you’re feeling worried about this” or “I can imagine this has been stressful for you.”

(continued)

- *Clarifying and confirming understanding:* Encouraging patients to restate key instructions or summarize their concerns ensures they feel heard and aligned with the care plan.
- *Inquiring beyond the obvious:* Asking open-ended questions to explore any hidden concerns, such as "Is there anything else you'd like to share?" helps patients feel fully supported.
- *Tone and pacing:* Speaking in a warm, calm voice and allowing pauses gives patients space to express their concerns without feeling rushed.

Impact of Empathy on Patient Outcomes

Research suggests that improving empathy in medical practice correlates with better patient outcomes, including improved treatment adherence, higher satisfaction, and even reductions in perceived pain (Neumann et al., 2007). In telephone consultations, verbal empathy techniques become especially important in compensating for the lack of visual interaction.

When GPs demonstrate empathy through clear communication and active listening, patients are more likely to feel recognized as individuals within the broader context of their lives. This not only strengthens the doctor–patient relationship but also encourages patients to engage meaningfully with their treatment plans.

6.3.2 Communication Setting for Telephone Consultations

In telephone consultations, the setting is essential for both the doctor and the patient. The lack of visual stimuli, human contact, and the perception of being in a physical space dedicated to a medical evaluation requires some precautions to ensure that the telephone evaluation can be complete and take place without obstacles or shortcomings. Therefore, the general practitioner needs to pay attention to certain aspects which are discussed as follows.

6.3.2.1 Key Considerations for Telephone Consultation Settings

The Key Considerations Include the Following

1. *Preparation and Accessibility*
   - *Equipment:* Make sure you have access to everything you need to conduct a telephone teleconsultation: telephone, PC, adequate connection where you are making the call, sufficient battery/access to a charging source, patient contact details.
   - *Connectivity:* Avoid technical/connection problems → use high-quality equipment (e.g., have a reliable telephone, a headset for clearer audio, use a silent keyboard).
2. *Minimizing Distractions*
   - *Quiet Environment for Patients:* Ensure an adequate environment that allows distractions to be minimized for both the doctor and the patient:

- Ensure that the patient is in a silent environment, free of audio interference (e.g., television on, children playing) and external stimuli.
- Ensure that the patient is in a private environment where he can speak freely without being overheard by others (and if not, ask him to find an appropriate environment).

- *Doctor's Environment:* Ensure that the doctor is in a silent environment; the presence of background noise cannot be accepted both because it is a clear obstacle to effective communication and because it could generate concerns in the patient about the safety of the conversation. If they can hear background noise, they will worry about who can hear them. A particularly intrusive noise that should be avoided is that of the keyboard also because the patient cannot see the hands typing on the keyboard as they can in a face-to-face consultation.

3. *Ensuring Privacy and Confidentiality*

Ensure that the doctor is in a private place that can maintain the confidentiality of the conversation → where other medical/nursing/secretarial staff or other people (including your family) cannot listen. This is as important as if you were in the room for surgery. Find a quiet place to ensure your patients' trust is maintained. If they can hear background noise, they will worry about who can hear them.

4. *Structured Call Management*
   - *Time Allocation:* Establish a clear structure for the consultation, allowing approximately 15 min per call. This timeframe enables focused discussions while providing ample opportunity for the patient to express concerns. At the beginning of the call, the doctor should introduce themselves, outline the consultation's purpose, and set expectations regarding the discussion flow.
   - *Systematic Approach:* Implement a systematic method for addressing the patient's concerns to minimize the likelihood of errors during the consultation. Ensure that key points are discussed and that any necessary follow-up actions are clearly communicated.
5. *Utilizing Electronic Medical Records (EMRs)*
   - *Pre-consultation Review:* Before the call, review the patient's electronic medical record (EMR) to familiarize yourself with their clinical history, medications, allergies, and any previous interactions. This preparation enhances the quality of care provided during the consultation [13].
   - *Documentation During the Call:* While speaking with the patient, make notes of relevant medical and surgical histories, including medication details and allergies. This practice not only aids in delivering comprehensive care but also provides accurate information for future reference.
   - *Post-Consultation Documentation:* After completing the consultation, document the discussion and any decisions made in the EMR. In addition, send a written summary of the consultation to the patient, reiterating important points discussed during the call. This follow-up helps reinforce understanding and ensures continuity of care.

6.4 Conclusion

This chapter has explored the distinctive elements of telephone teleconsultation within the realm of general medicine, aiming to equip practitioners with practical tools to enhance their implementation of this telemedicine modality. The future of telephone consultations remains uncertain; it is yet to be determined whether they will be overshadowed by the rise of video consultations—often viewed as superior—or if they will continue to thrive as a widely accepted method of healthcare delivery.

A significant challenge that persists is the inadequacy of training for general practitioners in conducting effective telephone consultations. Many healthcare professionals, including medical students, receive limited guidance on how to engage in telephone consultations effectively. This gap in training is critical, as it influences their ability to navigate the nuances of telemedicine. Comprehensive training should encompass several essential areas, including:

- *Verbal Communication Skills:* Practitioners need to develop sensitivity to verbal cues, enabling them to interpret patient emotions and concerns effectively, which is crucial in the absence of visual cues.
- *Focused History Taking:* Training should emphasize the importance of gathering pertinent information succinctly, allowing for a thorough understanding of the patient's condition within a limited timeframe.
- *Documentation Practices:* Proper documentation of telephone encounters is vital for maintaining accurate medical records, ensuring continuity of care, and complying with legal standards.
- *Recognizing Limitations:* Medical professionals must be trained to identify when telephone consultations may not be appropriate. For example, situations involving language barriers, complex medical conditions requiring physical examination, or instances where diagnostic tests are necessary should prompt a transition to in-person consultations.
- *Medico-Legal Awareness:* Understanding the legal implications of telephone consultations, including issues related to consent and liability, is essential for safeguarding both the patient and the healthcare provider [9].

Additionally, incorporating training on *clinical empathy* is crucial [17]. Empathy fosters effective communication and strengthens the doctor–patient relationship, even in remote settings. By ensuring that practitioners feel equipped to express empathy through their verbal communication, we can enhance patient satisfaction and improve overall health outcomes.

In summary, while telephone teleconsultation remains a vital aspect of modern healthcare delivery, addressing the current training deficiencies is imperative. By equipping general practitioners with the necessary skills and knowledge, we can optimize this telemedicine approach, ensuring that it continues to meet the evolving needs of patients.

References

1. Aronson SH. The lancet on the telephone 1876–1975. Med Hist. 1977;21(1):69–87.
2. Forte V, Vito C. Manuale di Medicina Generale e Cure Primarie. Guida teorico-pratica per MMG. Edises Università. 2022. ISBN: 9788836230501.
3. Carrillo de Albornoz S, Sia KL, Harris A. The effectiveness of teleconsultations in primary care: systematic review. Fam Pract 2022 Jan 19;39(1):168–182. https://doi.org/10.1093/fampra/cmab077. PMID: 34278421; PMCID: PMC8344904.
4. Salud. SAd. El SAS impulsa la consulta telefonica para pacientes de AtencionPrimaria. www.sspa.juntadeandalucia.es/servicioandaluzdesalud/todasnoticia/el-sas-impulsa-la-consulta-telefonica-para-pacientes-de-atencionprimaria. Published 2020. Accessed 05 Feb 21.
5. NHS. General practice in the context of coronavirus (COVID-19). NHS England; 2020.
6. Ministero della Salute. Covid-19, al via triage telefonico da parte dei medici di famiglia. http://www.salute.gov.it/portale/news/p3_2_1_1_1.jsp?lingua=italiano&menu=notizie&p=dalministero&id=4084. Published 2020. Accessed 05 February 21.
7. ALTEMS. Analisi dei modelli organizzativi di risposta al Covid-19. ALTEMS (Alta Scuola di Economia e Management dei Sistemi Sanitari), 2020.
8. Uscher-Pines L, Sousa J, Jones M, et al. Telehealth use among safety-net organizations in California during the COVID-19 pandemic. JAMA. 2021;325(11):1106–7.
9. Car J, Freeman GK, Partridge MR, Sheikh A. Improving quality and safety of telephone based delivery of care: teaching telephone consultation skills. Qual Saf Health Care. 2004 Feb;13(1):2–3. https://doi.org/10.1136/qshc.2003.009241. PMID: 14757786; PMCID: PMC1758049.
10. Car J, Sheikh A. Telephone consultations. BMJ. 2003;326:966–9.
11. British Medical Association, and General Practitioners Committee. Consulting in the modern world: guidance for GPs. BMA, General Practitioners Committee; 2001.
12. Downes MJ, Mervin MC, Byrnes JM, Scuffham PA. Telephone consultations for general practice: a systematic review. Syst Rev. 2017;6(1):128.
13. Iyengar K, El-Nahas W. A brief guide to telephone medical consultation. Br J Healthc Manag. 2020;26:1. https://doi.org/10.12968/bjhc.2020.0032.
14. Byambasuren O, Greenwood H, Bakhit M, Atkins T, Clark J, Scott AM, Glasziou P. Comparison of telephone and video telehealth consultations: systematic review. J Med Internet Res. 2023 Nov 17;25:e49942. https://doi.org/10.2196/49942. PMID: 37976100; PMCID: PMC10692872.
15. Greenhalgh T, Wherton J, Shaw S, Morrison C. Video consultations for covid-19. BMJ. 2020;368:m998.
16. RACGP. Guide to providing telephone and video consultations in general practice. The Royal Australian College of General Practitioners; 2020. https://www.racgp.org.au/FSDEDEV/media/documents/Clinical%20Resources/Guidelines/Guide-to-providing-telephone-and-video-consultations.pdf
17. Vennik J, Hughes S, Lyness E, McDermott C, Smith KA, Steele M, Bostock J, Howick J, Little P, Leydon G, Mallen C, Morrison L, Stuart B, Everitt H, Bishop FL. Patient perceptions of empathy in primary care telephone consultations: a mixed methods study. Patient Educ Couns. 2023 Aug;113:107748. https://doi.org/10.1016/j.pec.2023.107748. Epub 2023 Apr 12.
18. Reynolds WJ, Scott B. Empathy: a crucial component of the helping relationship. J Psychiatr Ment Health Nurs. 1999;6(5):363–70. https://doi.org/10.1046/j.1365-2850.1999.00228.x.
19. Mercer SW, Reynolds WJ. Empathy and quality of care. Br J Gen Pract. 2002;52(Suppl):S9.
20. Derksen F, Bensing J, Lagro-Janssen A. Effectiveness of empathy in general practice: a systematic review. Br J Gen Pract. 2013;63(606):e76–84. https://doi.org/10.3399/bjgp13X660814.
21. Howick J, Moscrop A, Mebius A, et al. Effects of empathic and positive communication in healthcare consultations: a systematic review and meta-analysis. J R Soc Med. 2018;111(7):240–52. https://doi.org/10.1177/0141076818769477.
22. Mistiaen P, van Osch M, van Vliet L, et al. The effect of patient-practitioner communication on pain: a systematic review. Eur J Pain. 2016;20(5):675–88. https://doi.org/10.1002/ejp.797.

Communication Settings and Skills for Video Consultation in Primary Care

7

Ulrik Bak Kirk, Kate King, and Rebecca Payne

7.1 Introduction

7.1.1 Video Consultation in Primary Care

Video consulting is not a recent health innovation. It has been used predominantly in secondary care and extreme remote locations for many years [1, 2]. However, its adoption accelerated during the COVID-19 pandemic, [3] with the rapid introduction of video consultations into general practice across the globe [4]. In many parts of Europe, video consultations soon became an additional method of primary care delivery, allowing family doctors to assess patients remotely while minimising the risk of infection [5–9]. The evolution of video consultation aligns with advancements in digital technology and changes in patient expectations. Internet connectivity and video technology have improved rapidly, just as access to internet-enabled devices has become widespread. This has made it feasible to conduct high-quality medical consultations remotely [10].

U. B. Kirk (✉)
Faculty Fellow, Department of Public Health, Aarhus University, Aarhus, Denmark

Digital Health, Research Unit for General Practice, Aarhus, Denmark
e-mail: ubk@ph.au.dk

K. King
Head of Academic Department of Military General Practice, Research & Clinical Innovation, Defence Medical Services, Lichfield, UK
e-mail: Kate.King415@mod.gov.uk

R. Payne
NIHR In-Practice Fellow, Nuffield Department of Primary Care Health Sciences, University of Oxford, Oxford, UK

North Wales Medical School, Bangor University, Bangor, UK
e-mail: rebecca.payne@bangor.ac.uk

J. Demurtas (ed.), *Remote Consultation in Primary Care*, TELe-Health,
https://doi.org/10.1007/978-3-031-89661-3_7

The foundation of primary care is the consultation. Traditionally conducted face to face, this has morphed as technology allows the use of other modalities such as telephone, messaging, e-mail and, most recently, video. Primary care consultation skills are based on face-to-face consultation with clinicians developing their skills over several years through training and beyond. Other modalities offer practical benefits for some patients at some times but are considered to lose something compared to the 'gold standard' face-to-face consultation [11]. The loss is often related to non-verbal communication that is inherently missing from non-visual modalities. Video theoretically offers this non-verbal communication while, at the same time, allowing patients and clinicians to benefit from remote consulting.

Unlike telephone and other remote consultations, video allows the visualisation of the patient, enabling the clinician to assess visual cues and conduct basic visual examinations [12]. This provides extra information about the patient and their current environment, contributing to a more thorough assessment than other remote modalities. In addition, video can offer a potential advantage over face-to-face consulting in that the clinician may be able to see the patient's home environment and thereby provide context and a more holistic understanding of the patient. Compared to telephone, video consulting can increase rapport between clinician and patient and so establish a more 'human' feel to the encounter [6].

However, video consulting is not a panacea. The rapid expansion in its use was followed, in many areas, by a rapid contraction, potentially because the technology was not implemented effectively, infrastructure was inadequate and there was inadequate training for users [13]. It is not just a face-to-face consultation done using some additional digital technology. Successful implementation of video consulting needs to be embedded into the primary care system in order to provide tangible benefits for clinicians and patients.

7.1.2 Aims of Video Consulting

Video consultation in primary care is increasingly being used as an alternative to face-to-face consultations, particularly when an in-person visit is not feasible or necessary. For some patients, it can be used to complete the entire consultation, but for others, it provides value even when a face-to-face consultation is still required.

The purpose of a video consultation is not merely to replicate an in-person visit but to provide a safe and effective remote consultation that meets the needs of both the patient and the clinician. Video can be used for the following:

- *Triage*: Determining whether a further in-person evaluation is required [5].
- *Assessment and management*: Conducting clinical assessments, discussing symptoms and managing ongoing conditions.
- *Patient education and support*: Offering guidance on self-management, medication use and lifestyle changes.
- *Follow-up care*: Monitoring progress after treatment or surgery, particularly when physical examinations are not required.

7.1.3 Peculiarities of Video Consulting

Video confers several advantages over other remote consultation modalities by incorporating visual communication, thereby enhancing the clinician's ability to observe non-verbal cues and, in some cases, allowing for patient examination. There are, however, some peculiarities to the modality which clinicians need to be aware of in order to undertake high-quality, safe, remote video consultations.

7.1.3.1 Impact of Connectivity and Technology Limitations on Communication

Good quality technology is essential for video consultations, but technology alone is insufficient. Both clinician and patient need to be able to use and have confidence in the platform. Various studies have shown that the ability to use and the confidence in the technology affect the quality of the consultation [8, 12]. The result of this can be shorter and more transactional consultations with the resultant risk of increased prescribing and referral rates.

Poor connectivity can lead to buffering or the link being lost entirely. Clinicians need to have agreed backup plans for loss of the connection, but also be cognisant of pauses and delays on the call which may interfere with the flow of the consultation. The use of silence to encourage patient contribution is useful in face-to-face consultations but can create uncertainty about the connection quality on video. The use of verbal listening strategies such as 'uh-huh' can cause the patient to feel interrupted in a video consultation [14].

7.1.3.2 Non-verbal Communication

The ability to see the patient helps to establish a more personal connection, which can enhance the therapeutic relationship and improve patient satisfaction. The video allows lip movements and gestures to be seen, reducing communication barriers for some patients, and the consultation can be supplemented with visual aids or the demonstration of techniques or exercises.

However, scrutiny of video as a modality has shown that it brings new communication challenges [15, 16]. Techniques such as maintaining eye contact, active listening and shared decision-making need to be adapted to the modality in order to be effective [14]. Video consulting needs to be taught to clinicians, just like any other consultation technique.

7.1.3.3 Accessibility

The obvious benefit of video consulting comes where there are geographical or physical barriers to the patient attending in person. Video can be used to replace a face-to-face consultation in some cases or help triage the patient to ensure travel is justified, particularly during adverse weather conditions or over long distances.

For many workers a video consultation can facilitate access to healthcare when it may otherwise be restricted due to working patterns. However, despite the abundance of internet-enabled devices, the infrastructure supporting connectivity is often worst in the most remote areas where it is arguably most needed [2].

If video is the predominant mode for consulting, there is a risk of digital exclusion for patients without the connectivity, device or the ability to use the technology. This digital poverty can widen pre-existing health inequalities.

7.1.3.4 Privacy and Confidentiality

All consultations require privacy and confidentiality. Maintaining these conditions can be challenging when video consulting. Staff or family members may inadvertently walk into a room where the clinician is consulting. Consideration should be given to locking the door or putting up a notice to prevent disturbances. If consulting from home, clinicians should be cognisant of what is visible to the patient and ensure personal information is off-camera.

Patients too require privacy, and some will not have thought about their environment when booking the appointment. The advantage of not needing to leave work, for example, means that the consultation may end up being conducted in a corridor or outside a school or workplace, with the patient distracted by who is around them, or limited in what information they are comfortable sharing.

One concern expressed by patients about video consultations is the security of the platform used and whether their data is safe from abuse [2]. Any video consultation platform used must comply with legal and ethical standards for patient confidentiality, ensuring that all communications are secure and encrypted.

7.1.3.5 Environmental Factors

The nature of any remote consultations means that they move the patient into their own environment rather than the clinician's environment. This has advantages to clinician and patient as described elsewhere, but it does mean that patients may be less ready to engage or distracted during the consultation. While waiting in a clinic environment, patients can rehearse their opening gambit and prepare for the consultation.

When we intervene in their lives through remote consulting, this opportunity is often missed. The time it takes the patient to transition into the consultation can result into the consultation becoming rushed. Video platforms that offer a virtual waiting room for patients can overcome some of this issue in a way that telephone consultations cannot.

7.2 A Systems Approach Promotes Safety

7.2.1 General Principles

A video consultation must be safe for both patients and clinicians. Any gains from the technology are undermined immediately if it leads to a patient safety incident. Patient and case selection through initial triage can improve the safety of remote consulting in general; however, additionally, video consulting needs to be embedded within the primary care system to minimise risk. Clinicians and patients need to be supported by processes that ensure patients receive consultation outputs such as prescriptions, letters and safety-netting information.

As with any form of remote care, video consultation is less suitable where a patient has multiple co-morbidities, vague symptoms or a condition that is worsening or not following the expected trajectory. Repeated video consultations about the same problem should trigger consideration of a face-to-face assessment.

7.2.2 Systems Approach

Video should be supported by practice processes so that all staff are able to respond to queries and when there are problems. Clear protocols for when video consultations are appropriate and ensuring that both clinicians and patients understand these guidelines means fewer rescheduled appointments and additional appointments for examinations. Ultimately, it means the patient gets the right care the first time.

Contingency plans should be established, and patients informed, in case of technical failures during the consultation. This might include reception rescheduling the appointment or the clinician switching to a telephone consultation. There should also be processes in case of emergencies such as a patient collapsing on the call.

Dealing with distressed mental health patients can be particularly challenging: There are many opportunities and ways to intervene with an upset, agitated or suicidal patient if they decide to abruptly leave a consulting room, but clicking 'leave' on a video call is quick and leaves no opportunity to assess the patient's safety. Systems should be in place to protect patients and staff in these situations.

Adequate training can be key to the technology being embraced by clinicians, staff and patients. Clinicians need training in video consultation techniques, including how to manage the technology, maintain patient rapport and conduct remote assessments effectively. Without this, there is a risk that the benefits of video are not maximised.

Patients need to know how to use the platform, what to expect and what the limitations are with video. Some guidance is needed on how to set themselves up to optimise lighting and best participate in the consultation, especially if being examined remotely. Patients should be able to participate in the consultation without having to hold their phone throughout. This will promote effective non-verbal communication.

Time management is critical when remote consulting. A good quality, non-transactional, video consultation is unlikely to be significantly shorter than a face-to-face one and may take longer if there are connectivity issues or patient factors that mean communication takes time to establish. If examination is required, additional appointment time will be needed to accommodate this and needs to be factored into the appointment system.

7.2.3 Clinician Safety

Remote consultations may be used to free up clinical examination rooms and allow clinicians to work flexibly. Video may allow the patient to glimpse into the clinician's home environment. While this can be advantageous to building rapport and trust, it also places the clinician in a more vulnerable position. The clinician needs to consider their own safety, making sure that personal information is not visible in the background. Workstations should be configured for comfort, ideally with a minimum of two screens and an external keyboard or mouse.

In addition, ensuring an optimal environment for remote consultations is essential. Avoiding excessive noise is crucial, as it may impair the quality of communication, and attention should also be paid to lighting, dress code and background colour, which can all influence the consultation's tone and professionalism. Adequate lighting improves visibility, neutral background colours help avoid distractions and a professional dress code helps maintain the formal nature of the consultation [17].

7.2.4 Patient Safety

Video offers a clear advantage over other modes of consulting when it allows the clinician a view of the patient's home environment. Signs of neglect or poverty can be seen. Abusive behaviour may be apparent if others are seen on screen, or bruising may be visible that would not have been seen if using a telephone [18]. A video consultation may not give all the information required to safely diagnose and treat a patient. This can lead to over-prescribing and over-investigation Clinicians should be careful to ensure that investigations and referrals are not done when bringing the patient in for a face-to-face appointment and examination would be more appropriate.

7.3 Conditions and Suitability for Video Consulting

7.3.1 General Principles

Video consultations have been used for a wide range of clinical presentations and conditions. There are some general principles for when video is most appropriate, but ultimately, clinical or personal need may determine the consultation modality, and it can be hard to prospectively decide which modality is best. Clinicians should always be free to change consultation mode when it becomes clear that it is necessary.

It is important to trust the clinician's gut feeling in such situations. If the clinician feels uncertain about whether video consultation can provide the necessary care, they should not hesitate to refer the patient or condition to the setting they find more appropriate. Trusting one's professional instincts ensures that patient care remains the priority, even if it means changing the consultation modality.

7.3.2 Patient Factors

The challenges with the transmission of non-verbal communication make video consultations easier when there is already an established relationship between clinician and patient. The uncertainty regarding the presenting complaint and need for examination makes it difficult to use for undifferentiated care and some initial triage can streamline patients appropriately.

However, rural areas especially, have been highly effective at using video in urgent and out-of-hours care settings where it is seen as reducing clinical risk for remote consultations. The additional visuals can support clinicians to recognise seriously unwell patients and escalate their care appropriately. Conversely, the use of video may also help to identify which patients can be safely managed without a face-to-face appointment.

Certain patient factors make video consults particularly helpful, such as for people of working age [7], children with autism spectrum disorders and deaf patients [6]. Video consultations can also help facilitate continuity of care for patients away from home, such as patients with chronic conditions. Another patient group that particularly benefits from video consultation includes students with acne, as they can avoid the distress of removing makeup during face-to-face consultations [6].

Facilitated consultations, where the patient is supported by a relative, carer or community-based healthcare professional, can provide valuable information to the clinician and improve the overall quality of the consultation. They can allow a fuller range of clinical observations to be taken, and remote healthcare professionals can contribute to the diagnostic process. In many cases, they can aid primary care clinicians in achieving clinical and legislative standards for patients unable to travel.

However, third-party consultations may also carry certain risks, such as potential miscommunication, privacy concerns or influence from the person facilitating the consultation. Despite these risks, facilitated consultations have notable advantages, including enhancing the clinician's ability to gather comprehensive information, supporting the diagnostic process and ensuring that clinical standards are met even when the patient cannot attend in person. The presence of an additional healthcare professional or caregiver can often provide reassurance and contribute to better outcomes.

7.3.3 Specific Clinical Conditions

The rurality of Scotland has resulted in video being embraced in primary and acute care. The national *Near Me* programme has compiled recommendations—reported in Table 7.1—for which consulting modality is suitable for which problem [19]. However, these offer guidance not rules. In some settings, such as in urgent care, video can be useful for 'eyeballing' a patient, even if they are then asked to travel for a subsequent in-person consultation.

Table 7.1 Modality recommendations from the 'Near Me Programme', Scotland [19]

Telephone	Video	In-person
Mental health	Mental health	Cancer (initial presentation)
Medication advice	Skin/nail problems	Abdo pelvic—New onset
Results (X Ray/Bloods)	Cellulitis	Type 1 diabetes—unwell
Review medication changes	Back pain if seen within last 2 weeks needs face to face	Headache—New onset
Memory impairment	Gout	Rectal bleeding
Contraception	Foot pain	Breast lump
BP if have BP monitor	Joint pain	Prostate/testicular
Menstrual problems	Sore throat	Altered bowel habit
Thyroid issues	Allergies	Post coital bleeding
Ear pain—Onset, if a returning issue/ worsening book face to face	Leg swelling	Abnormal weight loss
Post Natal—Contraception advice	Throat symptoms	
D&V—Onset if a returning issues/ worsening book face to face	Long term condition review	
Blood in urine	Rashes	
Vaginal discharge	Cough	
Abdo pains—Ongoing chronic		
Pelvic pains—Ongoing chronic		
Chest pain non cardiac if not 999		

- *Skin conditions:* Video consultations are particularly helpful for skin conditions, although there are limitations when picture quality is poor. Patients with skin conditions that they hide with makeup such as acne often really appreciate video as it avoids them needing to remove makeup in a setting where it cannot be easily re-applied. They can also be useful for anterior eye problems, particularly in differentiating between various causes of red eye [6].
- *Mental health conditions:* Video has been used extensively for delivering mental health therapies and many patients prefer the ability to be in their own environment when feeling psychologically vulnerable. Video confers benefits over the telephone with the gain of images helping build rapport and a better assessment of the patient's overall well-being, for example, showing if they are in dishevelled clothes or in an unsanitary environment [20].
- *Paediatrics:* Most clinicians will have encountered the child who is withdrawn and uncooperative in the clinic setting, but parents describe it as well at home. By assessing the child via video within their home environment, important additional information can be gathered about the child, for example, are they playing or just lying on the sofa, what is their respiratory rate and colour, are there any additional noises such as stridor when breathing? Children will often be more relaxed and chattier in their home environment, and even should they need a subsequent face-to-face assessment, they will often interact better with a clini-

cian that they have already seen on screen in their own home. However, acutely unwell infants under two should always be examined and video should be used as a tool to help determine the urgency and location of the face-to-face appointment [21].

7.3.4 Clinical Examination

The video enables the clinician to observe the patient's general physical condition, see visible discomfort and identify clinical signs, such as rashes and oedema. Various examinations can be conducted, at least in part, over video and these can be blended with information from patient-owned technology to provide more information to support diagnoses. Part consultations may allow the patient to be started on an initial management course before there is an opportunity for a face-to-face consultation to complete the examination and confirm the diagnosis. Where examinations are incomplete, clinicians must be confident that the absence of auscultation or palpation is justifiable, at least until the full examination is completed.

While some examinations are possible, it is not appropriate to conduct any intimate examinations using video due to the risk of breaching laws on sharing of intimate images [6]. As with any clinical encounter, at the end of the video consultation the clinician needs to be confident that they have gained sufficient information to address the problem. Where this is not the case, in-person assessment or further investigations or onward referral should be organised.

7.4 Techniques for Effective Video Consultations

Conducting an effective video consultation requires a blend of clinical skills and technical proficiency, and there is a consultation model published to support video consulting, as shown in Fig. 7.1 [14]. Written at the start of the pandemic, it describes the set-up before the consultation, covers various early requirements to ensure patient and clinician safety, and then details ways in which the video modality may interfere with the consultation and how to overcome this.

7.4.1 Preparation

- Ensure that all necessary equipment is functioning correctly and set-up appropriately before the consultation begins.
- Review the patient's medical history and any available data in the electronic medical record.
- Set up a quiet, private space with good lighting where you can focus on the consultation without interruptions. Remove distractions from the environment around you which could distract you or the patient.

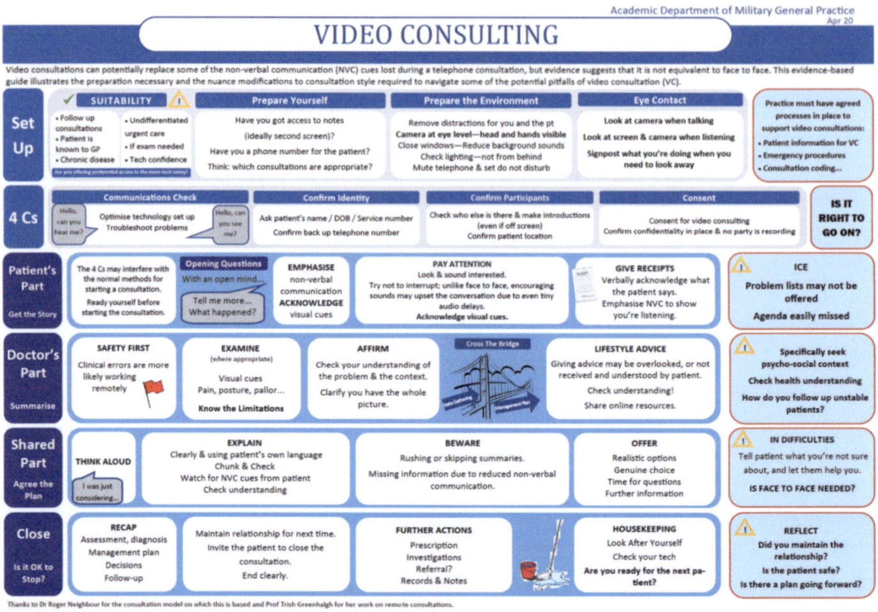
Academic Department of Military General Practice
Apr 20
VIDEO CONSULTING
Video consultations can potentially replace some of the non-verbal communication (NVC) cues lost during a telephone consultation, but evidence suggests that it is not equivalent to face to face. This evidence-based guide illustrates the preparation necessary and the nuance modifications to consultation style required to navigate some of the potential pitfalls of video consultation (VC).
Set Up
SUITABILITY
• Follow up consultations
• Patient is known to GP
• Chronic disease
• Undifferentiated urgent care
• If exam needed
• Tech confidence
Prepare Yourself
Have you got access to notes (ideally second screen)?
Have you a phone number for the patient?
Think: which consultations are appropriate?
Prepare the Environment
Remove distractions for you and the pt
Camera at eye level—head and hands visible
Close windows—Reduce background sounds
Check lighting—not from behind
Mute telephone & set do not disturb
Eye Contact
Look at camera when talking
Look at screen & camera when listening
Signpost what you're doing when you need to look away
Practice must have agreed processes in place to support video consultations:
• Patient information for VC
• Emergency procedures
• Consultation coding...
4 Cs
Communications Check
Hello, can you hear me?
Optimise technology set up
Troubleshoot problems
Hello, can you see me?
Confirm Identity
Ask patient's name / DOB / Service number
Confirm back up telephone number
Confirm Participants
Check who else is there & make introductions (even if off screen)
Confirm patient location
Consent
Consent for video consulting
Confirm confidentiality in place & no party is recording
IS IT RIGHT TO GO ON?
Patient's Part
Get the Story
The 4 Cs may interfere with the normal methods for starting a consultation.
Ready yourself before starting the consultation.
Opening Questions
With an open mind...
Tell me more... What happened?
EMPHASISE non-verbal communication
ACKNOWLEDGE visual cues
PAY ATTENTION
Look & sound interested.
Try not to interrupt; unlike face to face, encouraging sounds may upset the conversation due to even tiny audio delays.
Acknowledge visual cues.
GIVE RECEIPTS
Verbally acknowledge what the patient says.
Emphasise NVC to show you're listening.
ICE
Problem lists may not be offered
Agenda easily missed
Doctor's Part
Summarise
SAFETY FIRST
Clinical errors are more likely working remotely
EXAMINE
(where appropriate)
Visual cues
Pain, posture, pallor...
Know the Limitations
AFFIRM
Check your understanding of the problem & the context.
Clarify you have the whole picture.
Cross The Bridge
LIFESTYLE ADVICE
Giving advice may be overlooked, or not received and understood by patient.
Check understanding!
Share online resources.
Specifically seek psycho-social context
Check health understanding
How do you follow up unstable patients?
Shared Part
Agree the Plan
THINK ALOUD
I was just considering...
EXPLAIN
Clearly & using patient's own language
Chunk & Check
Watch for NVC cues from patient
Check understanding
BEWARE
Rushing or skipping summaries.
Missing information due to reduced non-verbal communication.
OFFER
Realistic options
Genuine choice
Time for questions
Further information
IN DIFFICULTIES
Tell patient what you're not sure about, and let them help you.
IS FACE TO FACE NEEDED?
Close
Is it OK to Stop?
RECAP
Assessment, diagnosis
Management plan
Decisions
Follow-up
Maintain relationship for next time.
Invite the patient to close the consultation.
End clearly.
FURTHER ACTIONS
Prescription
Investigations
Referral?
Records & Notes
HOUSEKEEPING
Look After Yourself
Check your tech
Are you ready for the next patient?
REFLECT
Did you maintain the relationship?
Is the patient safe?
Is there a plan going forward?
Thanks to Dr Roger Neighbour for the consultation model on which this is based and Prof Trish Greenhalgh for her work on remote consultations.

Fig. 7.1 Essential steps for video consultations [14]

- Ensure that the camera shows your head, shoulders and hand to promote physical communication. Cameras should be at eye level, not looking up or down at the patient. Consider whether a headset gives better audio quality for the patient by reducing background noise.

7.4.2 During the Consultation

- Speak clearly and slowly, ensuring that instructions and explanations are easy to follow, particularly in a potentially delayed or disrupted connection.
- Visual Engagement: Use the camera to establish a virtual connection with the patient, ensuring that you are making 'eye contact' by looking directly at the camera rather than the screen. This can help the patient feel more engaged and valued during the consultation.
- Begin by introducing yourself and confirming the patient's identity and the reason for the consultation. Ensure that you have a telephone number in case of technical difficulties and what the procedure is if there are issues.
- Establish the consultation structure, including the expected duration and goals.
- Use visual aids or screen sharing if necessary to explain concepts, demonstrate techniques or review test results.

- Pay close attention to the patient's visual cues, such as facial expressions, body language, and any physical signs of distress as non-verbal communication may not translate well over video.
- Signal to the patient or explain if you need to look away so that the patient understands that you are not disinterested or distracted.
- Summarise regularly. It acts as a safeguard against missed non-verbal cues and technical issues. Encourage the patient to ask questions and confirm their understanding of the discussion too. Thinking aloud is useful in face-to-face consultations and video provides an additional layer of security ensuring that clinician and patient agree with the issue and way forward.

7.4.3 At the End of the Consultation

- Document the consultation thoroughly in the electronic medical record, noting any observations made during the video call.
- Make any necessary follow-up arrangements and ensure that the patient is aware of how to access any consultation outputs such as prescriptions or letters.

7.5 Beyond the Video Consultation

Video is a useful modality for consulting in primary care and offers opportunities beyond the one-to-one consultation.

- *Blended consultations:* In conjunction with other communication modalities such as messaging and telephone, video can be used to help clarify diagnostic confusion or provide a visual support to the patient. Consultations do not have to be started and completed necessarily using video, especially when there is a pre-existing relationship between the clinician and patient. A blended consultation may start with asynchronous messaging and lead to a short video call to gain additional information before ending in an agreed way. Video, in this case, augments other consultation modes rather than being the focus.
- *Remote monitoring:* The pandemic led to many patients having medical technology, such as pulse oximeters or sphygmomanometers, in their own homes. Clinician-directed use of this technology, along with regular video check-ups, allows patients to be managed at home for chronic conditions and acute illness, optimising the timing of admission or avoiding it entirely [2].
- *Group consultations:* Patient education is a key tenet of self-management for chronic conditions. Group consultations can help with this and can easily be adapted to the video modality. Many platforms additionally allow the use of breakout rooms which can help patients discover a support network of people with similar medical challenges.

7.6 Conclusion

Video consultations are an increasingly important component of primary care, offering a versatile and effective way to deliver healthcare remotely. While they share some similarities with telephone consultations, video consultations allow for richer communication and more thorough patient assessments through visual interaction.

However, the success of video consultations hinges on the ability of clinicians to navigate the unique challenges they present—such as technological barriers, the absence of physical examination and the need for strong verbal and non-verbal communication skills. With proper training, preparation and attention to both the technical and interpersonal aspects of the consultation, video consultations can be a powerful tool in primary care.

As video consultations continue to evolve, ongoing research and experience will further refine best practices, ensuring that this mode of care remains safe, effective and patient-centred. Training in these areas is essential, as many clinicians may not yet be fully equipped to handle the nuances of video consultations. By developing these skills, general practitioners can provide high-quality care that meets the demands of modern healthcare environments. Ultimately, video consultations offer the ability to bridge the gap between the benefits of remote consulting and those of the face-to-face gold-standard primary care consultation.

References

1. Raven M, Butler C, Bywood P. Video-based telehealth in Australian primary health care: current use and future potential. Aust J Prim Health. 2013;19(4):283–6. https://doi.org/10.1071/PY13032.
2. Atherton H, Lasserson D. Technology. In: Cox J, Clark C, Sanders T, editors. Rural healthcare. 2nd ed. Boca Raton: CRC Press; 2023. p. 184–99.
3. Huibers L, Bech BH, Kirk UB, Kallestrup P, Vestergaard CH, Christensen MB. Contacts in general practice during the COVID-19 pandemic: a register-based study. Br J Gen Pract. 2022 Oct 27;72(724):e799–808. https://doi.org/10.3399/BJGP.2021.0703.
4. OECD. The COVID-19 pandemic and the future of telemedicine. Paris: OECD Health Policy Studies (OECD Publishing; 2023.
5. Murphy M, Scott LJ, Salisbury C, Turner A, Scott A, Denholm R, Lewis R, Iyer G, Macleod J, Horwood J. Implementation of remote consulting in UK primary care following the COVID-19 pandemic: a mixed-methods longitudinal study. Br J Gen Pract. 2021;71(704):e166–77. https://doi.org/10.3399/BJGP.2020.0948.
6. Payne RE, Clarke A. How and why are video consultations used in urgent primary care settings in the UK? A focus group study. BJGP Open. 2023;7(3):BJGPO.2023.0025. https://doi.org/10.3399/BJGPO.2023.0025.
7. Bak Kirk U, Høstrup Vestergaard C, Hammer Bech B, Bondo Christensen M, Kallestrup P, Huibers L. Video consultation in general practice during COVID-19: a register-based study in Denmark. BJGP Open. 2024 Jan 8:BJGPO.2023.0208. https://doi.org/10.3399/BJGPO.2023.0208.
8. Norberg BL, Johnsen TM, Kristiansen E, Krogh FH, Getz LO, Austad B. Primary care gatekeeping during the Covid-19 pandemic: a survey of 1234 Norwegian regular GPs. BJGP Open. 2023 Dec 13:BJGPO.2023.0095. https://doi.org/10.3399/BJGPO.2023.0095.

9. Dahlgren C, Dackehag M, Wändell P, Rehnberg C. Determinants for use of direct-to-consumer telemedicine consultations in primary healthcare—a registry based total population study from Stockholm, Sweden. BMC Fam Pract. 2021;22:133. https://doi.org/10.1186/s12875-021-01481-1.
10. Monteleone G, Terzulli G, Cefaloni F, Bonini M, Richeldi L. The impact of telemedicine during severe acute respiratory syndrome coronavirus 2 pandemic and future perspectives: a systematic review. Respiration. 2023;102(10):879–90. https://doi.org/10.1159/000533621.
11. Hammersley V, Donaghy E, Parker R, McNeilly H, Atherton H, Bikker A, Campbell J, McKinstry B. Comparing the content and quality of video, telephone, and face-to-face consultations: a non-randomised, quasi-experimental, exploratory study in UK primary care. Br J Gen Pract. 2019 Aug 29;69(686):e595–604. https://doi.org/10.3399/bjgp19X704573.
12. Byambasuren O, Greenwood H, Bakhit M, Atkins T, Clark J, Scott AM, Glasziou P. Comparison of telephone and video telehealth consultations: systematic review. J Med Internet Res. 2023 Nov 17;25:e49942. https://doi.org/10.2196/49942. PMID: 37976100; PMCID: PMC10692872.
13. Greenhalgh T, Ladds E, Hughes G, Moore L, Wherton J, Shaw SE, Papoutsi C, Wieringa S, Rosen R, Rushforth A, Rybczynska-Bunt S. Why do GPs rarely do video consultations? Qualitative study in UK general practice. Br J Gen Pract. 2022 Apr 28;72(718):e351-e360. https://doi.org/10.3399/BJGP.2021.0658. PMID: 35256385; PMCID: PMC8936181.
14. King K. Video consulting: not just a consultation plus tech. BJGP Life. 2000, May 15; https://bjgplife.com/video-consulting-not-just-a-consultation-plus-tech/.
15. Shaw S, Wherton J, Vijayaraghavan S, Morris J, Bhattacharya S, Hanson P, Campbell-Richards D, Ramoutar S, Collard A, Hodkinson I, Greenhalgh T. Advantages and limitations of virtual online consultations in a NHS acute trust: the VOCAL mixed-methods study. Southampton: NIHR Journals Library; 2018.
16. Seuren LM, Wherton J, Greenhalgh T, Shaw SE. Whose turn is it anyway? Latency and the organization of turn-taking in video-mediated interaction. J Pragmat. 2021 Jan;172:63–78. https://doi.org/10.1016/j.pragma.2020.11.005. PMID: 33519050; PMCID: PMC7819463.
17. Sandbæk A, Christensen LD, Larsen LL, Primholdt Christensen N, Kofod FG, Guassora AD, Merrild CH, Assing Hvidt E. Guidance for implementing video consultations in Danish general practice: rapid cycle coproduction study. JMIR Form Res. 2021 Nov 24;5(11):e27323. https://doi.org/10.2196/27323. PMID: 34821560; PMCID: PMC8663649.
18. Dixon S, Frost L, Feder G, Ziebland S, Pope C. Challenges of safeguarding via remote consulting during the COVID-19 pandemic: a qualitative interview study. Br J Gen Pract. 2022 Feb 24;72(716):e199–e208. https://doi.org/10.3399/BJGP.2021.0396. PMID: 35074797; PMCID: PMC8803093.
19. Near Me. Quick Start Guide for Practice Administrative Staff. 2023, August. https://tec.scot/sites/default/files/2023-08/Practice%20Admin%20Staff%20Quick%20Start%20Guide%20Aug2023.pdf.
20. Haun MW, van Eickels D, Tönnies J, Graue L, Ayoub-Schreifeldt M, Wensing M, Hartmann M, Szecsenyi J, Wild B, Friederich HC. An integrated mental health video consultations model for patients with somatic symptom disorder in primary care: the randomized VISION pilot trial. J Psychosom Res. 2024 Jul;182:111801. https://doi.org/10.1016/j.jpsychores.2024.111801. Epub 2024 May 14.
21. Castillo-Rodenas M, Vidal-Alaball J, Solanas-Bacardit N, Farràs-Company C, Fuster-Casanovas A, Miró Catalina Q, López Seguí F. Feasibility of a pediatric acute video consultation process among health care professionals in primary care in a rural setting: protocol for a prospective validation study. JMIR Res Protoc. 2024 Feb 1;13:e52946. https://doi.org/10.2196/52946. Erratum in: JMIR Res Protoc 2024 Mar 5;13:e57937. https://doi.org/10.2196/57937. PMID: 38300693; PMCID: PMC10870202.

8 Consultation Structure and Models

Rebecca Payne and Ulrik Bak Kirk

8.1 Introduction

8.1.1 Why Use a Consultation Model?

Using a consultation model provides valuable structure to any consultation, ensuring that all essential components are addressed. This structured approach enhances communication, leading to better patient satisfaction, improved recall, and more favorable outcomes [1]. It also mitigates the risk of a remote consultation becoming merely transactional [2], where important aspects such as health promotion, ongoing health issues, and the modification of health-seeking behaviors may be overlooked.

As both patients and clinicians adapt to new methods of conducting these crucial patient–doctor conversations, there is a risk that key elements of the consultation may be missed. Factors such as poor connection quality, the need to explain how the technology works, and external disruptions during the consultation add to the challenge. By following a consultation model, clinicians can stay focused and ensure that all critical points are covered.

While the twentieth century saw the development of numerous consultation models, most were designed for face-to-face interactions. Although the core

R. Payne (✉)
NIHR In-Practice Fellow, Nuffield Department of Primary Care Health Sciences, University of Oxford, Oxford, UK

North Wales Medical School, Bangor University, Bangor, UK
e-mail: rebecca.payne@bangor.ac.uk

U. B. Kirk
Faculty Fellow, Department of Public Health, Aarhus University, Aarhus, Denmark

Digital Health, Research Unit for General Practice, Aarhus, Denmark
e-mail: ubk@ph.au.dk

J. Demurtas (ed.), *Remote Consultation in Primary Care*, TELe-Health,
https://doi.org/10.1007/978-3-031-89661-3_8

principles remain relevant, not all aspects translate seamlessly to remote consultations. Remote consulting introduces new challenges, such as the lack of visual cues during telephone consultations, the potential for talking over a patient due to video call lag, difficulties with maintaining appropriate eye contact when using dual screens, and patients' unfamiliarity with the consultation format. Traditional consultation models often fail to account for these modern obstacles.

8.2 Key Components of a Primary Care Consultation

Whether a consultation is conducted remotely or face to face, it is crucial to consider what a primary care consultation should accomplish. While the patient may have their own agenda for seeking a consultation, primary care extends beyond simply addressing their immediate health concerns or preconceived needs.

8.2.1 Stott and Davis Model

The *Stott and Davis model* [3] highlights the potential in each primary care consultation, which clinicians should keep in mind. This model outlines four core elements: managing the presenting problem, modifying help-seeking behaviors, managing continuing health issues, and offering opportunistic health promotion.

The first priority in any consultation is managing the presenting complaint. Failure to address this effectively can quickly lead to the patient feeling unheard, which may cause frustration and break the rapport between clinician and patient. When technical disruptions occur, such as issues with a video or phone connection, it is vital to steer the conversation back to the presenting issue, signaling to the patient that the clinician cares and is committed to helping solve their problem.

Next, addressing help-seeking behavior is important, as it can empower the patient to self-manage their health when appropriate.

Managing ongoing or chronic problems is another key aspect of the consultation. Patients often appreciate inquiries into previously encountered issues, as this reinforces the relationship and shows that remote consultations are not merely a form of triage. In fact, remote consultations are particularly well suited to managing chronic conditions, sometimes more so than acute conditions.

However, the rise of telehealth during the COVID-19 pandemic largely focused on the assessment of acute or emergency conditions. With increasing demands on health systems—driven by an aging population requiring more care for complex conditions—efficient management of chronic conditions has become more critical than ever.

As healthcare shifts away from waiting rooms filled with patients reading leaflets or posters to remote consultations where interactions are more sporadic, it is essential that health promotion remains a consistent part of every patient-clinician interaction. This could involve providing advice on smoking cessation, reminders for health screenings, or education on making healthy lifestyle choices.

When patients are not physically present in the clinic, there is a risk that the final three components of the *Stott and Davis model* will be neglected. This can result in poorer health outcomes, both for individual patients and for the wider population. Furthermore, if doctors consistently deliver incomplete consultations during remote visits, patients may come to expect less from these consultations, which could fuel ongoing resistance to remote care among patients, clinicians, and society at large.

8.2.2 Smith–King Model for Video Consultations

Developed by British military GPs during the early stages of the pandemic, the *Smith–King model* [4] offers a structured approach to video consultations.

The model, shown in Fig. 8.1, emphasizes the importance of preparation before the consultation even begins. It starts with ensuring that the patient is appropriate for a video consultation, considering that some conditions and patients may be less suited to remote care. The clinician should also prepare by ensuring they have access to relevant information, such as the patient's medical records (ideally on a second screen) and their phone number in case of technical issues.

In addition, the environment should be optimized to reduce distractions—this includes placing the camera at eye level, muting phones and notifications, closing windows to reduce noise, and ensuring proper lighting. A crucial part of this preparation involves establishing appropriate eye contact, which includes looking directly

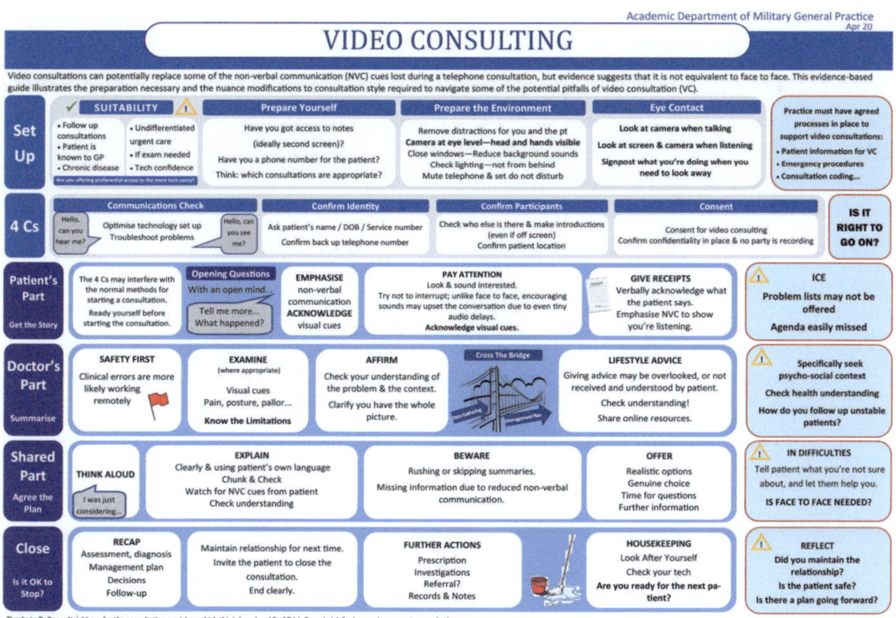

Fig. 8.1 Smith–King model for video consultations [4]

at the camera when speaking, alternating between the screen and camera when listening, and informing the patient if the clinician needs to look away (e.g., to check results on another screen). More on this is discussed in Chap. 7.

8.2.2.1 The 4 C's

Once setup is complete, the consultation begins with the 4 C's: *Communications check*, *Confirming the patient's identity*, *Confirming participants*, and gaining *Consent*. While these initial checks can seem cumbersome and might temporarily distract from establishing rapport, they are vital for ensuring the safety and security of the consultation.

The clinician should ensure the patient can both see and hear them, verify the patient's identity (name, date of birth), obtain a backup phone number, establish who else is present in the room, check the patient's location, and gain explicit consent for the consultation—especially regarding confidentiality and whether the consultation is being recorded.

8.2.2.2 Patient's Part

The next stage—*Patient's Part*—focuses on listening to the patient's story. Open-ended questions help encourage the patient to express their concerns in detail. Clinicians are reminded to pay special attention to nonverbal communication and to minimize interruptions, which can often be caused by technical lags. The term "give receipts" refers to offering verbal summaries of the patient's narrative and using nonverbal cues to assure them that they are being heard. This practice enhances both patient safety and satisfaction.

8.2.2.3 Doctor's Part

In the *Doctor's Part,* the clinician conducts any necessary examinations (limited by the video medium) and ensures they have a full understanding of the patient's problem and its broader context.

8.2.2.4 Shared Part

During the *Shared Part* of the consultation, the clinician shares their thought process to foster patient engagement and understanding. The "chunk and check" technique is recommended here: providing small pieces of information and checking the patient's understanding before moving on. Clinicians are cautioned not to rush or skip these summaries, as nonverbal cues are more limited in remote consultations.

This part concludes with the *Offer,* where the clinician presents the patient with realistic options, ensures they have time to ask questions, and offers genuine choices regarding their care.

8.2.2.5 Close

The model concludes with *Close,* which involves reviewing the assessment, diagnosis, management plan, and follow-up arrangements. The clinician is encouraged to end the consultation in a manner that maintains a positive rapport for future interactions.

The final step is *Housekeeping,* where the clinician takes time to ensure they are ready and focused for the next patient.

Although not formally part of the model, clinicians are reminded to consider the patient's psychosocial context, check the patient's understanding throughout the consultation, convert to face-to-face consultations when necessary, and ensure that a clear follow-up plan is in place.

The *Smith–King model* was specifically designed for video consultations and can be used without adaptation for remote settings. While the evidence base supporting this model is still developing, it has been widely and successfully applied in practice by the British military. The model builds on the principles of Roger Neighbour's well-known model [5] but is distinct in its application to video consultations. One limitation is that it does not explicitly include "safety-netting," so clinicians should ensure they incorporate this aspect when adopting the model.

8.2.3 Dr. Samosa

The *Dr. Samosa model* [6] was specifically designed for telephone consultations and incorporates components of more traditional consultation models, such as the Stott and Davis model [3]. The mnemonic "Dr. Samosa" serves as an easy-to-remember aide-mémoire, as shown in Fig. 8.2.

One notable aspect of this model is its emphasis on *documentation* at the very start of the consultation. This is unlike face-to-face consultations, where documentation typically happens afterward. In telephone consultations, documentation can be done throughout the conversation, as long as the clinician remains focused on the patient and avoids distractions. This approach can significantly speed up consultations by eliminating the need for extensive note-taking afterward. However, clinicians are advised to review their notes afterward to ensure that all important details are accurately captured.

The model also offers advice on *building rapport,* recommending the use of a warm and friendly tone, and even suggesting that clinicians smile while speaking, as this can make the interaction more welcoming. Since the patient may be feeling anxious, possibly after waiting for some time for the call, these simple strategies can help set a positive tone.

Fig. 8.2 The "Dr. Samosa" model for telephone consultations [6]

Box 1. DR SAMOSA consultation model.

D: Documentation

R: Rapport

S: Speaking clearly

A: Active listening

M: Mini-Management plan

O: Opportunistic health promotion

S: Summarise and Safety-net

A: Alternative Access

Active listening is emphasized, and since nonverbal cues are absent in a telephone consultation, verbal signals such as "uh-huh" or "okay" become crucial. Summarizing and repeating what the patient has said also helps to confirm understanding and build rapport.

The model introduces the concept of a *mini-management plan,* encouraging the clinician to consider the broader context of the patient's care. This might include the use of other consultation modalities such as video or face-to-face visits.

The model also stresses the importance of incorporating *opportunistic health promotion,* which can often be neglected in remote consultations [2].

A strong focus is placed on *summarizing* and *safety-netting.* Clinicians are reminded to ensure that patients understand what symptoms they should be wary of and what steps to take if those symptoms arise.

The model also advocates for educating patients about *alternative access,* meaning other available ways to seek support or care.

Ultimately, *the Dr. Samosa model* is simple, easy to remember, and highlights the importance of health promotion. Documenting as the consultation progresses can lead to more accurate and thorough notes, which not only saves time but also helps reinforce the consultation structure, potentially allowing more time with patients. However, a key weakness of the model is its omission of clinical examination, which remains one of the most essential pillars of any consultation.

8.2.4 Calgary–Cambridge Model

Although *the Calgary–Cambridge model* [7] was not originally designed for remote consultations, its principles can be applied effectively across various consultation formats. At its core, the model ensures that communication remains central to the consultation, reducing the risk of turning the interaction into a transaction of closed questions (see Fig. 8.3).

The model consists of five sequential steps, with two parallel themes that run throughout the consultation. Below, we offer advice on how to adapt the Calgary–Cambridge model to newer consultation methods.

The model begins with *initiating the session.* Similar to the Smith–King model [4], this includes setting up an appropriate environment and ensuring the technology is functioning properly. As the consultation begins, rapport-building is crucial, giving the patient the opportunity to outline their agenda [9].

The second step is *gathering information,* which involves exploring the patient's issues from both biomedical and patient-centered perspectives. The clinician must aim to understand the context of the problem, which can be more challenging during a remote consultation—especially if the clinician is unfamiliar with the patient or if it is their first encounter.

The model then moves to *physical examination,* which, of course, requires adjustments in a remote setting.

The fourth stage, *explaining and planning,* is where the patient is fully informed of their options, and a management plan is collaboratively developed, considering

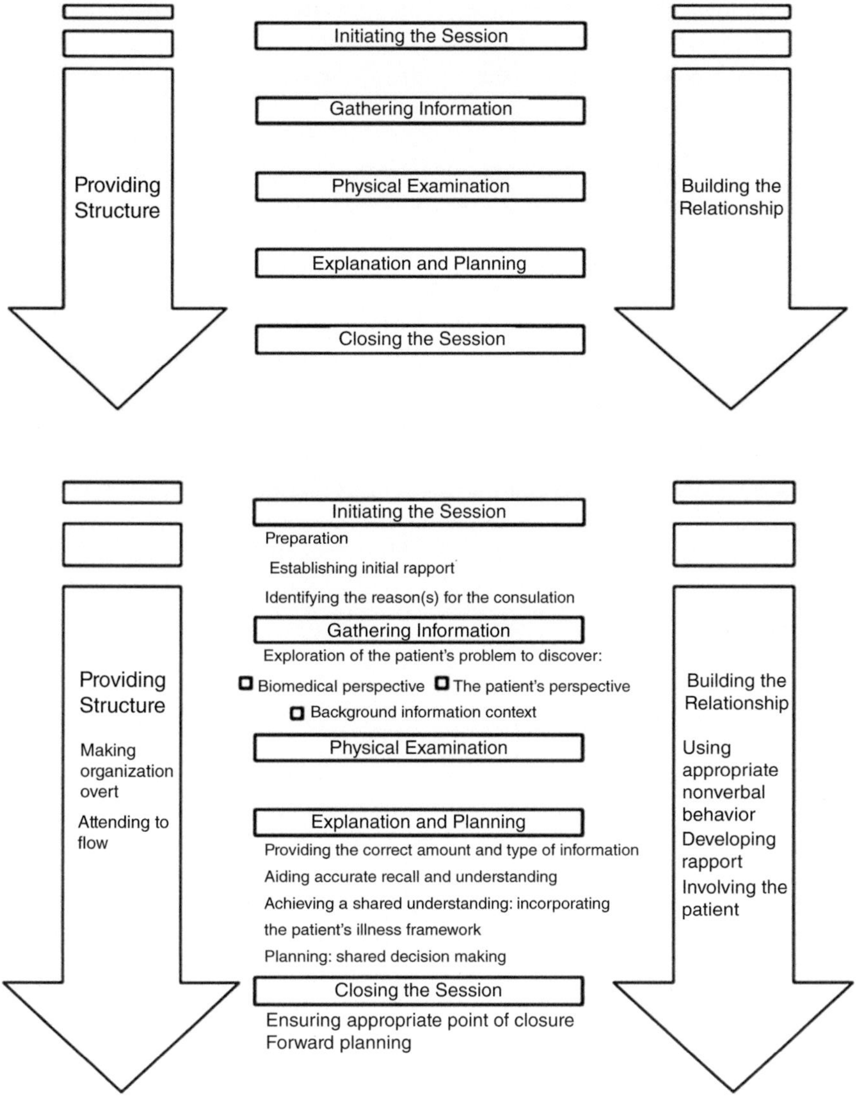

Fig. 8.3 Calgary–Cambridge model [8]

the patient's health and life realities. In remote consultations, extra effort is required to ensure the effectiveness of this stage. Information should be tailored to the patient's needs and delivered in a way that enhances recall and understanding.

Techniques such as *elicit-provide-elicit* or *chunk and check* are often used here [10]. For example, the clinician might ask, "Why do you think your chest is bad at the moment?" and follow up with, "I agree asthma could be a possibility – what do you know about asthma?." This approach helps achieve a shared understanding and facilitates shared decision-making.

Finally, the session concludes with *closing the session,* where plans for the next steps are agreed upon between the doctor and the patient.

The dual focus on content and process allows the clinician to fully understand the patient's symptoms, their impact, and context within a biomedical framework, while also gaining insight from the patient's perspective. This fosters relationship-building and creates an environment conducive to shared decision-making. These skills are vital, regardless of whether the consultation is remote or in person.

Although the Calgary–Cambridge model was not originally developed for remote consultations, it adapts well to this setting. However, it has some limitations. First, being developed in an analog world, it does not address the specific challenges posed by remote technologies, such as video call lag and the need for verbal rather than nonverbal expressions of empathy—points emphasized in the Smith–King model [4].

Clinicians should be aware that picking up and interpreting patient cues can be particularly difficult over the phone, and even video consultations are limited in comparison to face-to-face encounters. In addition, the model does not address key elements of primary care, such as health promotion, managing chronic illnesses, or modifying help-seeking behaviors [3].

8.3 Assessment Frameworks for Remote Consultations

A number of frameworks have been developed to assess the quality of telephone and video consultations, particularly in the out-of-hours setting. While these are not consultation models per se, they are useful for self-assessment, peer review, and audit. The selected examples include the KERNset tool and the RICE rating scale from the Netherlands, the Out-of-Hours Audit Toolkit from the UK's Royal College of General Practitioners, the Assessment of Quality in Telephone Triage (AQTT) tool from Denmark, and the Four Habits Coding Scheme (4-HCS) from the United States.

8.3.1 KERNset

KERNset [11], named after the Dutch word for "'core," was designed to assess the competency of telephone triage nurses in the Dutch out-of-hours system. It consists of 24 items, 13 of which focus on medical content and information gathering, while 10 relate to communication. One item spans both domains. Items are scored from 0 to 4, allowing areas of strength and weakness to be identified for individual clinicians. This tool is typically administered externally by a rater, who listens to a recording of the consultation.

8.3.2 RICE Rating Scale

The *RICE rating scale* [12] was initially developed to assess the competencies of clinical call handlers in the out-of-hours context in the Netherlands across four domains: reason for calling, information gathering, conclusion, and evaluation. As it is not intended for clinical assessment, it is more applicable for training nonclinical team members such as receptionists, rather than clinicians conducting telephone consultations.

8.3.3 RCGP Out-of-Hours Audit Toolkit

The *RCGP Out-of-Hours Audit Toolkit* is the most user-friendly tool for clinicians conducting remote consultations [13]. Each item is graded from 0 to 2, with 0 meaning "not achieved," 1 being "partially achieved," and 2 being "fully achieved." When applied across multiple consultations from the same clinician, recurring patterns can be identified, such as a consistent failure to provide safety-netting information. This helps target specific areas for improvement. However, it is important to note that the toolkit was designed for out-of-hours consultations and, thus, does not cover all aspects of the Stott and Davis model. Clinicians may want to adapt the score sheet to include additional elements from that model.

8.3.4 AQTT

The Dutch KERNset tool [11] was translated into Danish and enhanced with elements from other existing tools to develop the *Assessment of Quality in Telephone Triage* (AQTT) tool [14]. Face validity, content validity, and applicability in out-of-hours telephone triage were established through a two-round Delphi process that involved relevant stakeholders. The 24-item AQTT tool assesses communicative quality, health-related quality, and four overall quality dimensions in out-of-hours telephone triage performed by both nurses and general practitioners [15, 16].

8.3.5 Four Habits Coding Scheme (4HCS)

The *Four Habits Coding Scheme* (4HCS) is a standardized instrument developed to assess physicians' communication skills from the perspective of an external rater in the United States, using video-recorded primary care consultations [17]. The 4HCS integrates both evaluative and descriptive elements of physician communication behavior based on a conceptually driven teaching model. It holds significant potential for researchers, evaluators, educators, and clinicians alike. The 4HCS consists of 23 items divided into four subscales: [1] Invest in the Beginning, [2] Elicit the

Patient's Perspective, [3] Demonstrate Empathy, and [4] Invest in the End [18]. The 4HCS has been translated and validated in several languages, including German [19], Brazilian Portuguese [20], and French [21].

8.4 Conclusion

When conducting remote consultations in the primary care setting, it is beneficial to apply the *Stott and Davis model* to ensure that all key aspects of the consultation are covered. These include managing the presenting complaint, modifying health-seeking behavior, managing long-term conditions, and addressing ongoing health concerns. This model can be used in combination with other consultation models, such as the *Smith–King model* for video consultations, the *Dr. Samosa model* for telephone consultations, or the *Calgary-Cambridge model,* which can be adapted for both modalities. To assess the quality of remote consultations, frameworks such as KERNset, RICE, the RCGP Out-of-Hours Audit Toolkit, AQTT, and 4HCS can be employed for self-assessment, peer review, or audit, ensuring that a service's remote consultations meet high standards.

References

1. Ong LM, de Haes JC, Hoos AM, Lammes FB. Doctor-patient communication: a review of the literature. Soc Sci Med. 1995 Apr;40(7):903–18. https://doi.org/10.1016/0277-9536(94)00155-m.
2. Rosen R, Wieringa S, Greenhalgh T, Leone C, Rybczynska-Bunt S, Hughes G, Moore L, Shaw SE, Wherton J, Byng R. Clinical risk in remote consultations in general practice: findings from in-COVID-19 pandemic qualitative research. BJGP Open. 2022 Sep 28;6(3):BJGPO.2021.0204. https://doi.org/10.3399/BJGPO.2021.0204. PMID: 35487581; PMCID: PMC9680756.
3. Stott NC, Davis RH. The exceptional potential in each primary care consultation. J R Coll Gen Pract. 1979 Apr;29(201):201–5. PMID: 448665; PMCID: PMC2159027.
4. King K. Video consulting: not just a consultation plus tech. BJGP Life. 2000, May 15; https://bjgplife.com/video-consulting-not-just-a-consultation-plus-tech/
5. Neighbour R. The inner consultation: how to develop an effective and intuitive consulting style. Boca Raton/New York: CRC Press; 2005.
6. Mirza D. The need for new GP consultation models. InnovAiT. 2019;12(1):33–7. https://doi.org/10.1177/1755738018806931.
7. Kurtz SM, Silverman JD. The Calgary-Cambridge referenced observation guides: an aid to defining the curriculum and organizing the teaching in communication training programmes. Med Educ. 1996 Mar;30(2):83–9. https://doi.org/10.1111/j.1365-2923.1996.tb00724.x.
8. Kurtz S, Silverman J, Benson J, Draper J. Marrying content and process in clinical method teaching: enhancing the Calgary-Cambridge guides. Acad Med. 2003 Aug;78(8):802–9. https://doi.org/10.1097/00001888-200308000-00011.
9. McKinstry B, Hammersley V, Burton C, Pinnock H, Elton R, Dowell J, Sawdon N, Heaney D, Elwyn G, Sheikh A. The quality, safety and content of telephone and face-to-face consultations: a comparative study. Qual Saf Health Care. 2010 Aug;19(4):298–303. https://doi.org/10.1136/qshc.2008.027763. Epub 2010 Apr 29.

10. Frost KA, Metcalf EP, Brooks R, Kinnersley P, Greenwood SR, Powell CV. Teaching pediatric communication skills to medical students. Adv Med Educ Pract. 2015 Jan 16;6:35–43. https://doi.org/10.2147/AMEP.S68413. PMID: 25653569; PMCID: PMC4303365.
11. Smits M, Keizer E, Ram P, Giesen P. Development and testing of the KERNset: an instrument to assess the quality of telephone triage in out-of-hours primary care services. BMC Health Serv Res. 2017 Dec 2;17(1):798. https://doi.org/10.1186/s12913-017-2686-1. PMID: 29197376; PMCID: PMC5712191.
12. Derkx HP, Rethans JJ, Knottnerus JA, Ram PM. Assessing communication skills of clinical call handlers working at an out-of-hours Centre: development of the RICE rating scale. Br J Gen Pract. 2007 May;57(538):383–387. PMID: 17504589; PMCID: PMC2047013.
13. Royal College of General Practitioners, RcoPaCH, The College of Emergency Medicine. Urgent and Emergency Care Clinical Audit Toolkit 2011. Available online: https://heeoe.hee.nhs.uk/sites/default/files/urgentcaretoolkit.pdf.
14. Graversen DS, Pedersen AF, Carlsen AH, Bro F, Huibers L, Christensen MB. Quality of out-of-hours telephone triage by general practitioners and nurses: development and testing of the AQTT – an assessment tool measuring communication, patient safety and efficiency. Scand J Prim Health Care. 2019 Mar;37(1):18–29. https://doi.org/10.1080/02813432.2019.1568712. Epub 2019 Jan 28. PMID: 30689490; PMCID: PMC6454404.
15. Graversen DS, Christensen MB, Pedersen AF, Carlsen AH, Bro F, Christensen HC, Vestergaard CH, Huibers L. Safety, efficiency and health-related quality of telephone triage conducted by general practitioners, nurses, or physicians in out-of-hours primary care: a quasi-experimental study using the assessment of quality in telephone triage (AQTT) to assess audio-recorded telephone calls. BMC Fam Pract. 2020 May 9;21(1):84. https://doi.org/10.1186/s12875-020-01122-z. PMID: 32386511; PMCID: PMC7211335.
16. Graversen DS, Huibers L, Christensen MB, Bro F, Collatz Christensen H, Vestergaard CH, Pedersen AF. Communication quality in telephone triage conducted by general practitioners, nurses or physicians: a quasi-experimental study using the AQTT to assess audio-recorded telephone calls to out-of-hours primary care in Denmark. BMJ Open. 2020 Mar 26;10(3):e033528. https://doi.org/10.1136/bmjopen-2019-033528. PMID: 32220912; PMCID: PMC7170599.
17. Krupat E, Frankel R, Stein T, Irish J. The four habits coding scheme: validation of an instrument to assess clinicians' communication behavior. Patient Educ Couns. 2006 Jul;62(1):38–45. https://doi.org/10.1016/j.pec.2005.04.015. Epub 2005 Jun 17.
18. Park YS, Tekian A. Critical synthesis package: four habits coding scheme (4HCS). MedEdPORTAL. 2013;9:9611. https://doi.org/10.15766/mep_2374-8265.9611.
19. Scholl I, Nicolai J, Pahlke S, Kriston L, Krupat E, Härter M. The German version of the four habits coding scheme - association between physicians' communication and shared decision making skills in the medical encounter. Patient Educ Couns. 2014 Feb;94(2):224–229. https://doi.org/10.1016/j.pec.2013.10.006. Epub 2013 Oct 31.
20. Catani RR, Valadares EDS, Lacombe JB, Mendonça TMDS, Silva CHMD, Paro HBMDS. Cross-cultural adaptation of the four habits coding scheme (4HCS) for teaching and assessing patient-centered communication skills in Brazil. Cad Saude Publica. 2018 Nov 8;34(11):e00013918. https://doi.org/10.1590/0102-311X00013918.
21. Bellier A, Chaffanjon P, Krupat E, Francois P, Labarère J. Cross-cultural adaptation of the 4-habits coding scheme into French to assess physician communication skills. PLoS One 2020 Apr 16;15(4):e0230672. https://doi.org/10.1371/journal.pone.0230672. PMID: 32298278; PMCID: PMC7161987.

9 Clinical Prediction Rules in Remote Consultation

Jacopo Demurtas, Alberto Vaona, Luca Pasolli, Vinicius Anjos de Almeida, Deoclecio Avigo, and Mark H. Ebell

9.1 Background

Family physicians are asked every day to deal with uncertainty [1], relying on their gut feeling in many situations [2]. This is even more evident when it comes to triage and prioritizing interventions from remote locations.

It is noteworthy that while a single sign or symptom can often be misleading, the combination of several signs or symptoms can be much more helpful. General practitioners can rely during their consultations on statistics, evidence-based risk scores, and clinical prediction rules, which may help them deal with the challenge of remote consultations.

J. Demurtas
Clinical and Experimental Medicine PhD Program, University of Modena and Reggio Emilia, Modena, Italy

Family Medicine Department, USL Toscana Sud-Est, Capalbio, Italy

A. Vaona
ULSS 9 Scaligera, Primary Care, Verona, Italy

Italian Telemedicine Society, Verona, Italy

L. Pasolli
Department of Family Medicine Trento, University of Trento, Trento, Italy

School of Family Medicine, Trento, Italy

V. A. de Almeida · D. Avigo
University of São Paulo, São Paulo, Brazil
e-mail: vinicius.almeida@alumni.usp.br

M. H. Ebell (✉)
Department of Family Medicine, Michigan State University, East Lansing, MI, USA
e-mail: ebell@msu.edu; ebell@uga.edu

J. Demurtas (ed.), *Remote Consultation in Primary Care*, TELe-Health,
https://doi.org/10.1007/978-3-031-89661-3_9

Moreover, there are conditions in which objective examination done in a face-to-face consultation may be inappropriate, difficult (patients homebound, in very remote locations, or older people with relevant limitations) or impossible. For example, think of the first waves of COVID-19. In other situations, objective examination could be time-consuming and not influence the patient's outcome. It is in these cases that statistics may help, putting an evidence-based spin on the consultation.

Clinical prediction rules (CPR) can assist primary healthcare (PHC) professionals regarding the probability that a disease is present, the benefit of screening for potentially serious conditions, the likelihood that treatment is effective, and the risk of a patient developing more serious conditions such as hospital admission, myocardial infarction (MI), stroke, cancer, and premature death. They can be of great value in assisting clinical decision-making but should not be used indiscriminately. They are also not a substitute for clinical judgment. Their most appropriate use is as a check on clinical decisions: if the risk score provides a different answer than the physician's judgment, it is appropriate to carefully reconsider that decision.

Statistical models can address a much larger number of variables than the human brain. The human clinical model often results in inconsistencies, especially with less experienced practitioners. Resistance to the adoption of prediction models by health professionals may occur due to the large number of models available, their complexity, or lack of validation.

Many cardiovascular disease prevention guidelines advocate the use of cardiovascular risk calculators. There are more than 100 cardiovascular risk prediction models, but only about 25 of these models/calculators have been externally validated. However, disagreement is common in risk categorization. In part, this disagreement occurs because calculators vary depending on the database from which they are derived, when they were developed (as cardiovascular risk has declined over time), and the choice of clinical outcomes.

Healthcare professionals should use models derived from or calibrated for populations similar to their own. Ideally, calculators should provide absolute risks, a graphical representation, and an estimate of the benefit of key interventions to improve the shared decision-making process between doctor and patient [3]. Table 9.1 lists some CPRs used by PHC professionals [4].

Table 9.1 CPRs for GPs. (Adapted from "Clinical prediction rules in practice: review of clinical guidelines and survey of GPs")

List of clinical prediction rules (CPRs) included in a GP survey		
Clinical area	Clinical prediction rule	Description
Cardiovascular disease	QRISK[a] or QRISK2[b]	Ten-year risk of heart attack or stroke based on UK data.
	PREVENT risk score[c]	Cardiovascular risk assessment, based on US data
	Systematic coronary risk evaluation (SCORE) risk charts[d]	The European cardiovascular disease risk assessment model
	$CHADS_2$[e] or CHA_2DS_2[f]	Atrial fibrillation stroke risk
Anxiety and depression	Patient health questionnaire (PHQ)-9[g]	Nine-item depression module of the PHQ
	Generalized anxiety disorder screener (GAD)-7[h]	Seven-item anxiety measure
Cancer	Gail risk score	Breast cancer risk assessment tool
Infection	NICE traffic light system[i]	From the NICE guideline on feverish 39 illness in children
	Strep score (Centor)[j]	Diagnosis of streptococcal pharyngitis 3 in adults
	CRB-65 risk score[k]	Pneumonia prognosis in outpatients
General medical	California score[l]	Risk of stroke at 90 days
	Wells score (DVT)[m]	Risk of deep vein thrombosis
	WHO/FRAX algorithm[n]	Risk of osteoporotic fracture
Diabetes	Diabetes risk score Calculator[o]	Risk of type 2 diabetes mellitus
	ELSA-Brasil diabetes risk prediction[p]	Ten-year risk of developing diabetes [3]

[a] Hippisley-Cox J, Coupland C, Vinogradova Y, Robson J, May M, Brindle P et al. Derivation and validation of QRISK, a new cardiovascular disease risk score for the United Kingdom: prospective open cohort study *BMJ* 2007; 335: 136 https://doi.org/10.1136/bmj.39261.471806.55

[b] Collins G S, Altman D G. An independent and external validation of QRISK2 cardiovascular disease risk score: a prospective open cohort study *BMJ* 2010; 340: c2442 https://doi.org/10.1136/bmj.c2442

[c] Khan SS, Matsushita K, Sang Y, et al. Development and Validation of the American Heart Association Predicting Risk of Cardiovascular Disease EVENTs (PREVENTTM) Equations. Circulation 2023. https://doi.org/10.1161/CIRCULATIONAHA.123.067626 (link opens in new window)(link opens in new window)(link opens in new window).

[d] European Guidelines on CVD Prevention in Clinical Practice 2016 Eur J Prev Cardiol. 2016 Jul;23(11):NP1-NP96. https://doi.org/10.1177/2047487316653709

[e] Gage BF, Waterman AD, Shannon W, et al. Validation of clinical classification schemes for predicting stroke: results from the National Registry of Atrial Fibrillation. JAMA 2001; 285:2864.

[f] Lip GY, Nieuwlaat R, Pisters R, lane DA, Crijns HJ. Refining clinical risk stratification for predicting stroke and thromboembolism in atrial fibrillation using a novel risk factor-based approach: The euro heart survey on atrial fibrillation. Chest 2010, 137 (2): 263–72

[g] Arroll B, Goodyear-Smith F, Crengle S, et al. Validation of PHQ-2 and PHQ-9 to Screen for Major Depression in the Primary Care Population. Ann Fam Med 2010 8:348–353.

[h] Löwe B, Decker O, Müller S, Brähler E, Schellberg D, Herzog W, Herzberg PY. Validation and standardization of the generalized anxiety disorder screener (GAD-7) in the general population. Med care. 2008 Mar;46(3):266–74. https://doi.org/10.1097/MLR.0b013e318160d093. PMID: 18388841.

(continued)

Table 9.1 (continued)

[i] Clark A, Cannings-John R, Blyth M, Hay AD, Butler CC, Hughes K. Accuracy of the NICE traffic light system in children presenting to general practice: a retrospective cohort study. Br J Gen Pract. 2022 May 26;72(719):e398–e404. https://doi.org/10.3399/BJGP.2021.0633. PMID: 35577588; PMCID: PMC9119811.

[j] Centor RM, Witherspoon JM, Dalton HP, et al. The diagnosis of strep throat in adults in the emergency room. Medical Decision Making: An International Journal of the Society for Medical Decision Making 1981, 1 (3): 239–46

[k] McNally M, curtain J, O'Brien KK, Dimitrov BD, Fahey T. Validity of British Thoracic Society guidance (the CRB-65 rule) for predicting the severity of pneumonia in general practice: Systematic review and meta-analysis. Br J Gen Pract. 2010 Oct;60(579):e423–33. https://doi.org/10.3399/bjgp10X532422. PMID: 20883616; PMCID: PMC2944951.

[l] Bhatt A, Jani V. The ABCD and ABCD2 Scores and the Risk of Stroke following a TIA: A Narrative Review. ISRN Neurol. 2011;2011:518621. https://doi.org/10.5402/2011/518621. Epub 2011 Jul 21. PMID: 22389822; PMCID: PMC3263538.

[m] Wells PS, Anderson DR, Rodger M, Forgie M, Kearon C, Dreyer J, Kovacs G, Mitchell M, Lewandowski B, Kovacs MJ. Evaluation of D-dimer in the diagnosis of suspected deep-vein thrombosis. N Engl J Med. 2003 Sep 25;349(13):1227–35. https://doi.org/10.1056/NEJMoa023153. PMID: 14507948.

[n] Sophie Roux, François Cabana, Nathalie Carrier, Michèle Beaulieu, Pierre-Marc April, Marie-Claude Beaulieu, Gilles Boire, The World Health Organization Fracture Risk Assessment Tool (FRAX) Underestimates Incident and Recurrent Fractures in Consecutive Patients With Fragility Fractures, *The Journal of Clinical Endocrinology & Metabolism*, Volume 99, Issue 7, 1 July 2014, Pages 2400–2408, https://doi.org/10.1210/jc.2013-4507

[o] Lindstrom J, Tuomilehto J. The diabetes risk score: a practical tool to predict type 2 diabetes risk. Diabetes Care 2003; 26(3): 725–731.

[p] Comparison of machine-learning algorithms to build a predictive model for detecting undiagnosed diabetes—ELSA-Brasil: accuracy study Sao Paulo Med. J. 135 (03) • May-Jun 2017 https://doi.org/10.1590/1516-3180.2016.0309010217

9.2 Statistical Definitions

9.2.1 What Is a Clinical Prediction Rule?

Let us start with clinical prediction rules. These rules are designed to assist medical decision-making [5]; they may be useful for general practitioners while dealing with a patient, both in-person or remotely.

Clinical prediction rules are tools usually derived from multivariable analysis and either provide a probability of a disease or of an outcome, or suggest a diagnostic or therapeutic course of action [6].

They may also be called clinical decision rules or risk scores, and are based on physicians' experiences with large numbers of patients, distilled into simple rules using the most important predictors of the outcome [7].

To better understand clinical prediction rules, let us examine the concepts of sensitivity, specificity, predictive values, and likelihood ratios, before returning to how they apply to our rules.

9.2.2 Sensitivity and Specificity

Widely used to evaluate the performance of medical tests, sensitivity and specificity represent the core statistics used to describe the accuracy of a test [8]. In an ideal setting, a test should have a sensitivity and specificity of 1.0 or 100% [9].

Sensitivity represents the ability of the test to detect true positives (persons who have the disease) among those with a positive test and is expressed by the formula:

$$\text{Sensitivity} = \text{true positives} / (\text{false negatives} + \text{true positives})$$

Another way to state it is:

$$\text{Sensitivity} = \text{number with the disease} / \text{number with a positive test}$$

It is also sometimes called the true positive rate [10]. When sensitivity is very high (>95%), a negative test (or the absence of a clinical finding) provides good evidence that the disease is not present (SnNOut stands for a highly Sensitive test when "Negative Rules Out" disease).

Specificity represents the ability of the test to identify true negatives. It is expressed by the formula:

$$\text{Specificity} = \text{true negatives} / (\text{true negatives} + \text{false positives})$$

In other words.

$$\text{Specificity} = \text{number without disease} / \text{number with a negative test}$$

When the specificity is very high (>95%), a positive test provides good evidence that the disease is present (SpPIn STANDS FOR a highly Specific test when "Positive Rules In") [11].

9.2.3 Predictive Values

Positive and negative predictive values are more useful for the practitioners [5]. They are described as:

Positive Predictive Value: The proportion of patients who tested positive and have the disease [8].

Negative Predictive Value: The proportion of patients who tested negative and do not have the disease [8].

The usefulness of these statistics relies heavily on the pretest probability. If a disease is widespread in a population, that population has a higher pretest probability of disease. This implies that a positive diagnostic test does not change the clinician's hypothesis very much. Tests that are able to reduce the probability of disease significantly through a negative test are the most useful, since they have greater impact on clinical decision-making (Table 9.2).

Table 9.2 Predictive values for a disease using a test that is 80% sensitive and 80% specific

Pretest probability of disease	Positive predictive value	Negative predictive value
Rare (3%)	11.0%	99.2%
Common (50%)	80.0%	80.0%
Very common (97%)	99.2%	11.0%

9.2.4 Likelihood Ratios

The impact of a diagnostic test on the likelihood of disease is called the "likelihood ratio" (*LR*). It indicates the power of confirmation in the case of "positive likelihood ratio" or of exclusion in the case of "negative likelihood ratio."

Likelihood ratios describe how much our pretest probability will change once we have the test result. A positive likelihood ratio (*LR*+) is calculated as follows [11]:

$$LR+ = \frac{\text{Sensitivity}}{\left(1 - \text{Specificity}\right)}$$

A higher *LR*+ increases the probability of disease after a positive test and helps us confirm a diagnosis.

A negative likelihood ratio (*LR*−) is calculated as follows:

$$LR- = \frac{\left(1 - \text{Sensitivity}\right)}{\text{Specificity}}$$

A lower *LR*− decreases the probability of disease after a negative test and helps us rule out a diagnosis [9].

LR ranges from zero to infinity. There is no absolute rule for the interpretation of likelihood ratios. The positive or negative predictive value depends on *LR* as well as on the pretest probability of disease. A very rare condition needs a powerful diagnostic test to confirm it. However, there are some general rules of thumb for interpreting *LR*+ and *LR*−, as shown in Table 9.3 [7].

Another property of LRs is that they can report the accuracy of tests with more than two possible outcomes. For example, a risk score with low, moderate, and high-risk groups can have LRs of 0.1, 1.1, and 5.2 respectively. This allows for richer information to be reported by the risk score.

9.2.5 Receiver-Operating Characteristics Curves

If you are not familiar with this, do not panic. The performance of a test or clinical prediction rule changes depending on the cutoffs used. A test can be tuned to be more sensitive or specific depending on what is needed. For example, for a cancer screening test, you would favor sensitivity to avoid missing any cases of cancer. There is always a tradeoff: as sensitivity increases, specificity decreases, and vice

Table 9.3 Confirmation/exclusion power depending on the value of the "likelihood ratio" (LR)

Confirmation power		Exclusion power	
LR+ > 10	High confirmation power	**LR- < 0.1**	High exclusion power
LR+ 5 to 10	Moderate confirmation power	**LR- 0.1 to 0.2**	Moderate exclusion power
LR+ 2 to 5	Low confirmation power	**LR- 0.2 to 0.5**	Low exclusion power
LR+ 2 to 1	Minimal confirmation power	**LR- 0.5 to 1**	Minimal exclusion power

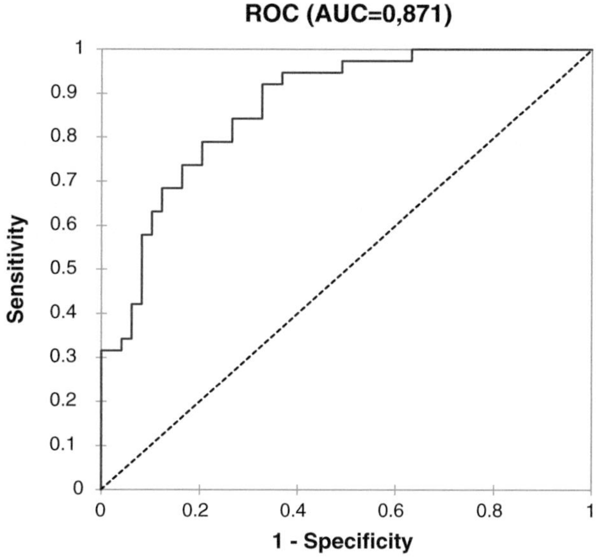

Fig. 9.1 An example of an ROC curve and AUC

versa. That association can be graphically represented by plotting the sensitivity on the *y*-axis and 100 minus specificity on the *x*-axis. This curve is known as receiver-operating curve (ROC) [5]. The area under the ROC is known as AUC (area under curve). It ranges from 0.5 (no predictive power) to 1 (perfectly categorizing all patients). A good test has an AUC of at least 0.7 [5] and an excellent test has an area of more than 0.85 [5]. Figure 9.1 is an example of a ROC curve with an AUC of 0.871.

9.3 Sample CPRs for Primary Care

To explain and exemplify how CPRs can work in practice, we will present two clinical prediction rules that are potentially useful for remote consultations: the Marburg Heart Score for evaluation of chest pain in primary care and the LOCH risk score that was derived and validated to identify the risk that primary care patients with COVID-19 will be hospitalized [9].

9.3.1 Marburg Heart Score

In primary care, according to the literature, approximately 40% of patients presenting with chest pain have musculoskeletal conditions, 12% have stable angina, 3% have acute cardiac ischemia (including myocardial infarction [MI]), and less than 1% have pulmonary embolism [13].

The "Marburg score" is a simple tool that physicians and nurses can use to rule out coronary artery disease as the cause of chest pain in primary care. It provides 1 point to each of these five characteristics: gender/age (over 65 for females and 55 for males), presence of known arterial disease (coronary, cerebral, peripheral), pain aggravated by physical exertion, pain not reproducible with palpation, and patient's belief that the pain is of cardiac origin [14].

If we consider the LR for this rule, it has a moderate positive likelihood ratio (6.7) for a score of 4 or 5; so additional testing is needed before ruling in CAD. The very low negative likelihood ratio (0.08) for a score of 0 or 1 makes the Marburg score very reliable for excluding a cardiac origin of the pain, which is especially useful for the primary care doctor who must decide whether to refer him or her to the emergency department and the hospital. So, if the score is 0–1, the probability of cardiac origin of the pain is <1%.

A recent study [15] compared the Marburg Heart Score and the INTERCHEST risk score for cardiac chest pain to standard telephone triage in the Netherlands based on the Netherland Triage Standard protocols. The results provided showed that both MHS and INTERCHEST outperformed standard telephone triage protocols.

9.3.2 The Leigh Outpatient COVID Hospitalization (LOCH) Risk Score

Many studies were developed based on observational retrospective or prospective data to assess COVID-19 severity and prognostic outcomes, but most relied on laboratory findings [16]. Only a few studies developed and validated tools that could be applied remotely to predict the risk of hospitalization in outpatients with COVID-19 in primary care.

The Leigh Outpatient COVID-19 Hospitalization (LOCH) risk score [12] was developed during the delta wave of the pandemic and has only three predictors: the presence of dyspnea, increasing age, and the presence of at least one of a list of comorbidities. Table 9.4 shows the results from the original study during the delta wave of COVID-19 when 4.4% of all outpatients with COVID-19 were hospitalized.

The AUC was 0.85, indicating excellent discrimination. An advantage of the risk score is that it has a low "data burden" and can be assessed remotely by telehealth consultation [9]. It is also notable that approximately half of all patients can be classified as low risk and can be cared for without need for close follow-up. However, with the milder omicron variant and immunity from both vaccination and previous

Table 9.4 LOCH risk score for COVID-19 prognosis in outpatients

Risk factor	Points	Risk group (points)	% hospitalized (delta wave
Dyspnea	1.5	Low: 0	15/1849 (0.8%)
Comorbidity[a]	1.0	Mod: 1 to 2.5	84/1623 (5.2%)
Age		High: ≥ 3	70/334 (21%)
<50 years	0		
50 to 59	1		
60 to 69	1.5		
70+	2.5		
Total (range 0 to 5)			

[a]One or more of diabetes mellitus, asthma, chronic obstructive lung disease, hypertension, cardiovascular disease, chronic kidney or liver disease, or cancer

Table 9.5 Application of the LOCH risk score to patients in the Omicron wave

Risk group (points)	Hospitalized/Total (%)	Recommended action
Vaccinated patients		
Low risk (0)	2/3136 (0.06%)	Care at home
Moderate risk (1 to 2.5)	13/4809 (0.27%)	Care at home
High risk (≥3)	54/1523 (3.4%)	Close follow-up + O_2 saturation
Total:	69/9468 (0.72%)	
Unvaccinated patients		
Low risk (0)	6/5294 (0.11%)	Care at home
Moderate risk (1 to 2.5)	68/3977 (1.7%)	Close follow-up + O_2 saturation
High risk (≥3)	51/523 (8.9%)	Refer to hospital
Total	125/9794 (1.26%)	

infection, the hospitalization rate has decreased. Was the LOCH risk score still valid with omicron, and what is the impact of vaccination?

Therefore, the researchers identified 19,456 new patients diagnosed between December 2021 and November 2022 when omicron was the dominant variant [17]. They also stratified the results by vaccination as shown in Table 9.5.

In this large omicron population, the risk score had a similar AUC (0.844) and identified three distinct risk groups:

Low risk (low or moderate risk vaccinated, low risk unvaccinated): 0.16% hospitalized, representing 68% of all patients. These patients can be safely managed at home with follow-up only as needed.

Moderate risk (high risk vaccinated or moderate risk unvaccinated): 2.2% hospitalized, representing 28% of the population. These patients can usually be sent home but should have close follow-up by phone or nurse visit.

High risk (high risk unvaccinated): 8.9% hospitalized, but only represents 2.6% of the population. Refer to hospital for further evaluation and possible hospitalization.

As expected, vaccinated patients had about half the risk of hospitalization as unvaccinated patients. This validation study illustrates the importance of revalidating risk scores as the patient population, disease, and factors like vaccines impact prognosis.

9.3.3 Research Gaps and Opportunities

With the increasing use of telemedicine in healthcare, a rigorous assessment of clinical prediction tools is needed. Before incorporating a new tool in clinical practice, it needs to be reliable across different contexts. A systematic review [18] analyzed studies about cognitive remote assessment methods for the diagnosis of dementia. Some studies had good results, but those results were inconsistent across different methods and settings and a meta-analysis could not be performed. For the diagnosis of dementia, it seems to not be accurate enough to be done through telemedicine.

Physical examination becomes more challenging in remote consultations and limits the evaluation of healthcare providers. Attempts to validate tools and strategies for remote physical and cognitive assessment show promising results, but the interrater reliability varies greatly and the sample sizes are small [19]. More studies are needed to determine the best tools for clinical practice.

Many machine learning algorithms are being developed as clinical prediction tools. Some show promising results and could be applied to remote consultations to aid clinical decision-making. As an example, an algorithm was developed focused on identifying patients with pneumonia through the cough sound [20]. Although the sample size was small and the results must still be replicated in different settings and with bigger samples, the algorithm achieved 90% sensitivity and 78.6% specificity. That corresponds to an $LR+$ of 4.21 and an $LR-$ of 0.13, a promising result that could be combined with other clinical information and help with the diagnosis of pneumonia remotely. Similar machine learning tools should be developed and tested in remote consultation settings as well.

9.4 Conclusions

In conclusion, clinical prediction rules (CPRs) offer invaluable support to healthcare professionals, especially in the context of remote consultations. By combining clinical intuition with evidence-based tools, CPRs enable physicians to navigate uncertainty, assess risk, and make informed decisions, even when direct patient examination is limited. The examples explored in this chapter, including the Marburg Heart Score and the LOCH risk score, illustrate how CPRs can enhance diagnostic accuracy and patient triage across various conditions. However, CPRs should be applied judiciously, complementing rather than replacing clinical judgment, to ensure the best outcomes. As remote healthcare grows and technology advances, continued development, validation, and adaptation of CPRs will be essential to meet the evolving needs of patient care.

References

1. O'Riordan M, Dahinden A, Aktürk Z, Ortiz JMB, Dagdeviren N, Elwyn G, Micallef A, Murtonen M, Samuelson M, Struk P. Dealing with uncertainty in general practice: an essential skill for the general practitioner. Qual Prim Care. 2011;19(3):175–81.
2. Alam R, Cheraghi-Sohi S, Panagioti M, Esmail A, Campbell S, Panagopoulou E. Managing diagnostic uncertainty in primary care: a systematic critical review. BMC Fam Pract. 2017;18:1–13.
3. Allan GM, et al. Comparison of cardiovascular disease risk calculators. Curr Opin Lipidol. 2014;25(4):254–65. https://doi.org/10.1097/MOL.0000000000000095.
4. Plüddemann A, et al. Clinical prediction rules in practice: review of clinical guidelines and survey of GPs. Br J Gen Pract. 2014;64(621):e233–42. https://doi.org/10.3399/bjgp14X677860.
5. Laupacis A, Sekar N. Clinical prediction rules: a review and suggested modifications of methodological standards. JAMA. 1997;277(6):488–94.
6. Ebell MH. Evidence-based diagnosis: a handbook of clinical prediction rules. Springer Science & Business Media; 2001.
7. Harris M, Taylor G. Medical statistics made easy. CRC Press; 2003.
8. Altman DG, Bland JM. Diagnostic tests. 1: sensitivity and specificity. Br Med J. 1994;308(6943):1552.
9. Shapiro DE. The interpretation of diagnostic tests. Stat Methods Med Res. 1999;8(2):113–34.
10. Harris M, Taylor G, Jackson D. Clinical evidence made easy. Scion Publishing Ltd; 2023.
11. McGee S. Evidence-based physical diagnosis e-book. Elsevier Health Sciences; 2021.
12. Ebell MH, Hamadani R, Kieber-Emmons A. Development and validation of simple risk scores to predict hospitalization in outpatients with COVID-19 including the omicron variant. J Am Board Fam Med. 2022;35(6):1058–64.
13. Ebell MH. Evaluation of chest pain in primary care patients. Am Fam Physician. 2011;83(5):603–5.
14. Bosner S, Haasenritter J, Becker A, Karatolios K, Vaucher P, Gencer B, Herzig L, Heinzel-Gutenbrunner M, Schaefer JR, Abu Hani M, Keller H, Sonnichsen AC, Baum E, Donner-Banzhoff N. Ruling out coronary artery disease in primary care: development and validation of a simple prediction rule. CMAJ. 2010;182(12):1295–300. https://doi.org/10.1503/cmaj.100212.
15. Manten A, De Clercq L, Rietveld R, Lucassen W, Moll van Charante E, Harskamp R. Evaluation of the Marburg heart score and INTERCHEST score compared to current telephone triage for chest pain in out-of-hours primary care. Neth Hear J. 2023;31(4):157–65.
16. Lagolio E, Demurtas J, Buzzetti R, Cortassa G, Bottone S, Spadafora L, Cocino C, Smith L, Benzing T, Polidori MC. A rapid and feasible tool for clinical decision making in community-dwelling patients with COVID-19 and those admitted to emergency departments: the Braden-LDH-HorowITZ Assessment—BLITZ. Intern Emerg Med. 2021;17(3):839–44.
17. Ebell MH, Hamadani R, Kieber-Emmons A. Prospective validation of a simple risk score to predict hospitalization during the omicron phase of COVID-19. J Am Board Fam Med. 2024;37:324–7.
18. Beishon LC, Elliott E, Hietamies TM, Mc Ardle R, O'Mahony A, Elliott AR, Quinn TJ. Diagnostic test accuracy of remote, multidomain cognitive assessment (telephone and video call) for dementia. Cochrane Database Syst Rev. 2022 Apr 8;4(4):CD013724. https://doi.org/10.1002/14651858.CD013724.pub2. PMID: 35395108; PMCID: PMC8992929.
19. Lu AD, Veet CA, Aljundi O, Whitaker E, Smith WB 2nd, Smith JE. A systematic review of physical examination components adapted for telemedicine. Telemed J E Health. 2022 Dec;28(12):1764–1785. https://doi.org/10.1089/tmj.2021.0602. Epub 2022 Apr 1.
20. Chung Y, Jin J, Jo HI, Lee H, Kim SH, Chung SJ, Yoon HJ, Park J, Jeon JY. Diagnosis of pneumonia by cough sounds analyzed with statistical features and AI. Sensors (Basel). 2021 Oct 23;21(21):7036. https://doi.org/10.3390/s21217036. PMID: 34770341; PMCID: PMC8586978.

Triage and Its Relevance to Remote Consultation in Primary Care

10

Jacopo Demurtas, Ulrik Bak Kirk, Andreas Meer, and Alberto Vaona

10.1 Introduction and Historical Roots

> [T]hose dangerously wounded must be attended first entirely without regard to rank or distinction and those less severely wounded must wait until the gravely hurt have been operated and addressed. The slightly wounded can go to the hospital in the first and second line, especially officers because the officers have horses….

Baron Dominique-Jean Larrey, Napoleon's chief surgeon during the French Revolutionary and Napoleonic wars [1].

Triage, an essential component of healthcare delivery, has gained renewed importance in the context of remote consultations, especially within primary care. Although its contemporary use is widespread, triage has military origins, designed

J. Demurtas
Clinical and Experimental Medicine PhD Program, University of Modena and Reggio Emilia, Modena, Italy

Family Medicine Department, USL Toscana Sud-Est, Capalbio, Italy

U. B. Kirk
Faculty Fellow, Department of Public Health, Aarhus University, Aarhus, Denmark

Digital Health, Research Unit for General Practice, Aarhus, Denmark
e-mail: ubk@ph.au.dk

A. Meer
CEO In4medicine Ltd., Berne, Switzerland
e-mail: a.meer@in4medicine.ch

A. Vaona (✉)
ULSS 9 Scaligera, Primary Care, Verona, Italy

Italian Telemedicine Society, Verona, Italy

J. Demurtas (ed.), *Remote Consultation in Primary Care*, TELe-Health,
https://doi.org/10.1007/978-3-031-89661-3_10

to prioritize care and manage resources effectively during crises or periods of overwhelming demand. The term itself comes from the French verb *trier*, meaning to sort or classify [2].

The concept of triage has been part of medical practice for centuries, with its earliest documented origins in military medicine during the Napoleonic Wars. These words are attributed to Baron Dominique-Jean Larrey, Napoleon's chief surgeon, who is credited with creating the first modern triage system on the battlefield and pioneering the concept of modern ambulances.

With his simple yet profound ideas, Baron Larrey introduced the foundational principles of prioritizing time to treatment and establishing the point of care, marking a significant turning point in medical history. He suggested that:

> The severely wounded soldiers must be treated first, independent of their military rank. Otherwise, they will not survive. The less severely wounded must wait until the severely wounded have been treated. The lightly wounded soldiers should be treated in hospitals further away from the battlefield.

Before Dr. Larrey introduced the concept of triage, wounded soldiers often faced grim prospects. Most were transported to hospitals long after sustaining injuries and then endured further delays before receiving treatment. However, the principle of triaging the wounded has proven to be the most effective method for organizing medical care for large numbers of casualties, whether during wartime or in natural disasters. To triage the injured effectively, the following key questions must be addressed:

1. Diagnosis: How serious are the injuries?
2. Prognosis: What are the chances of survival?
3. Logistics: What transport options are available?

Today, triage continues to be used to manage patient flow and minimize risks while awaiting definitive treatment, often with the assistance of artificial intelligence (AI)-powered tools and systems [3]. The objective of triage is to *assess the severity of a medical condition, determine the necessary type of care, and identify where and by whom this care should be provided.*

Since its military origins, triage has been a vital tool for conserving resources and ensuring timely care in the most appropriate settings. Centuries later, the prioritization of cases remains central to emergency medicine and widely utilized in primary care. The core principles of triage—prioritizing care based on urgency, balancing patient needs with available resources, and directing individuals to the appropriate level of care—have been adapted to civilian healthcare systems. Triage is fundamentally about determining which patients require immediate attention and defining the right time and place for the treatment of all cases assessed.

10.2 Triage: When? Where? By Whom?

Remote triage and consultation have become crucial in addressing healthcare needs, offering both economic and ecological alternatives to in-person consultations. The importance of this approach was underscored during the COVID-19 pandemic. Derkx, in his papers on the quality of telephone triage, highlights that it primarily depends on three factors: clinical skills, communication skills, and the ability to evaluate the gathered information [4–9]. As illustrated in Fig. 10.1, the triagist uses these skills to transform the question-and-answer phase into actionable information [4], allowing for the assessment of urgency and the determination of appropriate care advice:

In the reported experiences, notably the study published in the *BMJ* [5] using the methodology of incognito standardized patients [9], the importance of asking relevant questions (or failing to do so) became alarmingly evident [4].

A primary care professional working in out-of-hours settings and handling phone calls may forget or not know the crucial questions to ask in a particular scenario, which can compromise the advice given and lead to unsafe triage. Failing to ask the right questions at the right time can result in errors related to the timing of treatment and the appropriate point of care [4].

It is also worth noting that findings on training interventions aimed at improving telephone triage and consultations are scarce, with no specific evidence derived from studies on telephone consultations, as Vaona et al. report [10]. Greenhalgh et al. proposed a model for telephone and remote consultations during COVID-19 [11, 12], which, interestingly, follows the structure and recommendations provided by Derkx et al. [4–6].

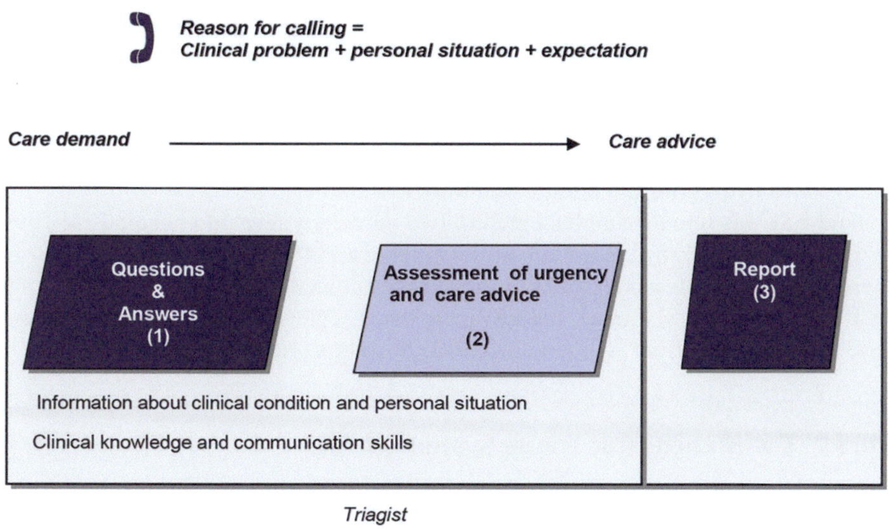

Fig. 10.1 Triage process. (Based on Derkx [4])

10.3 Triage Scores

Triage scores are codified to help identify emergencies. These scores can be applied in both face-to-face and remote consultations. Triage systems assist healthcare providers in evaluating cases, categorizing emergencies and urgent situations. This enables them to properly prioritize urgent cases, determine the sequence of interventions, and establish the appropriate point of care and timing for treatment [13]. Two main triage-scoring systems are widely used across the globe: the *Emergency Severity Index* (ESI) and the *Manchester Triage System* (MTS).

10.3.1 The Emergency Severity Index (ESI)

The Emergency Severity Index (ESI) was introduced by Dr. Richard Wuerz, Dr. David Eitel, and colleagues in 1998 as a tool for use in emergency department (ED) triage. The ESI triage algorithm offers a rapid, reproducible, and clinically relevant method of categorizing patients into five levels of care, ranging from level 1 (most urgent) to level 5 (least urgent) [14, 15]. The ESI categorizes patients based on both acuity and resource needs. Practically, it functions as an algorithm stream: ESI 1 indicates a patient who is likely dying and requires immediate attention, while ESI 5 corresponds to nonurgent cases with no anticipated resource needs. Resources, in this context, include laboratory tests, radiology, intravenous fluids, specialty consultations, procedures (simple or complex), and medications (intravenous, intramuscular, or nebulized).

Patients undergo a brief but thorough assessment by an experienced triage nurse, who assigns a numerical category based on the patient's expected resource utilization. This assessment considers the patient's symptoms and vital signs. Levels 3 through 5 are focused on resource allocation, while levels 1 and 2 are based on patient acuity. For instance, a 20-year-old patient presenting with abdominal pain, right lower quadrant tenderness, and nausea would likely be placed in ESI level 3, as the patient is expected to require two or more resources, such as blood work, intravenous hydration, and possibly radiological studies.

The ESI was initially implemented in two university teaching hospitals in 1999 and further refined in five additional hospitals in 2000, based on feedback from these sites. Several research studies have since evaluated the reliability, validity, and ease of use of the ESI. Today, the ESI is the most widely used triage system in the United States, employed by more than 3000 hospitals [16].

10.3.2 The Manchester Triage System (MTS)

Widely used in Europe, the Manchester Triage System (MTS) is a five-color triage scale (red, orange, yellow, green, and blue), with red indicating the need for immediate care and blue representing non-urgent care. The MTS includes 52 predefined conditions or presentation flowcharts that are combined with the patient's main complaint, which is recorded by a nurse [17, 18].

The risk of hospital admission is reported to be five times higher for high-priority patients (classified as red or orange) compared to low-priority patients, and the likelihood of death during hospitalization is 5.5 times greater for high-priority patients. However, the MTS has been found to occasionally misclassify patients with acute coronary syndrome (ACS) with ST-segment elevation [17].

In pediatric emergency care, the MTS demonstrated moderate validity compared to a reference standard, with 63% sensitivity for the "very urgent" classification. This means that 37% of patients who should have been seen within 10 min were not categorized as "urgent." Despite this, the MTS has shown to be a good discriminator for the use of diagnostic tools in the emergency department.

10.3.3 ESI Versus MTS

The performance of the two triage systems in emergency care has been evaluated by various comparative studies [19–22].

One study comparing the Emergency Severity Index (ESI) and the Manchester Triage System (MTS) revealed that both tools were predictive of hospital admissions. However, the ESI proved to be a stronger predictor of admission than the MTS. Mortality was also associated with urgency categories in both systems [19].

The comparison further highlighted that subtriage into the orange and yellow categories posed a significant issue with the MTS, particularly for older patients. Despite these challenges, the sensitivity and specificity for predicting hospital admission and mortality were similar for both systems [19, 20].

In a simulation study by Storm Versloot et al., both ESI and MTS showed similar validity, though the ESI had a higher rate of sub-triage (misclassifying more severe cases as less urgent) compared to the MTS [21]. The MTS under-triaged a smaller proportion of patients compared to the ESI (8.3% vs. 13.5%), but this came at the cost of a higher proportion of over-triage [21, 22]. While both systems generally perform reliably, they may under-triage certain conditions, such as acute coronary syndrome (ACS), and some patient groups.

10.4 Triage: A Question of Questions

As discussed in Chap. 9, many scenarios can be assessed remotely, and certain signs and symptoms have proven positive or negative predictive value. To effectively capture these scenarios through a triage system, specific key questions must be asked.

In most cases, the triagist will ask questions, some of which will help determine the appropriate time for treatment and the correct point of care. However, in some situations—such as when dealing with patients who are poor historians [23]—essential questions may be missed, compromising the quality of triage and putting both the triagist and patient at risk.

In an ideal system, computerized decision support software (CDSS), described further in Chap. 26, would ensure that all necessary questions for a safe and effective assessment are asked. However, how should these questions be posed? Several strategies have been explored to enhance triage questioning and reduce variability and errors:

Prominent experts advocate for a funnel model, starting with a broad question like, 'What is your main complaint?' and progressively narrowing to more specific questions [24, 25]. This method allows the triagist to gather detailed clinical information step by step, ensuring accurate determination of the patient's acuity and care needs [24, 26].

Another approach involves a branched questioning model, where subsequent questions depend on the answers to earlier ones. This model, often used in CDSS, follows different question trees based on the patient's main complaint.

It is crucial to remember that paraverbal communication plays a role equal to or greater than verbal communication. How a question is asked is just as important as what is asked. The way a question is phrased will inevitably influence the response. For instance, if the question implies a positive answer, patients are more likely to provide one, and similarly, framing a question to rule out a condition can steer responses in that direction.

The three most common questioning techniques used in remote consultation are as follows:

1. *Open-ended* questions.
2. *Closed* questions.
3. *Facilitative* questions.

By beginning with open-ended questions, followed by facilitative questions, and concluding with closed questions, we can interpret the funnel model as shown in studies on telephone triage quality [4], which emphasize the need for structured communication to ensure patient safety and effective clinical assessment.

Open-Ended Questions Used at the beginning of the conversation, open questions allow the patient to express themselves freely, providing insights into their condition, concerns, needs, and feelings. Examples include "Tell me about what you're experiencing," "How can I help you?" or "What is concerning you the most?"

Facilitative or Semi-Closed Questions These questions help probe further, enabling the triagist to gradually gather more detailed clinical information to assess the patient's acuity and disposition accurately. They are intermediate in nature, balancing between open and closed questions, often resembling multiple-choice queries. Examples include "Does the pain feel sharp or dull?" or "Is the urine yellow, red, or brown?"

Closed Questions Closed questions narrow the scope of the conversation, focusing on key details necessary to complete the triage process. These questions are typically used at the end of the conversation and require straightforward answers (yes/no, numbers, etc.) to cross-check information and confirm the overall clinical picture. Examples include "Is he short of breath?" or "Do you have chest pain?"

10.4.1 Probing and Pursuing

The skillful combination and transition between the three core questioning techniques—open, facilitative, and closed—used in remote triage allows the triagist to systematically extract necessary information while maintaining a structured and collaborative dialogue with the patient.

At the start of the conversation, the triagist often uses facilitative or semi-closed questions to gather essential details, giving the patient room to express themselves. If relevant information emerges, the triagist can explore it further by using a combination of semi-closed and closed questions.

The Derkx rating scale suggests that the prevalent use of facilitative questions is preferable to open questions, as this approach ensures that all necessary information is gathered and no concerns are overlooked [8]. Mastering this composite questioning technique is a core competency for any triagist, as it strikes the balance between obtaining comprehensive clinical information and allowing the patient to feel heard and understood.

10.5 Triage Applications in Modern Primary Care and Future Developments

In a healthcare system facing severe professional shortages, triage becomes essential for optimizing and reallocating resources. It can be effectively employed in rural settings, low-income countries, or areas with vast territories and limited facilities. Triage is indispensable in the management of emergencies and urgent care, as well as in out-of-hours and in-hours primary care [27–29].

As envisioned by Pope et al. in 2014, the future of triage will likely adopt a hybrid approach [30]. Triagists will operate in a meta-environment, supported by clinical decision support systems (CDSS) for guidance, with real-time connectivity to emergency services [31]. These systems may leverage 5G or 6G technology, enabling emergency responders to be alerted while the patient is still being assessed [32].

The emergence of technologies like ChatGPT highlights the need for healthcare professionals to engage with new and potentially disruptive innovations, which could play a significant role in improving patient care [33–35]. It is crucial to embrace these challenges and adapt to the evolving healthcare landscape, leveraging innovative technologies and integrating them into our current models to provide better care for patients.

10.6 Conclusions

Triage, with its deep-rooted history in military medicine, has evolved significantly over the centuries, becoming a cornerstone of both emergency and primary care [36]. From its origins on the battlefield to its modern-day applications in emergency departments and remote consultations, triage has consistently prioritized patient needs based on urgency, acuity, and resource allocation.

In today's healthcare landscape, the role of triage is more critical than ever. As the world faces professional shortages, resource constraints, and increasingly complex patient demands, triage remains essential for ensuring timely and effective care. Whether used in rural settings, low-income countries, or high-tech urban hospitals, the principles of triage—assessing urgency, determining resource needs, and guiding patients to the appropriate level of care—continue to be integral in managing patient flow and reducing risks.

The future of triage lies in its integration with advanced technologies, such as Clinical Decision Support Systems (CDSS) and real-time connectivity enabled by 5G or 6G. These innovations will allow triagists to work in a hybrid environment, enhancing their ability to deliver precise, timely care while maintaining human-centered patient interactions. Tools like ChatGPT and other AI-driven platforms will play a pivotal role in this evolution, offering new possibilities for improving care and overcoming the challenges faced by healthcare systems today.

As we move forward, embracing technological advancements while maintaining the foundational principles of triage will be key to improving patient outcomes and enhancing the efficiency of healthcare delivery. In doing so, healthcare professionals can continue to provide safe, effective, and compassionate care to all patients, regardless of the circumstances.

References

1. Iserson KV, Moskop JC. Triage in medicine, part I: concept, history, and types. Ann Emerg Med 2007 Mar;49(3):275–281. https://doi.org/10.1016/j.annemergmed.2006.05.019. Epub 2006 Jul 10.
2. Summersgill P. Review: telephone triage: a panacea for child and family health care? J Child Health Care. 1997;1(1):11–6. https://doi.org/10.1177/136749359700100103.
3. Meer A, Rahm P, Schwendinger M, Vock M, Grunder B, Demurtas J, Rutishauser J. A symptom-checker for adult patients visiting an interdisciplinary emergency care center and the safety of patient self-triage: real-life prospective evaluation. J Med Internet Res 2024 Jun 27;26:e58157. https://doi.org/10.2196/58157. PMID: 38809606; PMCID: PMC11240063.
4. Derkx HP. For your ears only: quality of telephone triage at out-of-hours centres in The Netherlands. Dissertation University of Maastricht; 2008.
5. Derkx HP, Rethans JJ, Muijtjens AM, Maiburg BH, Winkens R, van Rooij HG, Knottnerus JA. Quality of clinical aspects of call handling at Dutch out of hours centres: cross sectional national study. BMJ 2008 Sep 12;337:a1264. https://doi.org/10.1136/bmj.a1264. PMID: 18790814; PMCID: PMC2769520.
6. Derkx HP, Rethans JJ, Maiburg BH, Winkens RA, Muijtjens AM, van Rooij HG, Knottnerus JA. Quality of communication during telephone triage at Dutch out-of-hours centres. Patient

Educ Couns 2009 Feb;74(2):174–178. https://doi.org/10.1016/j.pec.2008.08.002. Epub 2008 Oct 8.

7. Derkx H, Rethans JJ, Muijtjens A, Maiburg B, Winkens R, van Rooij H, Knottnerus A. 'Quod scripsi, scripsi.' The quality of the report of telephone consultations at Dutch out-of-hours centres. Qual Saf Health Care 2010 Dec;19(6):e1. https://doi.org/10.1136/qshc.2008.027920. Epub 2010 Jun 27.
8. Derkx HP, Rethans JJ, Knottnerus JA, Ram PM. Assessing communication skills of clinical call handlers working at an out-of-hours centre: development of the RICE rating scale. Br J Gen Pract 2007 May;57(538):383–387. PMID: 17504589; PMCID: PMC2047013.
9. Derkx H, Rethans JJ, Maiburg B, Winkens R, Knottnerus A. New methodology for using incognito standardised patients for telephone consultation in primary care. Med Educ. 2009 Jan;43(1):82–8. https://doi.org/10.1111/j.1365-2923.2008.03177.x.
10. Vaona A, Pappas Y, Grewal RS, Ajaz M, Majeed A, Car J. Training interventions for improving telephone consultation skills in clinicians. Cochrane Database Syst Rev 2017 Jan 5;1(1):CD010034. https://doi.org/10.1002/14651858.CD010034.pub2. PMID: 28052316; PMCID: PMC6464130.
11. Greenhalgh T, Koh GCH, Car J. Covid-19: a remote assessment in primary care. BMJ. 2020 Mar 25;368:m1182. https://doi.org/10.1136/bmj.m1182.
12. Greenhalgh T, Wherton J, Shaw S, Morrison C. Video consultations for covid-19. BMJ. 2020 Mar;12(368):m998. https://doi.org/10.1136/bmj.m998.
13. Zachariasse JM, van der Hagen V, Seiger N, Mackway-Jones K, van Veen M, Moll HA. Performance of triage systems in emergency care: a systematic review and meta-analysis. BMJ Open 2019 May 28;9(5):e026471. https://doi.org/10.1136/bmjopen-2018-026471. PMID: 31142524; PMCID: PMC6549628.
14. Shelton R. The Emergency Severity Index 5-level triage system. Dimens Crit Care Nurs. 2009 Jan-Feb;28(1):9–12. https://doi.org/10.1097/01.DCC.0000325106.28851.89.
15. Gilboy N, Tanabe P, Travers DA, Rosenau AM, Eitel DR. Emergency Severity Index, version 4: implementation handbook, AHRQ Publication No. 05-0046-2. Rockville: Agency for Healthcare Research and Quality; 2005.
16. McHugh M, Tanabe P, McClelland M, Khare RK. More patients are triaged using the Emergency Severity Index than any other triage acuity system in the United States. Acad Emerg Med 2012 Jan;19(1):106–109. https://doi.org/10.1111/j.1553-2712.2011.01240.x. Epub 2011 Dec 23.
17. Azeredo TR, Guedes HM, Rebelo de Almeida RA, Chianca TC, Martins JC. Efficacy of the Manchester Triage System: a systematic review. Int Emerg Nurs 2015 Apr;23(2):47–52. https://doi.org/10.1016/j.ienj.2014.06.001. Epub 2014 Jun 18.
18. Mirhaghi A, Mazlom R, Heydari A, Ebrahimi M. The reliability of the Manchester Triage System (MTS): a meta-analysis. J Evid Based Med. 2017 May;10(2):129–35. https://doi.org/10.1111/jebm.12231.
19. van der Wulp I, van Baar ME, Schrijvers AJ. Reliability and validity of the Manchester Triage System in a general emergency department patient population in The Netherlands: results of a simulation study. Emerg Med J. 2008 Jul;25(7):431–4. https://doi.org/10.1136/emj.2007.055228.
20. van der Wulp I, Schrijvers AJ, van Stel HF. Predicting admission and mortality with the Emergency Severity Index and the Manchester Triage System: a retrospective observational study. Emerg Med J. 2009 Jul;26(7):506–9. https://doi.org/10.1136/emj.2008.063768.
21. Storm-Versloot MN, Ubbink DT, Chin a Choi V, Luitse JS. Observer agreement of the Manchester Triage System and the Emergency Severity Index: a simulation study. Emerg Med J. 2009 Aug;26(8):556–60. https://doi.org/10.1136/emj.2008.059378.
22. Storm-Versloot MN, Ubbink DT, Kappelhof J, Luitse JS. Comparison of an informally structured triage system, the emergency severity index, and the Manchester Triage System to distinguish patient priority in the emergency department. Acad Emerg Med. 2011 Aug;18(8):822–9. https://doi.org/10.1111/j.1553-2712.2011.01122.x.

23. Pygall SA. Telephone triage and consultation: are we really listening? London: Royal College of General Practitioners; 2017.
24. Christ M, Grossmann F, Winter D, Bingisser R, Platz E. Modern triage in the emergency department. Dtsch Arztebl Int. 2010 Dec;107(50):892–898. https://doi.org/10.3238/arztebl.2010.0892. Epub 2010 Dec 17. PMID: 21246025; PMCID: PMC3021905.
25. Fernandes M, Mendes R, Vieira SM, Leite F, Palos C, Johnson A, Finkelstein S, Horng S, Celi LA. Risk of mortality and cardiopulmonary arrest in critical patients presenting to the emergency department using machine learning and natural language processing. PLoS One. 2020 Apr 2;15(4):e0230876. https://doi.org/10.1371/journal.pone.0230876. PMID: 32240233; PMCID: PMC7117713.
26. Dugas AF, Kirsch TD, Toerper M, Korley F, Yenokyan G, France D, Hager D, Levin S. An electronic emergency triage system to improve patient distribution by critical outcomes. J Emerg Med. 2016 Jun;50(6):910–918. https://doi.org/10.1016/j.jemermed.2016.02.026. Epub 2016 Apr 25. Erratum in: J Emerg Med. 2016 Aug;51(2):224. https://doi.org/10.1016/j.jemermed.2016.08.004.
27. Kirk UB, Payne R, Tweedie JA, Huibers L. 'A tool for every job': use of video in urgent primary care. Br J Gen Pract. 2024 Sep 26;74(747):443–444. https://doi.org/10.3399/bjgp24X739473. PMID: 39327075; PMCID: PMC11441613.
28. Nebsbjerg MA, Vestergaard CH, Bomholt KB, Christensen MB, Huibers L. Use of video in telephone triage in out-of-hours primary care: register-based study. JMIR Med Inform. 2024 Apr 4;12:e47039. https://doi.org/10.2196/47039. PMID: 38596835; PMCID: PMC11007381.
29. Nebsbjerg MA, Bomholt KB, Vestergaard CH, Christensen MB, Huibers L. Reasons for encounter in video contacts at a Danish out-of-hours primary care service: a questionnaire study. BMJ Open. 2024 Oct 8;14(10):e086716. https://doi.org/10.1136/bmjopen-2024-086716. PMID: 39384244; PMCID: PMC11474727.
30. Pope C, Halford S, Turnbull J, Prichard J. Cyborg practices: call-handlers and computerised decision support systems in urgent and emergency care. Health Informatics J. 2014 Jun;20(2):118–26. https://doi.org/10.1177/1460458213486470.
31. Farshid M, Paschen J, Eriksson T, Kietzmann J. Go boldly! Explore augmented reality (AR), virtual reality (VR), and mixed reality (MR) for business. Bus Horiz. 2018 July;61(5):657–63. https://doi.org/10.1016/j.bushor.2018.05.009.
32. Nayak S, Patgiri R. A vision on intelligent medical service for emergency on 5G and 6G communication era. EAI Endorsed Trans Internet Things. 2020 July;6(22):e2.
33. Doshi RH, Bajaj SS, Krumholz HM. ChatGPT: temptations of progress. Am J Bioeth 2023 Apr;23(4):6–8. https://doi.org/10.1080/15265161.2023.2180110. Epub 2023 Feb 28.
34. Cascella M, Montomoli J, Bellini V, Bignami E. Evaluating the feasibility of ChatGPT in healthcare: an analysis of multiple clinical and research scenarios. J Med Syst. 2023 Mar 4;47(1):33. https://doi.org/10.1007/s10916-023-01925-4. PMID: 36869927; PMCID: PMC9985086.
35. Howard A, Hope W, Gerada A. ChatGPT and antimicrobial advice: the end of the consulting infection doctor? Lancet Infect Dis 2023 Apr;23(4):405–406. https://doi.org/10.1016/S1473-3099(23)00113-5. Epub 2023 Feb 20.
36. Skandalakis PN, Lainas P, Zoras O, Skandalakis JE, Mirilas P. "To afford the wounded speedy assistance": Dominique Jean Larrey and Napoleon. World J Surg. 2006 Aug;30(8):1392–9. https://doi.org/10.1007/s00268-005-0436-8.

Effective Safety Netting, Management Plan, and Ending the Call

11

Ulrik Bak Kirk, Almas Fatma, and Jacopo Demurtas

11.1 The Importance of Safety Netting in Remote Consultations

11.1.1 What Is Safety Netting?

(i) *Definition and Origins*: Safety netting refers to the medical advice provided to patients or their caregivers at the conclusion of a clinical consultation [1]. The term was first introduced by Roger Neighbour in 1987 as a tool for managing clinical uncertainty during consultations [2].

(ii) *Why It Matters in Remote Consultations*: This guidance aims to ensure that patients are aware of the need for further medical evaluation should their condition deteriorate or fail to improve over time. Despite its critical role in clinical practice, safety netting is often underemphasized in consultation skills training [3].

U. B. Kirk (✉)
Faculty Fellow, Department of Public Health, Aarhus University, Aarhus, Denmark

Digital Health, Research Unit for General Practice, Aarhus, Denmark
e-mail: ubk@ph.au.dk

A. Fatma
Family Physician & Certified Digital Health Professional at Alcura Family Clinic, Navi Mumbai, India

J. Demurtas
Clinical and Experimental Medicine PhD Program, University of Modena and Reggio Emilia, Modena, Italy

Department of Family Medicine, USL Toscana Sud-Est, Capalbio, Italy

J. Demurtas (ed.), *Remote Consultation in Primary Care*, TELe-Health,
https://doi.org/10.1007/978-3-031-89661-3_11

(iii) *Importance of Safety Netting in Remote Consultations:* Recent literature highlights that safety netting is arguably the most crucial element of any consultation, particularly in remote settings [4]. Effective safety netting safeguards both the patient and the physician by offering clear guidance that extends beyond simple follow-up suggestions.

To be truly effective, safety netting must be tailored to the individual patient's context, considering factors such as:

- Progression of their illness
- Accessibility to healthcare
- Health literacy of the patient

Essentially, safety netting involves providing the patient with a comprehensive plan detailing what actions to take after the consultation, especially if new symptoms arise or existing ones worsen.

(iv) *Key Research and Models:* Research indicates that the effectiveness of safety netting is heavily influenced by the clarity of communication during consultations. Smith et al. [5] advocate for integrating safety netting into patient-centered care models, such as the Calgary–Cambridge model, which underscores the significance of effective communication in clinical settings [6]. By aligning safety-netting strategies with these frameworks, healthcare providers can enhance their feasibility and efficacy. Moreover, Jones et al. recognize safety netting as a vital aspect of patient care but highlight the need for further research to identify the most effective techniques that improve patient outcomes, including reduced re-attendance rates and increased patient satisfaction [7].

11.1.2 When to Implement Safety Netting in Remote Consultations

In the realm of remote consultations, the implementation of safety netting is even more critical. Greenhalgh et al. define safety netting as a diagnostic strategy that guides patients on when to seek further medical advice amidst uncertainty [8]. The shift to remote consultations necessitates that GPs adapt their safety-netting strategies to ensure that patients receive adequate information despite the lack of face-to-face interaction.

11.1.2.1 Appropriate Scenarios

Safety netting is appropriate for all treatment outcomes. However, experts agree that it should be mandatory under specific circumstances, as outlined in Table 11.1.

Table 11.1 The various circumstances and considerations for implementing safety netting outlined. (Author, 2024)

Circumstance	Description	Considerations
Uncertain diagnosis	Safety netting is critical when a diagnosis is not definitive, and differential diagnoses include serious conditions that may progress rapidly	Assess the urgency of potential serious conditions Provide clear instructions for follow-up actions
Certain diagnosis with complications	When the diagnosis is clear but associated with known risks of serious complications, safety netting is essential to monitor potential adverse outcomes	Identify and communicate specific complications Establish a plan for monitoring and follow-up care
Increased risk patients	Patients who demonstrate increased susceptibility to serious illnesses or complications require robust safety netting to prevent adverse events	Evaluate risk factors (e.g., comorbidities, age, lifestyle) Tailor safety-netting advice to individual circumstances
Patient capabilities	It is vital to assess the patient's ability to understand and act on safety-netting advice, considering their legal competence and health literacy	Engage in shared decision-making Provide education tailored to the patient's understanding level

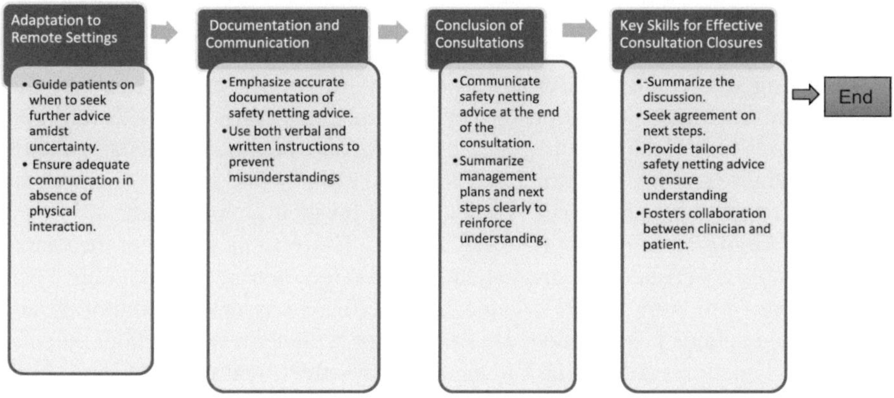

Fig. 11.1 Safety netting in remote consultations follows a structured approach to ensure patient safety. (Author, 2024)

11.1.2.2 Key Points of Safety Netting in Remote Consultations: Step-by-Step Process

To ensure patient safety, safety netting in remote consultations must follow a step-by-step process, as described in Fig. 11.1.

Table 11.2 Safety netting in remote consultations requires clear communication, thorough documentation, and a focus on follow-up actions [9, 10]

Aspect	Consideration
Lack of physical examination	Without direct physical exams, GPs rely heavily on patient-reported symptoms. Safety netting becomes crucial to guide patients on when to seek further medical attention if symptoms worsen
Limited patient monitoring	Remote consultations reduce the ability to continuously monitor patients. Emphasis on follow-up actions and clear instructions on red-flag symptoms is essential
Clarity in communication	Clear and concise safety-netting advice must be provided to avoid misunderstandings. Use of visual aids, summaries, and written instructions can reinforce understanding
Documentation	Accurate and thorough documentation of safety-netting advice ensures continuity of care and minimizes the risk of communication lapses in future follow-ups
Technology reliance	Remote settings rely on technology, and any technical issues can impede communication. Safety-netting advice should include steps to take if follow-up communication is interrupted

11.1.2.3 Considerations for Remote Settings

Safety netting in remote consultations requires clear communication, documentation, and follow-up actions, as outlined in Table 11.2.

11.1.3 Shared Responsibility in Safety Netting

- *GP's Role in Clear Communication*: The role of general practitioners (GPs) in delivering safety-netting advice is paramount. Silverston emphasizes that GPs must present this information clearly and understandably [11, 12]. Utilizing visual aids and checklists integrated into electronic health records can enhance clarity and retention. This structured approach ensures that patients comprehend the safety-netting instructions, which are vital for their ongoing care.
- *Patient Engagement and Active Participation:* Evans et al. highlight the shared responsibility between GPs and patients in the safety-netting process. Active participation from both parties is essential for effective symptom monitoring and follow-up actions [13], particularly for patients with serious conditions, such as cancer. Timely reconsultation can significantly affect treatment outcomes [14], reinforcing the need for collaboration in the safety-netting process.

11.1.4 Importance and Challenges of Safety Netting in Remote Consultations

Safety netting helps manage diagnostic uncertainty, especially in remote care, by offering structured follow-up plans and mitigating risks, as outlined in Table 11.3.

Table 11.3 Safety netting helps manage diagnostic uncertainty, especially in remote care, by offering structured follow-up plans and mitigating risks [2, 3, 9, 10, 15–17]

Aspect	Details
Uncertainty in diagnoses	Missed diagnoses are inevitable in general practice since no diagnostic test or clinical decision rule is 100% accurate For example, up to *50% of meningococcal disease cases in children* may go undetected in early consultations because hallmark symptoms have not yet appeared Similarly, complications such as *dehydration in gastroenteritis* or a *subdural hematoma* after head trauma may develop only after the initial visit
Safety netting as a strategy	Safety netting, conceptualized by Dr. Roger Neighbour in 1987, addresses diagnostic uncertainty by providing patients or caregivers with *advice on when to seek further medical attention* if symptoms change or worsen Safety netting ensures that patients know *what to monitor* and *how to act* if their condition deteriorates
Verbal communication and documentation	Clear *verbal communication and precise documentation* of safety-netting advice are essential for continuity of care *Edwards et al.* highlight that failing to document safety-netting advice can lead to *misunderstandings and poor outcomes* [3, 15, 16] Thorough documentation ensures patients have a clear plan for when to seek further help, reducing risks and improving safety
Ensuring continuity of care	In remote consultations, follow-ups may not involve the same clinician, increasing the need for *comprehensive documentation* Proper records enable seamless care transitions between healthcare providers and give patients *structured follow-up plans* [9] Scheduled callbacks or follow-ups also allow clinicians to *reassess symptoms*, reducing risks and enhancing patient satisfaction
Shared responsibilities and mitigating risks	Remote consultations often conclude without an in-person visit, which introduces *a degree of risk* A key question clinicians must address is: *'What might happen next, and who is responsible?'* Roland et al. [10] emphasize that safety-netting advice is essential to mitigate risks by ensuring patients know *when to escalate care* and how to recognize *worrying symptoms*
Impact of remote care	Ladds et al. [17] explore the challenges of remote care, noting that *continuity* is crucial for improved patient outcomes Remote consultations require special consideration of *contextual factors* to ensure safety-netting advice is effective and actionable
Safety netting as a mandate	Safety netting is not optional—it is a *mandatory aspect of patient care*, especially in remote settings Effective safety netting not only protects patients but also acts as a safeguard for clinicians, reducing the chances of *missed diagnoses* and adverse outcomes

Table 11.4 Remote consultations pose challenges in conveying nuanced advice, and structured frameworks can help manage cognitive load [3, 15, 16, 18]

Aspect	Details	Strategies to mitigate risks
Cognitive demands on clinicians	Managing *both remote and in-person consultations* increases cognitive load Reliance on *patient-reported symptoms* alone can lead to communication lapses *Multiple modes of interaction* (telehealth, video, in-person) can make it harder to convey *safety-netting advice* effectively [18]	Use *structured consultation frameworks* to streamline advice across all formats Maintain concise *patient notes* for easy handover and reference
Obstacles in conveying nuanced advice	Remote consultations limit *nonverbal observations* and *physical examinations* that are critical for assessing patient conditions It can be challenging to gauge *patient understanding* and identify *risks* without direct interaction [15, 16]	Provide *clear, jargon-free instructions* and use *teach-back methods* to confirm patient understanding Plan *follow-up calls* to reassess symptoms and ensure safety netting is effective [3]

11.1.4.1 Importance of Documentation

11.1.4.2 Unique Challenges in Remote Consultations

Structured frameworks can help manage cognitive load in remote consultations, as outlined in Table 11.4.

11.2 Strategies and Practical Guidance: Implementing Safety Netting and Managing Remote Consultations

11.2.1 Structuring Remote Consultations with Safety Netting

Safety netting should be tailored to the patient's condition and caregiver's reliability to enable better management and follow-up, as outlined in Table 11.5.

11.2.2 The Core of Safety Netting

Safety netting is a fundamental aspect of general practice, as identified by Dr. Roger Neighbour [2]. He framed this concept through three essential questions that guide clinicians in patient management, as outlined in Table 11.6.

A study by Almond et al. [20], referenced in Evans et al. [21], conducted a Delphi study to define the core elements of safety netting in clinical practice. The study involved NHS-based GP teachers, as well as pediatric and emergency department consultants, from Oxford Radcliffe Hospitals. These participants were asked to rate their level of agreement with several safety-netting statements, with the goal of deriving core guidelines for practice.

Table 11.5 Safety netting should be tailored to the patient's condition and caregiver's reliability, allowing for better management and follow-up in uncertain scenarios [19]

Aspect	Details
Establishing the baseline	*Gathering Initial Information:* Collecting thorough patient history and clinical details to guide the consultation *Tailoring Safety Netting to Context:* Safety-netting strategies should be adapted based on the patient's condition and caregiver's reliability *Example 1:* If a reliable caregiver (e.g., a nurse) is calm and caring for a 5-year-old child with a mild fever, a *simple follow-up plan* might be appropriate since the risk of complications is low *Example 2:* For situations with greater uncertainty (e.g., a child with a head injury), a *scheduled callback* in a few hours allows for reassessment and timely intervention [19]. If symptoms escalate, the clinician can initiate an *in-person visit* or *emergency referral*
Clinical frameworks	*Frameworks in Practice:* Clinicians should adopt structured frameworks to assess patient risks and guide remote consultations effectively These frameworks ensure *thorough documentation*, structured follow-ups, and timely escalations to in-person care when needed Clinicians must also assess the *patient's ability to comply* with the advice and proactively address potential challenges in following the care plan

Table 11.6 These three questions assist clinicians in evaluating their decisions and preparing for unexpected outcomes [4]

Questions	Purpose
1. If I'm right, what do I expect to happen?	Helps clinicians anticipate the expected progression of a patient's condition
2. How will I know if I'm wrong?	Encourages clinicians to consider indicators that may suggest a misdiagnosis or oversight
3. What would I do then?	Prepares clinicians to act decisively if the patient's condition does not align with expectations

In the initial round of the Delphi study, responses were gathered from:

- Twenty-eight out of 41 GPs (68.3%)
- Five out of 5 emergency department consultants (100%)
- Eight out of 12 pediatric consultants (66.6%)

Consensus was defined as achieving 75% of ratings in the ranges of 1 to 3 or 7 to 9 on a 9-point scale, with 1 representing strong disagreement and 9 indicating strong agreement. By this standard, consensus was reached on four out of the seven safety-netting statements.

The consensus statements from the Delphi study have been widely cited in the literature on safety netting in primary care [8, 15]. These core statements represent the foundational understanding of safety netting as a diagnostic tool in primary care, pediatrics, and emergency medicine, shaping clinical practices aimed at reducing diagnostic uncertainty and improving patient outcomes.

The Delphi study's findings underscore the importance of safety netting as a structured approach to patient management, ensuring that clinicians communicate clear, actionable guidance on what to monitor, when to seek further help, and whom to contact in the event of concerning changes in symptoms.

While safety netting plays a critical role in enhancing patient safety, it can sometimes create *unintended anxiety*. Clinicians must carefully *balance reassurance* with the need to provide accurate, actionable information. It is essential to ensure that most patients—who are likely to be well—feel reassured, while also *acknowledging the possibility of serious conditions.*

In this context, clinicians must avoid *shifting the burden of uncertainty onto patients*. The responsibility for diagnostic decision-making lies with healthcare professionals, and it is crucial to communicate uncertainty without causing confusion or stress. *Effective safety netting requires a nuanced approach* that combines:

- *Clear information* on what symptoms to watch for
- *Empathy* to reduce anxiety
- *Professional judgment* to avoid overloading the patient with unnecessary details

By *balancing transparency and reassurance*, clinicians can empower patients to act appropriately without feeling overwhelmed or anxious. This approach ensures better *public health outcomes and individual well-being*, minimizing the chances of missed diagnoses while maintaining trust and confidence in medical care [22].

11.2.3 The Core of Safety Netting: The "When" and "How"

An alternative model by Jones et al. [4] breaks down safety netting into the "Three W's," which help structure the advice given to patients, as outlined in Table 11.7.

By focusing on relevant symptoms while deprioritizing less critical ones, clinicians can provide targeted advice that minimizes the risk of overlooking serious complications.

Table 11.7 The Three W's framework helps guide patient advice systematically [4]

The three W's	Details
What	Identify specific symptoms or changes the patient should monitor, including concerning signs
When	Define when the patient should seek further help based on the clinician's evaluation
Whom	Specify the appropriate contact for assistance (e.g., their GP, out-of-hours services, A&E)

Table 11.8 SAFER components to guide patient assessment and safety netting. (Author, 2024)

SAFER components	Description
S: Serious illness risks	Identify serious illnesses and complications that the patient is at risk of developing
A: Alternative diagnoses	Recognize alternative diagnoses often missed with the presented symptoms
F: Findings	Distinguish between findings suggesting serious causes versus minor illnesses
E: Early signs	Highlight early and atypical signs of serious illness that may manifest
R: Flag symptoms	Inform the patient about red or amber flag symptoms that require immediate attention

11.2.4 The SAFER Approach to Safety Netting

The SAFER model, presented by Silverston et al. [23, 24], offers a comprehensive framework for exploring key aspects of safety netting, encapsulated in the following components, as outlined in Table 11.8.

11.2.5 Key Elements of Effective Safety-Netting Advice

- *Acknowledge Uncertainty:* Communicate any uncertainty in the diagnosis to the patient or their caregiver. This transparency empowers them to seek further consultation if needed.
- *Specify Warning Signs:* Outline the specific clinical features and red flags that indicate a risk of deterioration or complications. This helps patients understand what to monitor in their condition.
- *Provide Clear Help-Seeking Guidance:* Offer detailed instructions on how and where to seek further help. This includes information on contacting healthcare providers, emergency services, or other relevant resources.
- *Set Expectations for Illness Progression*: Include information about the expected time course of the illness when known. Emphasize that patients or caregivers should not hesitate to seek medical advice if they have concerns, regardless of the anticipated timeline.

11.2.6 Communication Techniques in Remote Consultations

Patient-friendly language and the teach-back method can enhance understanding during remote consultations. Table 11.9 clarifies essential strategies for effective communication and documentation in remote consultations, emphasizing the need for clear, patient-centered advice and thorough record-keeping.

Table 11.9 Patient-friendly language and the teach-back method can enhance understanding during remote consultations. (Author, 2024)

Aspect	Details
Communication techniques in remote consultations	Patient-Friendly Language: Use simple, jargon-free language to ensure clarity Teach-Back Method: Ask patients to repeat the advice in their own words to confirm understanding and correct misunderstandings in real time
Ensuring patient understanding	Tailor communication based on the patient's literacy and cognitive abilities Offer both written and verbal safety-netting advice to reinforce key points, especially for complex situations Visual aids or electronic summaries can improve comprehension
Recording safety-netting advice	Document safety-netting advice in the patient's medical records to ensure continuity of care between consultations Include specifics like symptoms to watch for, follow-up plans, and when to seek further help
Written vs. verbal communication	There is no strict consensus on whether safety netting should be communicated verbally or in writing Clinicians should assess patient preferences and the complexity of advice to determine the best mode of delivery
Challenges in documentation	Safety-netting advice may be overlooked or poorly documented, especially when multiple health issues are discussed in a single consultation Clinicians must prioritize safety netting, even during complex or lengthy consultations
Importance of documentation	Thorough documentation minimizes gaps in care and supports clinical decision-making in future consultations Accurate records ensure other healthcare professionals can seamlessly continue patient care if needed

11.2.7 Closing the Consultation: Ensuring Clarity and Understanding

The closing phase of a remote consultation is a critical, yet often underemphasized, part of the patient interaction. According to Derkx [25], this phase should include an evaluation of the patient's understanding of the advice provided, their willingness to follow it, and any limitations they may have in implementing those recommendations, as outlined in Table 11.10.

11.2.8 Key Considerations for Effective Remote Consultations

Table 11.11 provides a concise overview of essential components that general practitioners (GPs) should focus on to ensure patient safety, satisfaction, and continuity of care in remote consultations.

Table 11.10 Strategies for enhancing patient understanding and compliance, including confirming patient understanding through the teach-back method and planning for potential challenges. (Author, 2024)

Aspect	Details
Assessing understanding and agreement	Clinicians should confirm whether patients fully understand the instructions by asking them to *repeat* the advice in their own words This technique identifies misunderstandings and ensures accurate interpretation If confusion persists, rephrase instructions using *nontechnical language*
Planning for challenges	*Backup Plans:* It is essential to prepare alternative strategies if a mutually agreeable plan cannot be reached Pygall highlights the significance of having a backup plan for each consultation in case a mutually agreeable outcome cannot be reached [26]. It is essential to recognize that patients have the right to disregard advice Research shows that only *one-third of patients* adhere to advice fully, while others may follow it partially or ignore it altogether [27]
Addressing limitations to compliance	*Barriers to Compliance:* Some patients may face practical limitations, such as: Children relying on caregivers Young adults lacking transportation or funds Older adults with cognitive or mobility challenges Socially isolated individuals or those in care facilities *Solutions:* Include strategies like arranging transportation, engaging caregivers, or involving community services to overcome these obstacles [28]
Emphasizing patient-centered decision-making	Clinicians should ensure that patients are at the *center of decision-making*, enabling them to actively participate in their care plans Collaborative planning fosters adherence to recommendations and improves outcomes
Closing steps for remote consultations	Provide *clear next steps* based on the consultation's recommendations: *Home Visit Suggested:* Confirm the patient's *name and address* *Face-to-Face Appointment Recommended:* Share the practice's *address* and appointment details *Follow-Up Indicated:* Express openness to *further contact* and support if needed
Importance of quality communication	Closing the consultation with *clear guidance* enhances patient understanding and increases the likelihood of adherence The final moments of the interaction are crucial for setting expectations and reinforcing trust between the patient and clinician

11.2.9 Clinical Scenarios Requiring Safety Netting: Essential Guidance for Patient Management

Various clinical situations require safety netting. Table 11.12 highlights key points for effective patient guidance.

Table 11.11 Key components of effective patient consultation, highlighting the importance of safety-netting and management planning. (Author, 2024)

Component	Key focus	Best practice	Importance
Safety netting	Informing patients when to seek further help, especially in cases of diagnostic uncertainty	Provide clear, specific instructions on symptoms to monitor Document safety-netting advice in patient records Share patient education materials or relevant resources	Prevents missed diagnoses and ensures patient safety beyond the consultation
Management planning	Developing a structured care plan that patients can understand and follow	Clearly explain the diagnosis and treatment options Involve patients in shared decision-making Set realistic, achievable health goals	Promotes adherence to the care plan, leading to better health outcomes and patient engagement
Concluding the call	Ensuring patients leave the consultation informed, reassured, and prepared	Summarize key points such as diagnosis, treatment, and next steps Address any remaining questions Communicate availability for follow-ups	Builds trust, reduces patient anxiety, and ensures better adherence to care instructions

Table 11.12 Various clinical situations where safety netting is essential, highlighting key points for effective patient guidance. (Author, 2024)

Clinical situation	Why safety netting is important	Key points for safety netting
Unclear diagnosis	Symptoms may evolve, leading to a clearer diagnosis later	Advise on what to look out for and when to return
Mild viral illness	Could progress to more serious bacterial infections	Warn about red flag symptoms (e.g., high fever, persistent cough, breathing issues)
Chronic condition flare-ups	Condition could worsen despite initial treatment (e.g., asthma, diabetes)	Educate on symptoms that indicate deterioration and the need for urgent care
Unexplained abdominal pain	Potential for serious underlying issues (e.g., appendicitis, ectopic pregnancy)	Advise to return if pain worsens or other concerning symptoms (e.g., fever, vomiting)

(continued)

Table 11.12 (continued)

Clinical situation	Why safety netting is important	Key points for safety netting
Head injury (mild)	Risk of delayed complications like intracranial bleeding	Provide guidance on warning signs (e.g., confusion, vomiting, drowsiness)
Chest pain (non-cardiac)	Cardiac issues may still emerge even with an initial non-cardiac presentation	Advise immediate return if chest pain worsens, becomes persistent, or other symptoms arise
Children with fever	Risk of developing serious infections or complications	Emphasize monitoring for signs like rash, lethargy, or difficulty breathing.
Urinary tract infection (UTI)	Potential progression to pyelonephritis if untreated or symptoms worsen	Instruct to return if fever, back pain, or persistent symptoms develop.
Suspected minor fracture	Fractures can be missed in initial assessment	Encourage follow-up if pain, swelling, or function does not improve
New medications (e.g., antibiotics)	Risk of adverse reactions or medication inefficacy	Advise to report side effects or lack of improvement
Mental health concerns (mild anxiety/depression)	Symptoms could escalate or become more severe	Recommend seeking help if thoughts of self-harm or worsening emotional state occur
Vague neurological symptoms	Risk of more serious underlying neurological issues developing	Explain signs to watch for (e.g., weakness, slurred speech) and when to seek urgent care

11.3 Opportunities for Improvement and Common Pitfalls in Safety Netting

11.3.1 Key Areas for Improvement in Safety Netting

This section highlights key areas where safety-netting practices can be refined to improve patient outcomes, including talking about critical focus areas to be followed by actionable recommendations for clinicians, as outlined in Table 11.13.

Additional Insights

1. *Communicating Uncertainty*: Effective communication of diagnostic uncertainty is essential. Strategies that buy time may help conditions resolve or clarify; however, it is crucial to share this uncertainty with patients to prevent severe consequences.
2. *Re-accessing Care*: Evidence indicates that providing clear pathways for re-contact can improve follow-up rates. While specific mechanisms are explored mainly in chronic conditions, similar strategies should be adapted for acute care.

Table 11.13 Key recommendations for effective safety netting, highlighting the importance of clear guidance and patient empowerment. (Author, 2024)

Area of focus	Recommendations
Specific red flags and time frames	Provide clear red flags and specific follow-up timelines, avoiding vague reassurances such as "return if concerned [20, 24]
Written safety-netting advice	Offer written advice to reinforce verbal instructions, enhancing patient recall and comprehension [24]
Communicating uncertainty	Use strategies such as therapeutic trials or investigations to address diagnostic uncertainty, ensuring patients understand the uncertainty involved
Clear symptoms to monitor	Provide precise guidance on what symptoms to monitor, such as rapid breathing in respiratory infections and empowering patients and caregivers
Explicit care-seeking guidance	Legitimize follow-ups by encouraging patients to re-access care when needed and providing specific steps for re-contact
Precision in time course	Offer precise information about illness duration to manage patient expectations, e.g., symptoms of meningococcal disease beyond 48 h reduce complication risks

3. *Monitoring Illness Progression*: Key literature highlights the importance of knowing the expected time frames for conditions such as meningococcal disease, lower respiratory infections, and head injuries. Educating patients about these time frames can enhance safety-netting practices and help them recognize when to seek further medical advice.

11.3.2 Enhancing Safety Netting: A Structured Approach for Clinicians

Given the limited evidence available, clinicians should adopt practical strategies to improve safety-netting practices, which are essential in the diagnostic process due to the rarity of highly sensitive diagnostic strategies in primary care. However, the fragmentation of primary care can complicate these efforts. Table 11.14 suggests a structured approach for clinicians to improve patient care.

Detailed Considerations

- *What to Expect:* It is essential to help patients anticipate symptom progression and differentiate between manageable and critical symptoms. Patients often seek clarity on when to re-consult. Providing this information prevents unnecessary visits and promotes timely care.
- *What to Look out for:* Communicate both generic and specific safety-netting advice. Standardized templates can support effective communication, but personalized advice may be needed for vague symptoms.
- *Where and How to Seek Further Help:* Provide precise care-seeking instructions, avoiding vague phrases like "seek help if concerned." Direct patients to appropriate healthcare settings and define when urgent care is needed for red flags versus primary care for amber symptoms.

Table 11.14 Key areas and recommendations for improving patient care, emphasizing the importance of formal handovers and empowering patients. (Author, 2024)

Key areas	Recommendations
Establish a formal handover	Implement a handover to out-of-hours services for patients requiring urgent or follow-up care
Empower patients	Encourage self-monitoring and proactive health management
Set clear expectations	Explain what symptoms can be managed at home, offering reassurance where applicable, including reassurance about 'green flag' symptoms that can be safely managed at home
Clarify duration of symptoms	Provide guidance on the expected timeframe for recovery or worsening symptoms
Identify warning signs	Inform patients about specific red and amber flags to monitor (e.g., sepsis or cauda equina syndrome symptoms)
Use standardized resources	Utilize SMS templates or leaflets for consistent communication.
Provide care-seeking guidance	Clearly specify when, where, and how to seek further help
Communicate timelines for action	Educate patients on when urgent care is needed and distinguish between red and amber symptoms

11.3.3 Diagnostic Uncertainty in Patient Care (Table 11.15)

Table 11.15 Strategies for effective patient communication, emphasizing the importance of understanding diagnostic uncertainty and documenting patient decisions. (Author, 2024)

Strategy	Description
Understanding diagnostic uncertainty	Educate patients about the complexities of diagnosis and the role of time in clarifying conditions
Communicating the importance of time	Explain the significance of timelines in diagnosis to foster better understanding and reduce complaints
Encouraging patient compliance	Use prompts like "Based on what you've shared…" to clarify the need for follow-up
Utilizing the duty to terrify	In urgent cases, emphasize potential dangers to gain patient cooperation, e.g., "I can't rule out a heart attack; we need an ambulance"
Documenting patient decisions	Record refusals of care and the risks explained to protect both clinician and patient

11.3.4 Common Pitfalls in Safety Netting

- *Failure to Provide Advice*: Particularly in high-risk situations, neglecting to give safety-netting advice can lead to adverse outcomes.
- *Miscommunication*: Safety-netting advice may not be heard or understood by the patient, leading to confusion and missed opportunities for follow-up.
- *Insufficient Specificity*: Generic safety-netting advice, such as "Come back if you're not better," lacks clarity and may leave patients uncertain about what

actions to take. This can result in catastrophic delays in diagnosis and treatment, especially if a clinician offers inappropriate reassurance regarding serious symptoms [29].

11.3.5 Reporting Safety-Netting Advice

- *Documenting Patient Decisions:* When a patient rejects safety-netting advice, it is essential to document this decision clearly in the clinical record. This documentation should include a detailed explanation provided to the patient regarding the associated risks. Such clarity not only supports continuity of care but also serves as a legal safeguard for the clinician.
- *The Importance of Accurate Reporting:* A study by Derkx et al. [25] emphasized the critical role of accurate documentation throughout different stages of a consultation. It revealed that while reports often included thorough medical reasons for a call, they frequently lacked vital details about the patient's clinical history, expectations, and personal circumstances. Alarmingly, in most out-of-hours centers surveyed, trialists reported answers to mandatory questions that had not even been asked, with reporting variability ranging from 1 to 54%. Furthermore, subjective evaluations of the patient's condition appeared in only 12% of reports. This inconsistency highlights the necessity for meticulous documentation of safety-netting advice to ensure reasonable care and effective communication.
- *Enhancing Safety-Netting Practices:* The observed variation in safety-netting practices among clinicians likely stems from a general lack of research and explicit guidance on this topic. Evidence suggests that parental knowledge and satisfaction improve when written information accompanies verbal advice, particularly in pediatric cases. This practice could be equally beneficial for adult patients, especially considering potential memory impairments. As we strive to strengthen the evidence base for safety netting, all clinicians engaged in first-contact care should implement consensus recommendations derived from their clinical experiences. These recommendations can serve as core competencies for general practice (GP) trainees and others working in first-contact settings.

Key aspects of reporting safety-netting advice, emphasizing the importance of documenting patient decisions and improving safety-netting practices, is outlined in Table 11.16.

11.3.6 Summary of Safety-Netting Strategies

The definition of safety netting and key considerations, emphasizing the importance of shared responsibility between GPs and patients, are outlined in Table 11.17.

The importance of patient understanding and navigating diagnostic uncertainty in remote consultations, suggesting strategies to enhance compliance and access to appropriate care, is outlined in Table 11.18.

Table 11.16 Key aspects of reporting safety-netting advice, emphasizing the importance of documenting patient decisions and improving safety-netting practices. (Author, 2024)

Aspect	Description
Documenting patient decisions	Clearly record patient refusals and the risks discussed to ensure accountability
Accurate reporting	Include comprehensive clinical history and patient expectations in records. Avoid omissions that may affect care continuity
Improving safety-netting practices	Use both verbal and written advice to enhance patient comprehension, especially in pediatric or memory-impaired cases
Consensus recommendations	Implement best practices as part of core training for healthcare professionals engaged in first-contact care

Table 11.17 The definition of safety netting and highlights key considerations, emphasizing the importance of shared responsibility between GPs and patients. (Author, 2024)

Aspect	Description	Key considerations
Definition of safety netting	Advice given to patients or caregivers about when to seek further medical help	Aims to ensure understanding of potential health changes
When to implement	Situations of diagnostic uncertainty, known risks of complications, and increased patient risk	Consider patient's ability to understand and follow advice
Shared responsibility	Collaboration between GPs and patients in monitoring symptoms and follow-up	Both parties must engage actively for effective outcomes
Remote consultation challenges	Unique obstacles in conveying safety-netting advice without face-to-face interaction	Documentation and clarity of communication are crucial
Missed diagnoses	Addressing the risk of missed diagnoses in clinical practice	Safety netting serves as a strategy to manage uncertainty

Table 11.18 The importance of patient understanding and navigating diagnostic uncertainty in remote consultations, suggesting strategies to enhance compliance and access to appropriate care. (Author, 2024)

Key area	Importance	Strategies
Patient understanding	Ensures that patients grasp the advice provided, reducing misunderstandings, and enhancing compliance	Use clear language, ask patients to repeat instructions, and simplify complex medical jargon
Navigating diagnostic uncertainty	Helps patients understand the diagnostic process and the role of time in forming a diagnosis	Offer reassurance, explain safety-netting advice, and emphasize the importance of follow-up
Access to appropriate care	Ensures patients know how to seek further help if needed, preventing delays in treatment	Provide clear instructions on where to seek care, coordinate transportation if necessary, and involve caregivers or community resources

11.4 Conclusion

The evolving landscape of primary care, marked by an increasing reliance on remote consultations, necessitates a robust approach to patient safety and communication. Effective safety netting, structured management plans, and a thoughtful approach to concluding consultations are essential pillars in this new model. These elements not only mitigate diagnostic uncertainty but also empower patients to recognize when to seek further assistance, thereby enhancing overall care continuity and reducing risks.

Safety netting is foundational in guiding patients through the uncertainties that often accompany remote consultations. By providing clear, tailored instructions and identifying specific red-flag symptoms, healthcare providers can foster a proactive stance in patient care, particularly when in-person assessments are not feasible. The emphasis on patient understanding, combined with careful documentation, ensures that both patients and healthcare providers are aligned on the next steps, creating a safety net that supports patient autonomy while safeguarding clinical outcomes.

A well-structured management plan, integrated within each consultation, serves as a roadmap for both patient and provider. This planning is crucial not only for immediate symptom management but also for setting realistic expectations regarding illness progression and potential complications. Incorporating patient-centric communication techniques, such as the teach-back method, reinforces understanding and builds trust which are essential for adherence to advice and satisfaction with care.

Finally, a well-executed closing phase is key to ending each consultation on a reassuring note, with patients feeling informed and supported. By summarizing key points and clarifying follow-up options, clinicians can alleviate anxiety, ensuring that patients leave the consultation with confidence in their care plan.

In conclusion, by prioritizing effective safety netting, comprehensive management planning, and clear communication, healthcare providers can navigate the challenges of remote consultations. These practices not only enhance patient safety but also foster a sense of partnership and trust, which are crucial in the rapidly evolving digital healthcare environment.

References

1. Silverston P. Effective safety-netting in prescribing practice. Nurs Prescr. 2014;12(7):349–52.
2. Neighbour R. The inner consultation. MTP Press; 1987.
3. Edwards PJ, Silverston P, Sprackman J, Roland D. Safety-netting in the consultation. BMJ. 2022;378:e069094. https://doi.org/10.1136/bmj-2021-069094.
4. Jones D, Dunn L, Watt I, Macleod U. Safety netting for primary care: evidence from a literature review. Br J Gen Pract 2019 Jan;69(678):e70-e79. https://doi.org/10.3399/bjgp18X700193. Epub 2018 Dec 3. PMID: 30510099; PMCID: PMC6301356.
5. Friedemann Smith C, Lunn H, Wong G, Nicholson BD. Optimising GPs' communication of advice to facilitate patients' self-care and prompt follow-up when the diagnosis is uncertain: a realist review of 'safety-netting' in primary care. BMJ Qual Saf 2022 Jul;31(7):541–554.

https://doi.org/10.1136/bmjqs-2021-014529. Epub 2022 Mar 30. PMID: 35354664; PMCID: PMC9234415.
6. Kurtz S, Silverman J, Benson J, Draper J. Marrying content and process in clinical method teaching: enhancing the Calgary-Cambridge guides. Acad Med. 2003 Aug;78(8):802–9. https://doi.org/10.1097/00001888-200308000-00011.
7. Jones CH, Neill S, Lakhanpaul M, Roland D, Singlehurst-Mooney H, Thompson M. The safety netting behaviour of first contact clinicians: a qualitative study. BMC Fam Pract 2013 Sep 25;14:140. https://doi.org/10.1186/1471-2296-14-140. PMID: 24066842; PMCID: PMC3849506.
8. Greenhalgh S, Finucane L, Mercer CF, Selfe J. Safety netting; best practice in the face of uncertainty. Musculoskelet Sci Pract. 2020;48:102179. https://doi.org/10.1016/j.msksp.2020.102179.
9. Shupe R. Post-visit phone calls: reducing preventable readmissions and improving the patient experience. J Nurs Educ Pract. 2014 Jan;4(4) https://doi.org/10.5430/jnep.v4n4p45.
10. Roland D, Jones C, Neill S, Thompson M, Lakhanpaul M. Safety netting in healthcare settings: what it means, and for whom? Arch Dis Child Educ Pract Ed 2014 Apr;99(2):48–53. https://doi.org/10.1136/archdischild-2012-303056. Epub 2013 Oct 28.
11. Silverston P. The importance of teaching risk assessment and safety-netting skills in primary care. Prim Health Care. 2014;4:146. https://doi.org/10.4172/2167-1079.1000146.
12. Silverston P. Why, when and how to give safety-netting advice. InnovAiT. 2023;16(6):304–11. https://doi.org/10.1177/17557380231158129.
13. Evans J, Macartney JI, Bankhead C, Albury C, Jones D, Ziebland S, Nicholson BD. How do GPs and patients share the responsibility for cancer safety netting follow-up actions? A qualitative interview study of GPs and patients in Oxfordshire, UK. BMJ Open 2019 Sep 12;9(9):e029316. https://doi.org/10.1136/bmjopen-2019-029316. PMID: 31515421; PMCID: PMC6747661.
14. Black GB, van Os S, Renzi C, Walter FM, Hamilton W, Whitaker KL. How does safety netting for lung cancer symptoms help patients to reconsult appropriately? A qualitative study. BMC Prim Care. 2022 Jul 20;23(1):179. https://doi.org/10.1186/s12875-022-01791-y. Erratum in: BMC Prim Care 2022 Aug 4;23(1):195. Doi: 10.1186/s12875-022-01808-6. PMID: 35858826; PMCID: PMC9298706.
15. Edwards PJ, Ridd MJ, Sanderson E, Barnes RK. Safety netting in routine primary care consultations: an observational study using video-recorded UK consultations. Br J Gen Pract 2019 Nov 28;69(689):e878–e886. https://doi.org/10.3399/bjgp19X706601. PMID: 31740458; PMCID: PMC6863676.
16. Edwards PJ, Bennett-Britton I, Ridd MJ, Booker M, Barnes RK. Factors affecting the documentation of spoken safety-netting advice in routine GP consultations: a cross-sectional study. Br J Gen Pract 2021 Oct 28;71(712):e869–e876. https://doi.org/10.3399/BJGP.2021.0195. PMID: 34489251; PMCID: PMC8436774.
17. Ladds E, Khan M, Moore L, Kalin A, Greenhalgh T. The impact of remote care approaches on continuity in primary care: a mixed-studies systematic review. Br J Gen Pract 2023 Apr 27;73(730):e374–e383. https://doi.org/10.3399/BJGP.2022.0398. PMID: 37105731; PMCID: PMC10058181.
18. Payne R, Clarke A, Swann N, van Dael J, Brenman N, Rosen R, Mackridge A, Moore L, Kalin A, Ladds E, Hemmings N, Rybczynska-Bunt S, Faulkner S, Hanson I, Spitters S, Wieringa S, Dakin FH, Shaw SE, Wherton J, Byng R, Husain L, Greenhalgh T. Patient safety in remote primary care encounters: multimethod qualitative study combining Safety I and Safety II analysis. BMJ Qual Saf 2024 Aug 16;33(9):573–586. https://doi.org/10.1136/bmjqs-2023-016674. PMID: 38050161; PMCID: PMC11347200.
19. Borland ML, Dalziel SR, Phillips N, Lyttle MD, Bressan S, Oakley E, Hearps SJC, Kochar A, Furyk J, Cheek JA, Neutze J, Gilhotra Y, Dalton S, Babl FE; Paediatric Research in Emergency Department International Collaborative (PREDICT) group. Delayed Presentations to emergency departments of children with head injury: a PREDICT study. Ann Emerg Med 2019 Jul;74(1):1–10. https://doi.org/10.1016/j.annemergmed.2018.11.035. Epub 2019 Jan 14.

20. Almond S, Mant D, Thompson M. Diagnostic safety-netting. Br J Gen Pract 2009 Nov;59(568):872–874; discussion 874. https://doi.org/10.3399/bjgp09X472971. PMID: 19861036; PMCID: PMC2765844.
21. Evans J, Ziebland S, MacArtney JI, Bankhead CR, Rose PW, Nicholson BD. GPs' understanding and practice of safety netting for potential cancer presentations: a qualitative study in primary care. Br J Gen Pract 2018 Jul;68(672):e505–e511. https://doi.org/10.3399/bjgp18X696233. Epub 2018 May 8. PMID: 29739779; PMCID: PMC6014413.
22. Frostholm L, Fink P, Oernboel E, Christensen KS, Toft T, Olesen F, Weinman J. The uncertain consultation and patient satisfaction: the impact of patients' illness perceptions and a randomized controlled trial on the training of physicians' communication skills. Psychosom Med. 2005 Nov-Dec;67(6):897–905. https://doi.org/10.1097/01.psy.0000188403.94327.5b.
23. Silverston P. SAFER: a mnemonic to improve safety-netting advice. Pract Nurs. 2020 Jan 2;31(1):26–8. https://doi.org/10.12968/pnur.2020.31.1.26.
24. Silverston P. SAFER diagnosis: a teaching system to help reduce diagnostic errors in primary care. Br J Gen Pract 2020 Jun 25;70(696):354–355. https://doi.org/10.3399/bjgp20X710669. PMID: 32586822; PMCID: PMC7319682.
25. Derkx H, Rethans JJ, Muijtjens A, Maiburg B, Winkens R, van Rooij H, Knottnerus A. 'Quod scripsi, scripsi.' The quality of the report of telephone consultations at Dutch out-of-hours centres. Qual Saf Health Care 2010 Dec;19(6):e1. https://doi.org/10.1136/qshc.2008.027920. Epub 2010 Jun 27.
26. Pygall SA. Telephone triage and consultation: are we really listening? Royal College of General Practitioners; 2017.
27. Donovan JL, Blake DR. Patient non-compliance: deviance or reasoned decision-making? Soc Sci Med. 1992 Mar;34(5):507–13. https://doi.org/10.1016/0277-9536(92)90206-6.
28. Udonwa NE, Ogbonna UK. Patient-related factors influencing satisfaction in the patient-doctor encounters at the general outpatient clinic of the University of Calabar teaching hospital, Calabar, Nigeria. Int J Family Med. 2012;2012:517027. https://doi.org/10.1155/2012/517027. Epub 2012 May 20. PMID: 22675629; PMCID: PMC3363396.
29. Richards MA, Smith P, Ramirez AJ, Fentiman IS, Rubens RD. The influence on survival of delay in the presentation and treatment of symptomatic breast cancer. Br J Cancer 1999 Feb;79(5–6):858–864. https://doi.org/10.1038/sj.bjc.6690137. PMID: 10070881; PMCID: PMC2362673.

12 Leveraging Patient Views for Optimal Remote Care

Luís Pinho Costa, Ana Luís Pereira, Liliana Amorim, and Liliana Coelho

12.1 Introduction

The population requiring healthcare services is growing faster than the capacity of our present healthcare delivery methods. Thus, appropriate integration of remote consultation in health systems has become increasingly important, especially when considering that patients often view telehealth based on their own experiences, expectations, worries and illnesses. For many people, especially the elderly and those in technologically deprived areas, this is a path less walked upon as far as remotely accessing health services is concerned. Nonetheless, in general, patients appreciate being able to get medical attention at home since it can greatly reduce appointment waiting time, satisfying their social and medical needs while aiding in personalizing care. Yet, privacy breaches or security threats can be obstacles to effective use of such services by patients, as are other impediments like the lack of technological infrastructure and of human touch (and warmth), among others. Throughout this chapter, we will leverage patient perspectives on remote care to develop strategies for delivering patient-centered remote care effectively.

L. P. Costa (✉) · A. L. Pereira
HSC – Healthy Smart Cities, Santa Maria da Feira, Portugal
e-mail: luispinhocosta@healthysmartcities.pt; analuispereira@healthysmartcities.pt

L. Amorim
P5 Digital Medical Center, Braga, Portugal
e-mail: liliana.amorim@p5.pt

L. Coelho
Teladoc Health, Lisbon, Portugal
e-mail: lcoelho@teladochealth.com

J. Demurtas (ed.), *Remote Consultation in Primary Care*, TELe-Health,
https://doi.org/10.1007/978-3-031-89661-3_12

12.2 How Can Medical Doctors Align with Patients' Perspectives, Expectations, and Perceived Facilitators for Remote Consultations?

Our success as medical doctors and healthcare professionals in the realm of remote consultations largely depends on our understanding and alignment of patient expectations and perceived facilitators. By immersing ourselves in their perspective, we can effectively tailor our approach to remote consulting so that it is congruent with what patients wish for.

Patients perceive that telemedicine offers them a chance to reach healthcare providers anytime they need, without the need to travel or attend costly unscheduled providers [1–5]. As such, it provides an easy way of accessing services at their convenience, thereby reducing time wastage, costs and other logistical hassles associated with traditional face-to-face visits (e.g., traveling costs or unscheduled expensive visits paid to caregivers, organizing leave days off from work) [1–14]. This is particularly true for individuals living in rural areas where travel may be inconvenient or too costly [15]. Notwithstanding, this appreciation extends also to those who find it difficult to attend physical meetings due to disability as well as employment obligations or family responsibilities [1].

In order to meet these expectations, we can make our telehealth services easily accessible and usable by giving clear instructions on how to schedule a remote appointment and access virtual platforms, while considering the value of our patients' time. To this end, providers can reduce waiting times, inform patients when appointments are running late, have less paperwork for them to complete, and offer them convenient visit slots/times and flexible appointment booking options that are compatible with their lives. By removing the necessity of taking time off work or from school, we can allow them to remain healthy without compromising other responsibilities. Furthermore, the administrative staff may also help in organizing trial sessions for telehealthcare users, given that they are often anxious to use an unfamiliar platform, and this promotes their familiarity with it in a guided manner, before they have to starting using it for remote consultations [16].

Patients enjoy remote care for many reasons, one of which is its ability to overcome some of the barriers specific groups have with in-person visits [1]. For instance, some patients may struggle to communicate verbally due to hearing loss, finding it easier to communicate with their doctor by writing. Others might have mental health conditions that cause them to be anxious during face-to-face conversations with medical professionals. In these cases, being able to talk through a screen can drastically improve equity and satisfaction with care. If we want to take equitable healthcare delivery even further, we can organize outreach programs or virtual clinics to reach underserved communities. Many people in rural or remote areas do not have access to specialist care, so having an option that does not involve long or costly trips can be life-changing [1, 7, 15]. As accessibility is a major selling point for patients who like having timely responses for their inquiries and need specialists' consultation, telehealth teams and technology can be used to streamline referral to specialist advice so that care is delivered fast [7, 15]. The telehealth platforms can also be used for communication across multidisciplinary care teams, ensuring comprehensive and coordinated care plans that provide immediate solutions to every aspect regarding the health status of the patient.

Remote consultations also offer relief from the physical and emotional burden attached to traveling for diagnosis, treatment, or follow-up, for both patients and their finances [14, 16]. During remote appointments, acknowledging patients' pains by showing them empathy will go a long way in their eyes. In addition, some patients value having family members present during consultations [16]; so if they do want someone listening alongside them over the phone or computer, we should accommodate that.

Finally, another major plus of remote consultations is the continuity of care they may foster [14]. Patients appreciate being able to consistently see the same doctors, nurses, and other healthcare professionals because it strengthens the patient-provider relationship while instilling trust in the quality of care received [1, 14, 16]. To maintain that level of continuity throughout all appointments—virtual or not—keeping accurate records is crucial. Transitioning between digital and personal meetings as seamlessly as possible should be a priority for us as well when planning these appointments so there are no hiccups along the way for patients who rely on this care model more than others do [1].

By having a patient-first mindset, physicians can reap a host of benefits. Outranking the bunch are things like good back-and-forth with patients and privacy guarantees. It is important that we speak to our patients clearly and concisely, especially in the age of virtual health care visits. That means using everyday words when describing complicated medical concepts and treatments. Lacking the face-to-face nature of regular appointments, our remote checkups should still make patients feel powerful. We can do this by getting them actively involved in their own care decisions, encouraging questions during video calls, and simply making sure they know they've got some control over their health journey. Sharing educational resources also does not hurt.

To build on our consulting skills—which will no doubt be vital well into the future—we need to ask for feedback about our telehealth approach so far and find out what works (and what does not), then put any changes into action. That should not be done just for show, either; if you set expectations and then meet them every time, people will respect you more and more. This level of respect leads to better outcomes across the board, from patient satisfaction right down to good old-fashioned results.

12.3 How Can Medical Doctors Address Patient Concerns and Overcome Barriers about Remote Consultations?

The literature reveals a series of worries and anxieties from patients when it comes to teleconsultations. It is critical that healthcare professionals recognize these concerns and confront them head on to ensure that remote care works effectively. By understanding what stops patients, medical doctors are able to tackle the problem at its roots preventing future, similar problems. This approach will build trust in the process which is essential for a strong doctor-patient relationship.

Patients often express their concerns over the lack of traditional physical examination in teleconsultations [7, 16]. They worry about things like potential prescription errors, misdiagnoses, and safeguarding issues. To confront these issues, medical doctors must focus on maintaining high standards of care. A growing body of literature provides advice for safe remote consultations which should be referred to as much as possible.

Medical professionals need to clearly communicate the limitations of remote assessments (and prescriptions) with patients while offering alternative methods to gather information about their health. In applicable scenarios, we should elucidate that a thorough evaluation can still be achieved through medical history and indirect indicators obtainable via teleconsultation, including photographs or videos that could potentially provide just enough information for an accurate decision.

Patients must also be made aware of how the absence of a conventional physical examination affects their diagnosis and treatment plan. There are instances where teleconsultation just is not the best option for their specific case, and this needs to be acknowledged by both parties involved so issues can be avoided entirely—including possible litigation and medico-legal problems. Medical professionals must remain vigilant of symptoms that are hard to verify without face-to-face contact because failure to do so increases the risk of misdiagnosis [17].

With all this in mind, it is crucial to evaluate the appropriateness of a teleconsultation ideally before the scheduling and even when in progress. To analyze if a teleconsultation is appropriate, we need to consider whether a physical examination is needed or not. In case one is required, teleconsultations should be out of question. We must also think about possible emergencies. If so, it is advisable to triage rapidly during preliminary consultation stages. Even after starting a teleconsultation, doctors should reevaluate potential red flags before moving forward. International guidelines suggest that patients be asked several questions depending on the clinical context for initial emergency screenings [18]. These could include, but are not restricted to the following:

- Do you feel chest pain or palpitations?
- Are you having trouble breathing? Do you have shallow breaths and wheezes or are you coughing severely?
- Do you have newly developed abdominal pain?
- Are your ears hurting or discharging pus? Is your hearing altered in any way that worries you?
- Are your face, arm, or leg numb or feeling weak?
- Have you suddenly had difficulty walking, felt dizzy, or lost balance without reason?
- Are there sudden changes in vision bothering you? Or eye pain?
- Have your legs swollen up suddenly?
- Did recent accidents or assaults take place involving yourself?

- Are you concerned that your symptoms require immediate face-to-face consultation or may be an emergency?

When available, providers should also look at the patient's medical data and recent health records to better understand what treatment and plan of care they need. To effectively gather, store and share patient data, healthcare providers should adopt secure and interoperable electronic health record (EHR) systems. EHRs not only improve decision-making but offer a whole view on each patient's background. Integrating data from other sources such as wearables and remote monitoring devices can further enhance our understanding of a patient and enable prompt interventions when necessary.

Privacy and security are other primary concerns when talking about remote consultations, since patients expect their personal health information to be treated with absolute confidentiality. The literature clearly highlights the crucial need for maintaining privacy standards equivalent to in-person consultations. Patients expect their sensitive health data to be guarded and protected, emphasizing the importance of secure communication channels and robust data protection measures [9, 17, 19]. This aspect becomes particularly critical when sensitive topics are discussed, such as mental health, gynecological or urological issues, where patients rely on teleconsultations to ensure the most privacy and confidentiality.

A related set of issues that trouble patients are the potential risks of privacy breaches and unauthorized access to their health data during or after teleconsultations [14, 17]. However, these concerns can be addressed with a few changes in how we go about things. It starts with healthcare professionals adopting stringent security measures and adhering to established privacy and digital safety guidelines. The sharing of information should always take place through appropriate platforms and secure means, to build patient trust and mitigate any risks associated with unauthorized access to medical information. These same measures should be discussed at length with the patient as well, along with any other participants in the remote consultations. By doing so, healthcare professionals will have reassured patients about the confidentiality and integrity of their health information, thereby enhancing trust and confidence in remote care delivery. What's more, utilizing platforms specifically designed for care delivery can help us maintain clear boundaries between work and personal life, addressing patients' increasing demand for immediate responses without time constraints.

In addition, creating an appropriate physical environment and establishing robust technological infrastructure plays a significant role in ensuring telemedicine appointments are effective from the patient's perspective [17]. When conducting telemedicine sessions, medical doctors should ensure that both they and the patient are in a suitable location where no one can hear or interrupt them. Good lighting is important so that not only patients can see their provider clearly, but also the provider can view the patient accurately during any examinations. Both must be reminded of the consultation's formality, and it should be made clear that a remote consultation is indeed a medical consultation with the same intentions as those conducted in-person.

As some patients appreciate having access to an audio recording of their appointments [11], clinicians must take into account that remote consultations may be recorded without their consent. This poses legal and ethical problems; however, in many jurisdictions, legal action is to no avail unless there is public use of such recordings. In light of this, consent to record could prove beneficial to both parties and encouraging it might be worth considering [6].

Moreover, reliable technology and internet connection are necessary components to ensure online/video consultations go smoothly without interruption. If these conditions cannot be reliably met, it may be prudent to reconsider utilizing online consultations. Technological barriers are indeed vastly documented in the literature—including difficulties setting up or joining video calls and poor sound or video quality during remote consultations—and can affect access and engagement of patients during these sessions, as well as the message the provider intended to deliver, thus increasing risks of errors occurring. These issues may occur even when video demonstrations, prior testing and technical support are available, which reduces patients' confidence in this type of consultation and may compromise its effectiveness [6, 14, 16, 20]. Therefore, besides going the extra mile to establish whether everyone participating in the online consultation has access to a fast internet connection and to technology that permits convenient remote consultations, we should make arrangements for a backup plan that allows us to reach the participants through other means in case things go awry—for instance, a mobile number we can otherwise use. Telephone calls require nothing more than a basic mobile phone or landline, eliminating the need for high-speed internet and computer or smartphone access. Most patients are familiar with using a phone, so there is no learning curve associated with navigating new technology, making it a much less stressful experience for them.

Patients' digital literacy must also be taken into account when considering them for remote consultations. Their cognitive and mental state, sight and hearing capabilities as well as language or other barriers to understanding medical information should be assessed. Depending on the situation, the patient may need assistance from a family member or another healthcare professional. It is important to record the presence of a third person in the medical records and, if such a person is another practitioner, the remote consultation can be dealt with as teleassistance [16]. Extra attention must be paid toward patients with disabilities, ensuring the technical features of the platform, as well as the remote care service altogether, responds appropriately to their specific needs.

Finally, it is worth noting that in remote consultations, similar to in-person appointments, communication is key. It is particularly important that providers are sensitive to cultural and emotional cues when physical cues are less obvious. On the other hand, phone calls allow both patient and provider to focus on their voices, which can be more personal and less distracting than video calls. For patients who might not feel confident with their appearance or video skills, audio-only consultations can reduce stress and make the consultation more comfortable. Especially over the phone, but also in video consultations, patients may feel more at ease to address sensitive topics (if confidentiality is ensured) [16]. This requires medical doctors to be prepared to adequately manage such topics and related medical conditions, for instance, sexually transmitted diseases that they seldom are asked about in their in-person consultations.

That being said, some patients still prefer in-person consultations to virtual ones. Many patients feel that they have a closer relationship with their medical doctor during in-person appointments and that communication is more effective this way [11, 15]. Recognizing this is crucial, as is developing a successful patient-centered approach: one where patients understand that our aim is to help them achieve better health and quality of life in a way that is most comfortable for them—be it remote and/or in-person. Equally important is increasing patients' self-efficacy by empowering them to take charge of their health. To achieve it, we must equip ourselves with the skills to empower patients, providing consistent and constructive feedback.

12.4 Concluding Remarks on Pioneering Remote Care that Puts Patients First

Remote care models can be extremely beneficial when it comes to reducing healthcare costs, getting patients engaged, and improving health outcomes. However, the journey toward widespread remote care adoption is not as straightforward as it may seem. The journey to patient-centered remote care starts with understanding patient expectations, addressing their concerns and being proactive in implementing strategies that are well aligned with their perspectives.

Although there is still work to be done, primary care physicians have a role to play in revolutionizing healthcare delivery by bringing high-quality remote care to everyone, no matter where they're located. Collaboration between them and other healthcare professionals, patients, technologists and policymakers, as well as interdisciplinary research, will be needed to come up with new scalable remote solutions. Strengthening these relationships is vital, with patients at the center.

References

1. Darley S, Coulson T, Peek N, Moschogianis S, van der Veer SN, Wong DC, et al. Understanding how the design and implementation of online consultations affect primary care quality: systematic review of evidence with recommendations for designers, providers, and researchers. J Med Internet Res. 2022;24 https://doi.org/10.2196/37436.
2. Gupta T, Gkiousias V, Bhutta MF. A systematic review of outcomes of remote consultation in ENT. Clin Otolaryngol. 2021;46:699–719. https://doi.org/10.1111/COA.13768.
3. DeWyer A, Scheel A, Kamarembo J, Akech R, Asiimwe A, Beaton A, et al. Establishment of a cardiac telehealth program to support cardiovascular diagnosis and care in a remote, resource-poor setting in Uganda. PLoS One. 2021;16:e0255918. https://doi.org/10.1371/JOURNAL.PONE.0255918.
4. Conway MP, Forristal MT, Treacy MP, Duignan ES. Investigating the role of optometrists in Teleophthalmology and the implications of increasing access to advanced imaging techniques and digital referral: a systematic search and review. Telemed J E Health. 2020;27:974–81. https://doi.org/10.1089/TMJ.2020.0284.

5. Mclaughlin EJ, Ellett LC, Readman E, Mooney S. Telehealth for gynaecology outpatients during the COVID-19 pandemic: patient and clinician experiences, vol. 62; 2022. p. 553. https://doi.org/10.1111/ajo.13510.
6. Tsampras N, Craciunas L, Dearden M, Sood A, Mathur R. Video consultations in reproductive medicine: safety, feasibility and patient satisfaction. Eur J Obstet Gynecol Reprod Biol. 2023;286:35–8. https://doi.org/10.1016/j.ejogrb.2023.05.013.
7. Osman MA, Schick-Makaroff K, Thompson S, Bialy L, Featherstone R, Kurzawa J, et al. Barriers and facilitators for implementation of electronic consultations (eConsult) to enhance access to specialist care: a scoping review. BMJ Glob Health. 2019;4 https://doi.org/10.1136/bmjgh-2019-001629.
8. Almathami HKY, Than Win K, Vlahu-Gjorgievska E. Barriers and facilitators that influence telemedicine-based, real-time, online consultation at patients' homes: systematic literature review. J Med Internet Res. 2020;22 https://doi.org/10.2196/16407.
9. Ruiz-Romero V, Torres-Domínguez Y, Acón-Royo D, De Toro-Salas A, Cruz-Villalón F, Rivera-Sequeiros A, et al. Evaluación de la satisfacción del paciente en la teleconsulta durante la pandemia por COVID-19 (*). Rev Esp Salud Pública. 2021;95:16–7.
10. Gupta T, Bowles P, Bhutta MF. Effectiveness, perceptions and environmental benefits of remote consultation for adults referred with recurrent tonsillitis, vol. 106; 2024. p. 173. https://doi.org/10.1308/rcsann.2022.0098.
11. Damery S, Jones J, Francischetto EOC, Jolly K, Lilford R, Ferguson J. Remote consultations versus standard face-to-face appointments for liver transplant patients in routine hospital care: feasibility randomized controlled trial of myVideoClinic. J Med Internet Res. 2021;23:23. https://doi.org/10.2196/19232.
12. Hakim N, Longmore P, Hu VH. Patient experience survey in a corneal service conducted by remote consultation. Clin Ophthalmol. 2021;15:4747–54. https://doi.org/10.2147/OPTH.S331622.
13. Haider Z, Aweid B, Subramanian P, Iranpour F. Telemedicine in orthopaedics during COVID-19 and beyond: a systematic review. J Telemed Telecare. 2022;28:391–403. https://doi.org/10.1177/1357633X20938241/FORMAT/EPUB.
14. Maria ARJ, Serra H, Heleno B. Teleconsultations and their implications for health care: a qualitative study on patients' and physicians' perceptions. Int J Med Inform. 2022;162:162. https://doi.org/10.1016/j.ijmedinf.2022.104751.
15. Joschko J, Liddy C, Moroz I, Reiche M, Crowe L, Afkham A, et al. Just a click away: exploring patients' perspectives on receiving care through the Champlain BASE TM eConsult service. Fam Pract. 2018;35:93–8. https://doi.org/10.1093/fampra/cmx073.
16. Bradwell H, Baines R, Edwards KJ, Stevens S, Atkinson K, Wilkinson E, et al. Exploring patient and staff experiences with video consultations during COVID-19 in an English outpatient care setting: secondary data analysis of routinely collected feedback data. JMIR Form Res. 2022;6 https://doi.org/10.2196/30486.
17. Bhat KS, Jain M, Kumar N. Infrastructuring telehealth in (in)formal patient-doctor contexts. Proc ACM Hum Comput Interact. 2021;5:1. https://doi.org/10.1145/3476064.
18. Florea M, Gindrovel D, Iancu A, Alexiu S, Deleanu A, Motea O, et al. A guide to telemedicine in primary healthcare. 2022.
19. Sulaman H, Akhtar T, Naeem H, Ara Saeed G, Fazal S. Beyond COVID-19: Prospect of telemedicine for obstetrics patients in Pakistan. Int J Med Inform. 2022;158:104653. https://doi.org/10.1016/j.ijmedinf.2021.104653.
20. Bowman M, Jalink M, Sharpe I, Srivastava S, Wijeratne DT. Videoconferencing interventions and COPD patient outcomes: a systematic review. J Telemed Telecare. 2023; https://doi.org/10.1177/1357633X231158140/SUPPL_FILE/SJ-DOCX-1-JTT-10.1177_1357633X231158140.DOCX.

Part III

Main Clinical Scenarios

Remote Assessment of the Respiratory and Cardiovascular Systems 13

Roberto Tonelli, Giulia Bruzzi, Alessandro Marchioni, and Enrico Clini

13.1 General Introduction

The respiratory and cardiovascular systems are intricately interconnected, with any disturbances in one system often affecting the other. Early detection of respiratory or cardiovascular issues through remote consultations can lead to timely intervention, minimizing the risk of complications and hospitalizations. These assessments are particularly valuable for individuals with chronic conditions, where regular evaluations are essential to prevent exacerbations and optimize treatment outcomes. By integrating patient-reported symptoms, visual observations, and shared data from medical devices, healthcare providers can gain comprehensive insights into the patient's health status, enabling informed decision-making and tailored interventions.

R. Tonelli (✉) · E. Clini
Respiratory Diseases Unit, University Hospital of Modena, Modena, Italy

Department of Surgical and Medical Sciences of Motherhood and Child, University of Modena and Reggio Emilia, Modena, Italy
e-mail: enrico.clini@unimore.it

G. Bruzzi
Respiratory Diseases Unit, University Hospital of Modena, Modena, Italy

Department of Surgical and Medical Sciences of Motherhood and Child, University of Modena and Reggio Emilia, Modena, Italy

Clinical and Experimental Medicine PhD Program, University of Modena Reggio Emilia, Modena, Italy

A. Marchioni
Respiratory Diseases Unit, University Hospital of Modena, Modena, Italy
e-mail: marchioni.alessandro@unimore.it

J. Demurtas (ed.), *Remote Consultation in Primary Care*, TELe-Health,
https://doi.org/10.1007/978-3-031-89661-3_13

Consider the following steps when approaching the remote assessment of respiratory and cardiovascular system.

1. *Patient history and symptoms assessment*: begin by gathering a comprehensive medical history, including previous diagnoses, medications, allergies, and lifestyle factors. Inquire about symptoms related to respiratory distress (e.g., breathlessness, cough) and cardiovascular concerns (e.g., chest pain, palpitations).
2. *Technological tools and remote devices*: leverage technology to your advantage. Encourage patients to use home devices like pulse oximeters to provide objective data during the consultation.
3. *Visual observations*: utilize video calls (rather than phone calls) to observe visual cues such as the patient's general appearance, skin color, and respiratory rate. Pay attention to any signs of distress, cyanosis, or peripheral edema.
4. *Patient education*: educate patients on proper usage of remote assessment tools, as well as the importance of consistent data recording. Provide guidance on recognizing and reporting any significant changes in symptoms or readings.
5. *Patient-reported outcome measures*: incorporate validated patient-reported outcome measures and scales particularly related to breathlessness. These tools help quantify symptom severity and provide standardized data for assessment.

13.2 Respiratory Rate

13.2.1 Introduction

The remote assessment of respiratory rate (RR) through video consultation has been found to be reliable and feasible for use in primary care settings [1]. Remote monitoring devices, such as wearable fitness trackers or remote monitoring apps, can also provide accurate real-time RR data [2]. Bae et al. showed that the remote measurement of RR using a smartphone camera-based technique was accurate, thus indicating the feasibility of this approach [3]. Awareness of monitoring appears to reduce RR, and shorter monitoring durations yield systematically lower RR estimates [4]. As such, strategies should be implemented to perform the remote assessment with the patient unaware of the evaluation and with adequate length of the RR count. Remote assessment of RR requires video consultation. If unavailable and telephone consultation is the only option, a family member should be instructed on how to perform the evaluation.

13.2.2 Evaluation

To evaluate RR, it may be of help to tell the patients to rest and not talk for 1 min because after that preparation a test of their breathing is going to be performed. The normal RR ranges between 12 and 20 breaths per min (brpm) for a resting adult, being slightly higher for older adults [5]. To assess the RR while the patient is waiting for the breathing test to be performed, provide the following instructions:

1. Instruct the patient to sit or lie comfortably in a quiet and relaxed environment.
2. Instruct the patient to place one hand on their chest or abdomen to help you see the rise and fall of the chest more clearly.
3. Explain that they should breathe normally during the 1-min preparation phase and avoid any forced or exaggerated movements.

Count the number of breaths they are taking in that 1-min preparation. Avoid observation period lasting less than 1 min. Ask a family member to do this in case of telephonic consultation.

13.2.3 Warning Signs

1. *RR ≥ 20 bpm*: it could be a sign of respiratory distress, infection, fever, anxiety, or other medical conditions requiring attention.
2. *RR ≤ 10 bpm*: it might suggest respiratory depression, drug overdose, or neurological issues.
3. *Self-reported recent changes in RR: consider* potential triggers such as infections, allergies, or exacerbations of preexisting respiratory conditions.

13.2.4 Special Conditions

13.2.4.1 Pediatrics

Instruct the caregiver/parent to identify anatomical landmarks on the child's body for counting respiratory rate. The two common areas are the chest and abdomen. For chest counting, ask the caregiver/parent to focus the camera on the child's chest and observe the rise and fall of the chest with each breath. Instruct them to count the number of breaths the child takes in 1 min (a full cycle of inhaling and exhaling). For abdomen counting, if the chest movement is difficult to see or if the child is predominantly breathing with their abdomen, instruct the caregiver/parent to focus the camera on the child's abdomen and count the number of abdominal movements in 1 min. The normal ranges of respiratory rate for children can vary depending on their age. The approximate normal respiratory rate ranges for children aged 0 to 14 years old are [6]:

1. Newborns (0–28 days): 30 to 60 breaths per min (brpm).
2. Infants (1–12 months): 24 to 40 brpm.
3. Toddlers (1–2 years): 22 to 34 brpm.
4. Preschoolers (3–5 years): 20 to 30 brpm.
5. School-age children (6–12 years): 18 to 25 brpm.
6. Adolescents (13–14 years): 12 to 20 brpm.

13.3 Heart Rate and Peripheral Blood Saturation

13.3.1 Introduction

Performing a remote assessment of heart rate (HR) and peripheral blood oxygen saturation (SpO_2) involves using specific devices. Choose remote monitoring devices that are designed to measure HR and SpO_2. The two commonly used devices are:

1. Pulse oximeter: it is a noninvasive device that measures SpO_2 and by clipping onto a person's fingertip, earlobe, or toe. Some advanced models can be used on other body parts like the wrist or forehead. A study by Buekers et al. demonstrated the feasibility and reliability of wearable finger pulse oximeters to continuously measure SpO_2 during daily home routines of chronic obstructive pulmonary disease (COPD) patients and assess natural SpO_2 fluctuations [7].
2. Wearable devices: certain smartwatches and fitness trackers can estimate HR and may provide some indication of SpO_2. Regarding HR, a growing body of evidence indicates that smartwatch-derived HR variability provides a practical alternative with excellent accuracy compared with ECG-based HR variability [8]. However, caution is warranted, and further studies are needed to validate this technique. A recent study by Jiang and coworkers investigated the accuracy of SpO_2 measurements in common consumer smartwatches. The authors reported that there were statistically significant differences in accuracy between devices [9]. Further, it is known that pulse oximeters underperform under circumstances of low perfusion [10]. Thus, to date there is no sufficient data to validate wearable devices (i.e., smartphones or smartwatches) to monitor SpO_2.

Several studies, as well as expert consensus, indicate that the normal adult resting HR values lie between 60 and 90 beats per min (bpm). For most healthy individuals at sea level, a normal SpO_2 level is typically considered to be 95–96% or higher [11].

Be aware that when conducting remote HR and SpO_2 assessments, you should consider the limitations of the technology used and the potential impact of environmental factors, signal disruptions, and user compliance.

13.3.2 Evaluation

For HR evaluation, ensure that the device is properly positioned on the body, typically on the wrist, chest, or finger, depending on the type of device used. Instruct the patient to start the HR monitoring process on the device or app. Depending on the device, this may involve tapping a button or activating a specific feature.

For SpO_2 evaluation, guide the patient in starting the SpO_2 monitoring process on the device by placing it on a fingertip, earlobe, or toe for measurement. Be aware of the interference of nail polish when assessing SpO_2 evaluation on a fingertip.

13.3.3 Warning Signs

1. *$SpO_2 \leq 90\%$*: a 90%-SpO_2 is most commonly recommended as a clinical threshold for detecting a significant hypoxic episode [12].
2. *HR ≤ 50 bpm*: Spodick et al. identified the level of 50 bpm as the lowest normal limit of heart rate, but there is no indication from the literature that a heart rate below that limit is really hazardous in the absence of sinoatrial dysfunction [13].
3. *HR ≥ 85 bpm*: although official upper normal limits for resting heart rate are not yet available, the data of the literature are sound and indicate that these limits should be set well below 100 bpm, the threshold currently used to define tachycardia, particularly in those patients suffering from cardiac disease [14].

13.3.4 Special Conditions

13.3.4.1 Pediatrics

The normal values of HR can vary depending on factors such as age, activity level, fitness, and overall health. Here are approximate normal heart rate ranges for different age groups [6]:

1. Newborns (0–28 days): 100–160 beats per min (bpm).
2. Infants (1–12 months): 90–160 bpm.
3. Toddlers (1–2 years): 80–130 bpm.
4. Preschoolers (3–5 years): 80–120 bpm.
5. School-age children (6–12 years): 70–100 bpm.
6. Adolescents (13–18 years): 60–100 bpm.

13.4 Blood Pressure

13.4.1 Introduction

Performing the evaluation of blood pressure within a remote consultation requires collaboration with the patient and the utilization of appropriate equipment. Although remote assessments have limitations compared to in-person evaluations, they can still provide valuable information [15].

13.4.2 Evaluation

Guide the patient to expose their upper arm and place the blood pressure cuff on it. The lower edge of the cuff should be about 1 inch above the elbow crease. Ensure the tubing is aligned with the brachial artery. Instruct the patient to turn on the blood pressure monitor and follow the device's prompts to start the measurement. Advise the patient to remain still and refrain from talking during the measurement. Recommend taking multiple readings for accuracy, allowing a brief rest period between measurements.

13.4.3 Warning Signs

Unusual symptoms: patients may describe dizziness, lightheadedness, shortness of breath, or chest discomfort during or after the measurement. These symptoms could indicate underlying health issues that need immediate attention.

13.5 Pulse Taps

13.5.1 Introduction

The accuracy of the self-measured radial pulse has been investigated by Suzuki et al. in a population of 496 nonmedical participants (schoolteachers) between 2016 and 2018. The authors reported that nonmedical persons showed high accuracy in detecting and measuring respiration and radial pulse, although they did not accurately determine radial pulse strength for the early recognition of cardiopulmonary arrest [16].

13.5.2 Evaluation

To guide a patient in remote pulse tap assessment, consider the following steps [17]:

1. Positioning and comfort: instruct the patient to sit or lie down in a comfortable position. If possible, have them rest their arm on a flat surface, such as a table or their lap.
2. Locating the pulse: guide the patient on how to locate their pulse on their wrist, neck, or another location. Common pulse points include the following:
   (a) Radial pulse (wrist): instruct the patient to place the index and middle fingers on the palm side of the wrist, just below the base of the thumb.
   (b) Carotid pulse (neck): place the fingers on the side of the neck, just below the jawline and to the side of the windpipe.
3. Light pressure: advise the patient to apply gentle, consistent pressure with their fingers to feel the pulse. Pressing too hard can compress the blood vessels and affect the accuracy of the pulse reading.
4. Counting the pulse: instruct the patient to count the number of beats they feel in a specific time period, usually for 1 min. Alternatively, they might be asked to say "tap" each time they feel the pulse. The number of "taps" must then be counted while keeping track of the time.

5. Focus on regular rhythm: encourage the patient to focus on the rhythm of their pulse and count the beats in a regular pattern. If the rhythm is irregular, they should mention it during the evaluation.
6. Use a timer or clock: suggest using a timer, clock, or the second hand of a watch to accurately measure the pulse for the desired time period.

13.5.3 Warning Signs

1. *Irregular rhythm.*
2. *Weak or thready pulse.*
3. *Pulsus paradoxus:* a significant decrease in pulse strength during inhalation may be a sign of severe respiratory distress or cardiac tamponade.
4. *Pulsus alternans:* regular alternation of strong and weak pulses may suggest severe left ventricular dysfunction.
5. *Excessively fast or slow change in pulse tap:* abrupt changes during the assessment may indicate underlying nervous system dysfunction.
6. *Pain or discomfort during assessment.*
7. *Severe dizziness or fainting:* if the patient experiences severe dizziness or fainting during or immediately after pulse assessment, it may indicate a drop in blood pressure or other cardiovascular issues.

13.6 Sit–Stand Test

13.6.1 Introduction

Performing the sit–stand test (STS) during a remote consultation can be a useful way to assess a patient's respiratory function and functional capacity. The sit–stand test evaluates how well a person can perform repetitive sit-to-stand movements, which can provide insights into their potential respiratory limitations cardiovascular fitness and lower body strength [18]. Being a validated measure of the functional outcome in COPD patient, the STS test could also be considered a surrogate for the walking test [19–21].

The median number of repetitions ranged from 50/min (25–75th percentile 41–57/min) in young men and 47/min (39–55/min) in young women aged 20–24 years to 30/min (25–37/min) in older men and 27/min (22–30/min) in older women aged 75–79 years [22].

13.6.2 Evaluation

To guide the patient in performing a correct STS consider the following steps [17]:

1. Clear the space: ensure the patient has a safe and open area to perform the test. The space should be free from obstacles and provide enough room for the patient to stand and sit without any hindrance.
2. Chair setup: instruct the patient to sit on a sturdy chair with their feet flat on the floor, shoulder-width apart. The chair height should be standard, allowing their knees to form a 90-degree angle when seated.
3. Check SpO_2 of the resting patient.
4. Demonstration: perform a demonstration of the sit-stand test for the patient to observe the correct technique. Emphasize the importance of maintaining good posture and breathing throughout the test.
5. Instructions: provide clear instructions on how to perform the STS:
   (a) Start in a seated position with both feet flat on the floor and hands resting on the thighs or crossed over the chest.
   (b) Use their arms, if necessary, for balance and support, but encourage them to rely on their lower body strength to stand up.
   (c) Rise from the chair to a full standing position.
   (d) Return to the seated position in a controlled manner.
6. Test rounds: have the patient perform the sit-stand test for a specific duration, such as for 1 min. During this time, the patient should complete as many sit-to-stand repetitions as they can comfortably manage.
7. Check SpO_2 of the patient soon after STS has been concluded.

13.6.3 Warning Signs

1. *$SpO_2 \leq 90\%$ or desaturation $\geq 4\%$* needs a referral to secondary care [23].
2. *SpO_2 fluctuations*: significant fluctuations in SpO_2 levels ($\geq 4\%$) during the test, especially if they occur rapidly and repeatedly, can be concerning and warrant further evaluation.
3. *Inability to complete the test for excessive respiratory distress.*
4. *Prolonged recovery of SpO_2:* after completing the sit-stand test, if the individual's SpO_2 levels take an extended period to return to baseline (namely more than 5 min), it may suggest delayed recovery and impaired cardiovascular function.

13.7 Breathing Pattern

13.7.1 Introduction

During remote consultation, healthcare providers can carefully observe the patient's breathing pattern, chest movements, and use of accessory muscles. Patients can also be asked to take a deep breath and then cough to provide additional insights into lung function and potential airway obstruction [24].

13.7.2 Evaluation

To assess breathing, consider the following steps:

1. Ask the patient to sit in a comfortable position with their back straight and shoulders relaxed. Make sure there are no obstructions to their chest or abdomen that could affect breathing.
2. Pay attention to the following aspects:
   (a) Breathing depth: observe whether the patient's breathing is shallow or deep.
   (b) Breathing rhythm: note the regularity and rhythm of their breaths. Look for any irregularities, such as rapid, slow, or irregular breathing patterns.
   (c) Chest versus abdominal breathing: observe whether the patient predominantly uses chest or abdominal breathing.
   (d) Use of accessory muscles: look for signs of increased effort, such as the use of neck, shoulder, or rib muscles during breathing and increased flaring nostrils [25, 26].

13.7.3 Warning Signs

During a remote consultation focused on breathing pattern assessment, it is important to monitor for signs that could indicate underlying respiratory issues or the need for immediate referral to emergency department. Here are some warning signs to address:

1. *Rapid or labored breathing:* rapid breathing (tachypnea) or labored breathing (dyspnea) involving accessory muscles are highly suggestive of a lung-related issue and need direct medical evaluation.
2. *Changes in breathing pattern:* a sudden change in breathing pattern, such as shallow breathing becoming deep or vice versa, could signal distress and should be referred to the emergency department.
3. *Unusual breathing sounds:* wheezing, crackling, rattling, or other abnormal sounds heard during breathing might indicate conditions such as asthma, bronchitis, or pneumonia.
4. *Frequent coughing*: frequent or persistent coughing during breathing assessment, especially if it is accompanied by sputum production, could indicate bronchial inflammation and lung restriction.
5. *Chest pain or tightness:* chest pain or tightness associated with breathing might point to issues indicating pleural involvement such as pleuritis, pulmonary embolism, and pneumonia.
6. *Sudden dizziness or confusion*: feeling lightheaded, dizzy, or confused in conjunction with breathing difficulties could suggest inadequate oxygenation.
7. *Excessive fatigue during breathing.*

13.8 Breathlessness

13.8.1 Introduction

Dyspnea is a debilitating symptom that affects the quality of life [27]. However, the mechanisms of dyspnea remain not completely understood, being a subjective experience whose objective measurements still challenge clinicians. Further, like reports of pain, the description of dyspnea may be influenced by cultural and linguistic factors [28, 29]. Quantifying breathlessness during a remote consultation can be even more challenging, but there are several tools and scales that can help healthcare professionals to assess the severity of breathlessness experienced by patients [30, 31]. These tools rely on patient-reported outcomes and subjective assessments. Commonly used tools to quantify breathlessness are as follows:

1. Modified Borg scale: the modified Borg scale is a simple numerical scale that allows patients to rate their perceived breathlessness on a scale from 0 to 10, with 0 indicating no breathlessness and 10 indicating the most severe breathlessness. This scale is often used during exercise testing or other activities that induce breathlessness [32].
2. Medical Research Council (MRC) dyspnea scale: the MRC dyspnea scale is commonly used to assess breathlessness in patients with chronic respiratory conditions. It categorizes breathlessness into five levels based on how activities affect the patient's breathing [33].
3. Baseline dyspnea index (BDI) and transition dyspnea index (TDI): these indices assess the impact of breathlessness on various activities and also measure changes in breathlessness over time. BDI focuses on baseline breathlessness, while TDI assesses changes after interventions [34].

An objective variable to use and monitor that reflects the real respiratory effort experienced by the patient may help healthcare providers identify patients at major risk for respiratory deterioration. Recent studies have shown how the real-time noninvasive assessment of nasal pressure is and can predict the clinical evolution of patients with hypoxic respiratory failure, being significantly correlated with perceived dyspnea [25, 26]. Further studies on nasal pressure manometry may warrant an easy-to-use tool to quantify breathlessness in an objective manner.

13.8.2 Evaluation

Assessing the presence of dyspnea (shortness of breath) by asking a patient to complete full sentences can provide valuable insights into their breathing difficulties. This method is often used to gauge the impact of breathlessness on daily activities. The following steps indicate how to perform this assessment:

1. Ask the patient to speak: instruct the patient to speak full sentences about a specific topic, such as their recent activities or interests. Encourage them to speak naturally and without rushing.
2. Observe and listen: as the patient speaks, closely observe their breathing pattern, rhythm, and any signs of breathlessness. Listen for pauses, gasping for breath, or other signs that the patient is struggling to complete sentences.
3. Assessing effort and distress: pay attention to the patient's facial expressions, body language, and any signs of effort or distress while speaking. Note if the patient appears fatigued, pauses frequently, or takes shallow breaths during the activity.
4. Ask about perceived difficulty: after the patient has completed a few sentences, ask them how difficult it was for them to speak without becoming breathless. Using tools to quantify breathlessness during remote consultations requires clear instructions for patients and effective communication. Describe each tool by illustrating the level of breathlessness and then ask the patient to rate their breathlessness based on their perception during specific activities or at rest (Borg and BDI), to identify the level that best matches their current breathlessness (MRC) and to assess changes in breathlessness after an intervention (TDI).

13.8.3 Special Conditions

For COPD patients, besides Borg, MRC, and BDI/TDI, tools such as the COPD Assessment Test (CAT) and the Breathlessness, Cough, and Sputum Scale (BCSS) are commonly used to assess breathlessness and overall health status.

1. CAT: while primarily used to assess overall health status in COPD patients, the CAT questionnaire includes an item on breathlessness. Patients rate the impact of breathlessness on their daily life [35].
2. BCSS is used to assess and quantify the impact of chronic cough and sputum production on patients' lives. It includes items related to breathlessness [36].

13.8.4 Warning Signs

1. *Inability to complete a full sentence.*
2. *A sudden increase in Borg or MRC* scale rating during a specific activity or exercise compared to previous assessments.
3. *Borg ratings 8–10 and MRC rating 3–5* for mild activities.
4. *Rapid deterioration of baseline BDI* scores over a short period.
5. *CAT scores rating above 20–25.*

13.9 Body Peripheries

13.9.1 Introduction

Assessing general physical appearance as part of the evaluation of the respiratory system during a remote consultation involves observing physical indicators that could provide insights into the patient's overall health and potential respiratory or circulatory issues.

13.9.2 Evaluation

1. *Clubbing of fingers*: ask the patient to extend their arms and fingers in front of the camera. Observe the angle between the nail bed and the fingertip. Clubbing (widening and rounding) of fingertips might indicate chronic respiratory conditions [37].
2. *Cyanosis and pallor*: observe the patient's lips, nail beds, and the skin around their mouth for cyanosis (bluish discoloration) or pallor (paleness), which could suggest poor oxygenation or circulatory issues.
3. *Neck veins*: ask the patient to tilt their head slightly to the side to expose their neck. Observe the jugular venous pulsations, if visible. Elevated jugular venous pressure may indicate fluid overload.
4. *Capillary refill*: ask the patient to hold their hand at heart level for a few seconds and then press on a fingernail. Release and observe the speed of capillary refill, which should occur within 2 s.
5. *Peripheral edema*: instruct the patient to show their hands and arms to the camera. Look for signs of peripheral edema, such as swelling in the hands, arms, or fingers.

13.10 Significance of Telemonitoring in Patients with Chronic Respiratory Disease

13.10.1 Introduction

Remote consultation holds profound significance in the care and management of patients grappling with chronic respiratory diseases. Chronic respiratory conditions, such as chronic obstructive pulmonary disease (COPD) and asthma, necessitate vigilant monitoring to ensure timely intervention and optimal management. Telemonitoring leverages technology to remotely observe patients' vital signs, oxygen levels, symptoms, medication adherence, and device usage. This real-time data transmission facilitates healthcare professionals in making informed decisions, tailoring treatment plans, and detecting early signs of exacerbations.

13.10.2 Pharmacological Treatment Adherence

Poor adherence to inhaler therapy in patients with asthma and COPD can lead to increased access to the emergency room and hospitalization rates with consequent deaths, worsening outcomes, and increasing costs [38, 39]. Further, guidelines on the management of patients with asthma highlight the importance of assessing compliance in uncontrolled asthma before proceeding to upgrade pharmacological therapy [40, 41]. As causes of low adherence are complex, targeted interventions are required. Digital health technologies and telemonitoring might contribute to improving personalized patient care. In this scenario, electronic methods might be a helpful tool to enhance adherence to inhaler drugs and include several options such as electronic monitoring devices (EMD) and mHealth (text messaging services) [38]. EMD records daily usage of the inhaler and showed the most promising results in terms of adherence.[4] Electronic devices are connected to the inhaler (such as smart inhaler, propeller health, and aero chamber) and transmit details on drug usage to a smartphone [38, 42].

The use of EMD proved to be feasible and might lead potential improvement in inhaler technique up to 30% [42]. Other clinical interventions include mHealth and message services with the aim of sending educational messages and reminders of therapy.

Telemedicine has proved to be useful in follow up visits, especially in patients living in remote areas. A study by Portnoy et al. compared 169 children residing in two remote locations offering telemedicine and in person consultation demonstrating a comparable grade of asthma control in the two groups [1]. A recent Cochrane analysis by Chan demonstrated that digital interventions may result in a significant increase in adherence (low certainty evidence) and might reduce asthma exacerbations; however, further studies are needed to explore the benefit–cost ratio [43].

13.10.3 Long-Term Home Ventilation

Telemonitoring might also find its application in patients with long-term home noninvasive ventilation. Patients affected by various respiratory conditions can benefit from the use of home ventilation including neuromuscular diseases and COPD [44]. Monitoring noninvasive ventilation (NIV) usage can help in evaluating compliance and hours of application; it might also contribute to early detection of issues such as asynchronies, unintentional leaks, and upper airway obstruction that affect the quality of ventilation [45]. As NIV requires at least 5 h of usage to be effective in COPD patients, the assessment of daily usage is the easiest way to monitor NIV compliance [46]. Daily usage is an easy screening tool that does not require special training of the operator to investigate compliance and might suggest a need for settings change. However, it only gives an approximative information on quantity of usage. Since it cannot investigate all the reasons for a reduction in usage (e.g., asynchronies), it might not be sufficient for accurate and thorough monitoring. An interpretation of pressure and flow of waveforms can help in examining upper airway obstructions and patient–ventilator asynchronies. Moreover, telemonitoring might also detect the onset of air leaks, thus forecasting the interface deterioration. Telemonitoring of patients under home NIV could include nocturnal pulse oximetry and capnography, which can assess precisely nocturnal exchanges and possible persistence of undetected hypoventilation in patient with normal daily gas exchanges [47].

Telemonitoring of ventilator usage has reduced access to healthcare utilization in patients with neuromuscular disease on long-term home ventilation (e.g., patients with amyotrophic lateral sclerosis) [48, 49]. Whereas a benefit in the reduction of hospitalizations for acute exacerbation of COPD has been demonstrated only for long-term home oxygen, some studies have suggested a reduction in acute exacerbations when home NIV usage is frequently assessed [50]. In this line, larger studies are necessary to understand the potential role and the extent of benefits in telemonitoring home NIV in patients with COPD.

13.11 Conclusions

The comprehensive approach to remote assessment of respiratory and cardiovascular diseases is transforming patient outcomes, particularly for those managing chronic conditions. By integrating detailed patient history with advanced remote technologies and structured patient guidance on self-monitoring practices, healthcare providers can gather critical data at a distance and intervene at the earliest indication of concern. This approach not only facilitates timely detection and treatment of emerging health issues but also enables a continuity of care that minimizes the likelihood of hospital admissions and supports optimized long-term management.

Remote consultations have proven effective in enabling ongoing monitoring of vital metrics such as respiratory rate, heart rate, blood oxygen saturation, and blood pressure. By equipping patients with wearable devices and guiding them in symptom self-assessment, healthcare professionals can gain insights that were once only accessible through in-person visits. This data empowers clinicians to provide personalized interventions and detect early changes in a patient's condition before they progress, reducing the need for emergency interventions and enhancing overall quality of care. In this line, integrating telemonitoring into chronic condition management provides an essential structure for ensuring adherence to treatments, particularly in patients with respiratory diseases like COPD and asthma, where medication and ventilation adherence directly impact disease progression. Remote monitoring enables tracking of daily habits and therapeutic compliance, alerting providers to any deviations that may signal declining health or the need for treatment adjustments. This dynamic feedback loop not only enhances a proactive approach to healthcare but also builds a stronger, more collaborative relationship between patients and their care teams, promoting greater patient engagement and self-efficacy.

The future of remote assessment holds the promise of expanded capabilities, including the potential for predictive algorithms to anticipate complications before they arise. As technology continues to advance, remote monitoring will increasingly allow for a model of care that rebuilds patient management from reactive interventions to proactive, preventive healthcare.

Conflict of Interest Disclosure Roberto Tonelli, MD, PhD.

Respiratory Intermediate Care Unit, University Hospital of Modena, Modena, Italy.

RT declares patent N. 102021000007478 "APPARATO PER IL RILEVAMENTO ED IL MONITORAGGIO DELLA PRESSIONE NASALE" released on March 28th 2023 by the Italian Ministry of Enterprises and Made in Italy.

RT is co-founder of IREC ltd (VAT 02959080355), Reggio Emilia (Italy).

RT received travel support and fees from GSK, SEDA, Guidotti, United HealthCare Services.

Giulia Bruzzi, MD,

Respiratory Intermediate Care Unit, University Hospital of Modena, Modena, Italy.

GB declares no conflict of interest.

Alessandro Marchioni, MD, PhD.

Diagnostic and Interventional Bronchoscopy, University Hospital of Modena, Modena, Italy.

AM declares patent N. 102021000007478 "APPARATO PER IL RILEVAMENTO ED IL MONITORAGGIO DELLA PRESSIONE NASALE" released on March 28th 2023 by the Italian Ministry of Enterprises and Made in Italy.

AM is co-founder of IREC ltd (VAT 02959080355), Reggio Emilia (Italy).

Enrico Clini, MD, PhD.

Head of the Respiratory Disease Unit, University Hospital of Modena, Modena, Italy.

EC declares patent N. 102021000007478 "APPARATO PER IL RILEVAMENTO ED IL MONITORAGGIO DELLA PRESSIONE NASALE" released on March 28th 2023 by the Italian Ministry of Enterprises and Made in Italy.

EC is co-founder of IREC ltd (VAT 02959080355), Reggio Emilia (Italy).

References

1. Portnoy JM, Waller M, De Lurgio S, Dinakar C. Telemedicine is as effective as in-person visits for patients with asthma. Ann Allergy Asthma Immunol. 2016;117(3):241–5.
2. Ali M, Elsayed A, Mendez A, Savaria Y, Sawan M. Contact and remote breathing rate monitoring techniques: a review. IEEE Sensors J. 2021;21(13):14569–86.
3. Bae S, Borac S, Emre Y, Wang J, Wu J, Kashyap M, et al. Prospective validation of smartphone-based heart rate and respiratory rate measurement algorithms. Commun Med. 2022;2(1):40.
4. Hill A, Kelly E, Horswill MS, Watson MO. The effects of awareness and count duration on adult respiratory rate measurements: an experimental study. J Clin Nurs. 2018;27(3–4):546–54.
5. Rodríguez-Molinero A, Narvaiza L, Ruiz J, Gálvez-Barrón C. Normal respiratory rate and peripheral blood oxygen saturation in the elderly population. J Am Geriatr Soc. 2013;61(12):2238–40.
6. Fleming S, Thompson M, Stevens R, Heneghan C, Plüddemann A, Maconochie I, et al. Normal ranges of heart rate and respiratory rate in children from birth to 18 years of age: a systematic review of observational studies. Lancet. 2011;377(9770):1011–8.
7. Buekers J, Theunis J, De Boever P, Vaes AW, Koopman M, Janssen EV, et al. Wearable finger pulse oximetry for continuous oxygen saturation measurements during daily home routines of patients with Chronic Obstructive Pulmonary Disease (COPD) over one week: observational study. JMIR Mhealth Uhealth. 2019;7(6):e12866.

8. Theurl F, Schreinlechner M, Sappler N, Toifl M, Dolejsi T, Hofer F, et al. Smartwatch-derived heart rate variability: a head-to-head comparison with the gold standard in cardiovascular disease. Eur Heart J Digit Health. 2023;4(3):155–64.
9. Jiang Y, Spies C, Magin J, Bhosai SJ, Snyder L, Dunn J. Investigating the accuracy of blood oxygen saturation measurements in common consumer smartwatches. Rush B, editor. PLOS Digit Health. 2023;2(7):e0000296.
10. Louie A, Feiner JR, Bickler PE, Rhodes L, Bernstein M, Lucero J. Four types of pulse oximeters accurately detect hypoxia during low perfusion and motion. Anesthesiology. 2018;128(3):520–30.
11. Nitzan M, Romem A, Koppel R. Pulse oximetry: fundamentals and technology update. Med Devices Evid Res. 2014;7:231.
12. Jubran A. Pulse oximetry. Crit Care. 2015;19(1):272.
13. Spodick DH, Raju P, Bishop RL, Rifkin RD. Operational definition of normal sinus heart rate. Am J Cardiol. 1992;69(14):1245–6.
14. Palatini P. Need for a revision of the normal limits of resting heart rate. Hypertension. 1999 Feb;33(2):622–5.
15. Paterson C, Jack E, McKinstry B, Whyte S, Denison FC, Cheyne H. Qualitative evaluation of rapid implementation of remote blood pressure self-monitoring in pregnancy during Covid-19. Buttigieg SC, editor. PLoS One. 2023;18(3):e0278156.
16. Suzuki K, Sakaniwa R, Endo N, Kubota M, Nakazawa M, Narikawa K, et al. Accuracy of breathing and radial pulse assessment by non-medical persons: an observational cross-sectional study. Sci Rep. 2023;13(1):1800.
17. Avolio AP, Butlin M, Walsh A. Arterial blood pressure measurement and pulse wave analysis–their role in enhancing cardiovascular assessment. Physiol Meas. 2010;31(1):R1–47.
18. Vaidya T, De Bisschop C, Beaumont M, Ouksel H, Jean V, Dessables F, et al. Is the 1-minute sit-to-stand test a good tool for the evaluation of the impact of pulmonary rehabilitation? Determination of the minimal important difference in COPD. Int J Chron Obstruct Pulmon Dis. 2016;11:2609–16.
19. Ozalevli S, Ozden A, Itil O, Akkoclu A. Comparison of the Sit-to-Stand Test with 6min walk test in patients with chronic obstructive pulmonary disease. Respir Med. 2007;101(2):286–93.
20. Jones SE, Kon SSC, Canavan JL, Patel MS, Clark AL, Nolan CM, et al. The five-repetition sit-to-stand test as a functional outcome measure in COPD. Thorax. 2013;68(11):1015–20.
21. Fernandes AL, Neves I, Luís G, Camilo Z, Cabrita B, Dias S, et al. Is the 1-minute sit-to-stand test a good tool to evaluate exertional oxygen desaturation in chronic obstructive pulmonary disease? Diagnostics. 2021;11(2):159.
22. Strassmann A, Steurer-Stey C, Lana KD, Zoller M, Turk AJ, Suter P, et al. Population-based reference values for the 1-min sit-to-stand test. Int J Public Health. 2013;58(6):949–53.
23. Núñez-Cortés R, Rivera-Lillo G, Arias-Campoverde M, Soto-García D, García-Palomera R, Torres-Castro R. Use of sit-to-stand test to assess the physical capacity and exertional desaturation in patients post COVID-19. Chron Respir Dis. 2021;18:147997312199920.
24. Boulding R, Stacey R, Niven R, Fowler SJ. Dysfunctional breathing: a review of the literature and proposal for classification. Eur Respir Rev. 2016;25(141):287–94.
25. Tonelli R, Cortegiani A, Marchioni A, Fantini R, Tabbì L, Castaniere I, et al. Nasal pressure swings as the measure of inspiratory effort in spontaneously breathing patients with de novo acute respiratory failure. Crit Care. 2022;26(1):70.
26. Tonelli R, Cortegiani A, Fantini R, Tabbì L, Castaniere I, Bruzzi G, et al. Accuracy of nasal pressure swing to predict failure of high-flow nasal oxygen in patients with acute hypoxemic respiratory failure. Am J Respir Crit Care Med. 2023;207(6):787–9.
27. Laviolette L, Laveneziana P. on behalf of the ERS Research Seminar Faculty. Dyspnoea: a multidimensional and multidisciplinary approach. Eur Respir J. 2014;43(6):1750–62.
28. Cortegiani A, Crimi C, Noto A, Helviz Y, Giarratano A, Gregoretti C, et al. Effect of high-flow nasal therapy on dyspnea, comfort, and respiratory rate. Crit Care. 2019;23(1):201.

29. Vilaça M, Aragão I, Cardoso T, Dias C, Cabral-Campello G. The role of noninvasive ventilation in patients with "do not intubate" order in the emergency setting. Staffieri F, editor. PLoS One. 2016;11(2):e0149649.
30. Barros-Leite BRAF, Lima MRDO, Caminha M, Santos K, Cunha CBCD, De Andrade LB. Short-term functional changes after hospital discharge by COVID-19 through teleconsultation at a reference service in Northeast Brazil: a cross-sectional study. J Med Virol. 2022;94(3):994–1000.
31. Greenhalgh T, Thompson P, Weiringa S, Neves AL, Husain L, Dunlop M, et al. What items should be included in an early warning score for remote assessment of suspected COVID-19? Qualitative and Delphi study. BMJ Open. 2020;10(11):e042626.
32. Kendrick KR, Baxi SC, Smith RM. Usefulness of the modified 0-10 Borg scale in assessing the degree of dyspnea in patients with COPD and asthma. J Emerg Nurs. 2000;26(3):0216–22.
33. Bestall JC, Paul EA, Garrod R, Garnham R, Jones PW, Wedzicha JA. Usefulness of the Medical Research Council (MRC) dyspnoea scale as a measure of disability in patients with chronic obstructive pulmonary disease. Thorax. 1999;54(7):581–6.
34. Witek TJ, Mahler DA. Minimal important difference of the transition dyspnoea index in a multinational clinical trial. Eur Respir J. 2003;21(2):267–72.
35. Houben-Wilke S, Janssen DJA, Franssen FME, Vanfleteren LEGW, Wouters EFM, Spruit MA. Contribution of individual COPD assessment test (CAT) items to CAT total score and effects of pulmonary rehabilitation on CAT scores. Health Qual Life Outcomes. 2018;16(1):205.
36. McCarroll ML, Pohle-Krauza RJ, Volsko TA, Martin JL, Krauza ML. Use of the Breathlessness, Cough, and Sputum Scale (BCSS©) in pulmonary rehabilitation§. Open Respir Med J. 2013;7(1):1–5.
37. Sarkar M, Mahesh D, Madabhavi I. Digital clubbing. Lung India. 2012;29(4):354.
38. Almutairi M, Marriott JF, Mansur A. Effect of monitoring adherence to regular inhaled corticosteroid (ICS) alone or in combination with a long-acting β2-agonist (LABA) using electronic methods on asthma outcomes: a narrative systematic review. BMJ Open. 2023;13(8):e074127.
39. Van De Hei SJ, Kim CH, Honkoop PJ, Sont JK, Schermer TRJ, MacHale E, et al. Long-term cost-effectiveness of digital inhaler adherence technologies in difficult-to-treat asthma. J Allergy Clin Immunol Pract. 2023;11:3064. S221321982300716X
40. Jansen EM, van de Hei SJ, Dierick BJH, Kerstjens HAM, Kocks JWH, van Boven JFM. Global burden of medication non-adherence in chronic obstructive pulmonary disease (COPD) and asthma: a narrative review of the clinical and economic case for smart inhalers. J Thorac Dis. 2021 Jun;13(6):3846–64.
41. Global Initiative for Asthma – GINA [Internet]. [cited 2023 Sep 4]. 2023 GINA Main Report. Available from: https://ginasthma.org/2023-gina-main-report/
42. Dierick BJH, Achterbosch M, Eikholt AA, Been-Buck S, Klemmeier T, Van De Hei SJ, et al. Electronic monitoring with a digital smart spacer to support personalized inhaler use education in patients with asthma: the randomized controlled OUTERSPACE trial. Respir Med. 2023;218:107376.
43. Chan A, Simoni AD, Wileman V, Holliday L, Newby CJ, Chisari C, et al. Digital interventions to improve adherence to maintenance medication in asthma. Cochrane Database Syst Rev [Internet]. 2022; [cited 2023 Sep 8];2022(6). Available from: https://www.readcube.com/articles/10.1002%2F14651858.cd013030.pub2
44. Ergan B, Oczkowski S, Rochwerg B, Carlucci A, Chatwin M, Clini E, et al. European Respiratory Society guidelines on long-term home non-invasive ventilation for management of COPD. Eur Respir J. 2019;54(3):1901003.
45. Arnal JM, Oranger M, Gonzalez-Bermejo J. Monitoring Systems in Home Ventilation. J Clin Med. 2023;12(6):2163.
46. Struik FM, Lacasse Y, Goldstein RS, Kerstjens HAM, Wijkstra PJ. Nocturnal noninvasive positive pressure ventilation in stable COPD: a systematic review and individual patient data meta-analysis. Respir Med. 2014;108(2):329–37.

47. Georges M, Nguyen-Baranoff D, Griffon L, Foignot C, Bonniaud P, Camus P, et al. Usefulness of transcutaneous PCO2 to assess nocturnal hypoventilation in restrictive lung disorders. Respirology. 2016;21(7):1300–6.
48. Réginault T, Bouteleux B, Wibart P, Mathis S, Le Masson G, Pillet O, et al. At-home noninvasive ventilation initiation with telemonitoring in amyotrophic lateral sclerosis patients: a retrospective study. ERJ Open Res. 2023;9(1):00438–2022.
49. Pinto A, Almeida JP, Pinto S, Pereira J, Oliveira AG, De Carvalho M. Home telemonitoring of non-invasive ventilation decreases healthcare utilisation in a prospective controlled trial of patients with amyotrophic lateral sclerosis. J Neurol Neurosurg Psychiatry. 2010;81(11):1238–42.
50. Vitacca M, Paneroni M, Grossetti F, Ambrosino N. Is there any additional effect of tele-assistance on long-term care programmes in hypercapnic COPD patients? A retrospective study. COPD J Chronic Obstr Pulm Dis. 2016;13(5):576–82.

Remote Cardiovascular Consultations: Bridging Distances in Primary Care

14

Marco Solari, Alberto Vaona, Francesca Menichetti, Vildan Mevsim, Hans Heguia, Yasemin Özkaya, and Fiona Ecarnot

Abbreviations

BP	Blood pressure
ECG	Electrocardiogram
ED	Emergency department
GPs	General practitioners
HCPs	Healthcare providers
ILR	Implantable loop recorder

M. Solari (✉) · F. Menichetti
Cardiology Unit, Azienda USL Centro, S. Giuseppe Hospital, Empoli, FI, Italy
e-mail: solari.m@tiscali.it; marco.solari@uslcentro.toscana.it; francesca.menichetti@uslcentro.toscana.it

A. Vaona
ULSS 9 Scaligera, Primary Care, Verona, Italy

Italian Telemedicine Society, Verona, Italy

V. Mevsim · Y. Özkaya
Department of Family Medicine, Faculty of Medicine, University of Dokuz Eylul, Izmir, Turkey
e-mail: vildan.mevsim@deu.edu.tr

H. Heguia
PhD Candidate in AI, Member WONCA Working Party – eHealth, Member Dansk Selskab for Almen Medicine and Dansk Selskab for Digital Sundhed, Member SEMERGEN Working Party IT and Digital Health, Prof. Col. Master eHealth Universitat Oberta de Catalunya, Barcelona, Spain
e-mail: heguia@uoc.edu

F. Ecarnot
SINERGIES, University of Franche-Comté, Besançon, France

Department of Cardiology, University Hospital Besançon, Besançon, France
e-mail: fiona.caulfield@besancon-cardio.org

J. Demurtas (ed.), *Remote Consultation in Primary Care*, TELe-Health,
https://doi.org/10.1007/978-3-031-89661-3_14

LHR	Likelihood ratio
LOC	Loss of consciousness
PC	Primary care
TLOC	Transient loss of consciousness

14.1 Introduction

The field of cardiovascular medicine lends itself particularly well to the use of telehealth, since many forms of cardiovascular diseases are chronic, and therefore, necessitate regular follow-up and monitoring. Risk factor monitoring is one such area that is well suited to telehealth, and virtual contact with a healthcare provider can increase patient engagement. Similarly, issues with medications and symptoms can also be dealt with in a virtual health encounter, such as checking vital signs, laboratory results, treatment compliance, up-titrating medications, deprescribing or providing lifestyle counselling for smoking cessation, diet and exercise. A plethora of applications, websites and portals exist for these purposes and make it possible for general practitioners (GPs) and other physicians to dispose of large amounts of data about their patients, in real time or asynchronously.

Despite the clear advantages, there are also a number of challenges to the use of telehealth that have been pinpointed by the recent COVID-19 pandemic and that need to be kept in mind by GPs planning to use telehealth solutions to deliver care in the primary care (PC) setting.

In the specific context of cardiovascular medicine, telehealth is useful as a form of forward-triage, whereby GPs may perform a virtual electrocardiogram (ECG) that could be forwarded to an on-call cardiologist, to enable prehospital diagnosis and activate the catheterization laboratory, where necessary. Several studies have investigated the utility of this form of collaboration. In one study in Italy, 200 GPs were equipped with a portable electrocardiograph that could transmit a 12-lead ECG to an on-call cardiologist for interactive teleconsultation [1]. It was shown that the telecardiology service thus provided had sensitivity of 97.4%, specificity of 89.5% and diagnostic accuracy of 86.9% for chest pain, and 74% of all cases could be managed by the GP alone. This underlines the utility of supportive telehealth services for forward triage, thereby minimizing unnecessary use of hospital-based services. Elsewhere, a systematic review and meta-analysis reported that telemedicine was beneficial and associated with a reduction in all-cause mortality and heart failure-related hospitalizations and mortality in patients with heart failure [2]. Rehabilitation and lifestyle interventions can also be enhanced by virtual health encounters, and nowadays, the wide availability of connected devices to monitor steps, heart rate or even glycemia can generate large amounts of data that can be used to inform telehealth visits in PC [3].

Against this background, and keeping all these issues in mind, we will now provide pointers for performing telehealth encounters in four common clinical cardiovascular situations, namely chest pain, tachycardia, dyspnoea and syncope.

14.2 Clinical Situations in Cardiovascular Disease

14.2.1 Chest Pain

GPs often deal with patients complaining of chest pain, almost always without diagnostic instruments, far from equipped health facilities and compelled to make decisions on a symptomatologic presentation often nuanced and far from the classic scenarios, with unpredictable risk that the clinical situation could precipitate at any moment.

The help that comes from most chest pain management guidelines is limited because the perspective in which they were developed is that of hospital management and they assume the availability of equipment that the PC physician context does not have.

According to NICE Guidance and ESC/AHA Guidelines, classical chest pain could be defined as discomfort in the chest and/or other areas (i.e. other chest areas, epigastric, the arms, back or mandibular) lasting longer than 15 minutes. These symptoms could be associated with nausea and vomiting, marked sweating, breathlessness or a combination of these and may be also associated with signs or symptoms of hemodynamic instability [4].

The clinical presentation is extremely variable and could include ischemic equivalent symptoms such as dyspnoea or fatigue; moreover, the discomfort is sometimes diffuse or not localized, nor positional, nor affected by movement of the region.

These symptoms, however, are not cardiac specific and can be observed in gastrointestinal, neurological, pulmonary or musculoskeletal diseases.

Finally, myocardial ischemia may present with palpitations or cardiac arrest, or even without symptoms.

The most clinical prediction rules (combinations of signs and symptoms) are intended for hospital use (HEART, TIMI) and require data that GPs cannot obtain.

In literature, two prediction rules could be applied in PC. Gencer et al.'s results have shown the combination of gender and age (2 points for age over 55 for males and 65 for females), coronary risk factors (2 points if one or more risk factors are present), history of cardiovascular disease (2 points if history is positive), pain duration (1 point if duration is greater than 60 minutes), pain characteristics (2 points if described as retrosternal), whether the pain was precipitated by physical movement (1 point if confirmed) and the absence of tenderness on palpation of the chest (1 point if no tenderness). A value of more than 3 of these clinical prediction rules indicates a very high positive likelihood ratio LHR, but also a high negative LHR, which makes the rule reliable in confirmation but not in exclusion [5].

The second rule, known as the "Marburg score," provides for the assignment of 1 point to each of these five characteristics: gender/age (over 65 for females and 55 for males), presence of known arterial disease (coronary, cerebral, peripheral), pain aggravated by physical exertion, pain not reproducible with palpation and belief of the patient that the pain is of cardiac origin [6]. Also in this case, the rule was evaluated on the cut-off of 3 which resulted in having a moderate positive likelihood ratio

(6.7) and a very low negative likelihood ratio (0.08): these data make the Marburg score very reliable especially in the phase of exclusion of the cardiac origin of the pain (element of greatest interest for the PC doctor who must decide whether or not to subject the patient to immediate tests).

Although clinical prediction rules are not mentioned in the guidelines, their use in the rapid assessment of a patient with chest pain in PC appears reasonable.

The ESC and ACCA/AHA guidelines almost completely ignore the role of the PC physician and the pre-hospital management of the patient, focusing in this regard only on the organization of the territorial system for the purpose of reducing the delay in the patient's arrival at the hospital.

In particular, the ESC guidelines state that "in most settings, a consultation with the PC physician, rather than the emergency service, increases pre-hospital delay. For this reason, the population—in case of chest pain—should be educated to call the emergency service rather than the PC doctor."

In contrast, NICE guidelines provide a number of recommendations on pre-hospital management: a summary of the recommendations in this document is provided below.

14.2.1.1 Initial Evaluation and Decision to Call Emergency Medical Systems

1. Clarify as soon as possible if the patient is in pain now or if he was in the previous 12 hours.
2. Decide if the pain may be of cardiac origin based on:
   (a) The history of pain.
   (b) Location of the pain (e.g. in the chest or in other areas such as in the back, arms or jaw).
   (c) Duration more than 15 minutes.
   (d) Related symptoms such as nausea or vomiting, profuse sweating, dyspnoea or a combination.
   (e) Hemodynamic instability (check for: SBP <90 mmHg, HR >110 bpm, impaired cognitive status).
   (f) Cardiovascular risk factors.
   (g) History of previous ischemic heart disease.
   (h) Previous tests for chest pain.
3. Do not use nitrates response as a diagnostic element.
4. Do not use the patient's gender or race as a diagnostic element.

- Immediately refer the patient to the emergency services if:
  - The pain is ongoing.
  - The pain is currently absent but has occurred within the last 12 hours, and a 12-lead resting ECG is still not available or there are electrocardiographic abnormalities.
- If there are no indications for immediate referral to the emergency services, send the patient the same day if:

  - The pain has occurred within the last 12 hours but the resting 12-lead ECG is normal.
  - The pain occurred more than 12 hours before the contact.
- Send the patient to the emergency department (ED) if the pain has resolved but there is suspicion of complications (e.g. dyspnoea) using clinical common sense to establish whether the referral should be done in emergency or during the day.
- If pain of cardiac origin is not suspected, consider other serious causes of life-threatening chest pain.

14.2.1.2 Immediate Pain Management

1. Pain control should begin as soon as possible without delaying the transfer to the ED.
2. Pain control should include, if available for the patient, the administration of short-acting nitrates. A 300 mg dose of ASA should be offered to the patient, unless an allergy to this drug is known. The administration must be reported on the report sent by the patient to the ED.
3. Do not routinely administer oxygen even if available for the patient; use oxygen only below 94% saturation with the aim of bringing the level to 94–98% (88–92% in patients with chronic respiratory failure).

14.2.1.3 Communication with the Patient

1. It is mandatory to provide the patient an explanation of the possible causes of the pain without using clinical jargon and most of all, always keeping in mind the importance of triaging, avoiding delays and providing safety netting for the patient.
2. Patient's concerns, expectations and preferences about the situation should be dealt with, without causing delay.

14.2.2 Dyspnoea

There are currently no established and validated tests for remote assessment of breathlessness in an acute PC setting. The Roth score has been validated for face-to-face assessment in hospitalized patients with suspected hypoxia; its effectiveness in PC and via telephone consultations has not yet been determined, despite its potential usefulness in remote settings [7]. A quick survey of 50 healthcare providers (HCPs) who frequently assess patients over the phone showed some varying opinions. While most clinicians rejected the use of the Roth score, which times how long it takes for a patient to take a breath while speaking, some did not agree as it has not been validated in the acute setting and could potentially lead to misleading results. However, there was consensus among respondents around the following advice [8]:

- Ask the patient to describe the problem with their breathing in their own words, and assess the ease and comfort of their speech. Ask open ended questions and listen to whether the patient can complete their sentences:

  - "How is your breathing today?"
  - "Are you so breathless that you are unable to speak more than a few words?"
  - "Are you breathing harder or faster than usual when doing nothing at all?"
  - "Are you so ill that you've stopped doing all of your usual daily activities?"
- Focus on change. A clear story of deterioration is more important than whether the patient currently feels short of breath. Ask questions such as:
  - "Is your breathing faster, slower or the same as normal?"
  - "What could you do yesterday that you can't do today?
  - "What makes you breathless now that didn't make you breathless yesterday?"
- Interpret the breathlessness in the context of the wider history and physical signs. For example, a new, audible wheeze and a verbal report of blueness of the lips in a breathless patient are concerning.
  - There is no evidence that attempts to measure a patient's respiratory rate over the phone would give an accurate reading, and experts do not use such tests. It is possible, however, to measure the respiratory rate via a good video connection. More generally, video may allow a more detailed assessment and prevent the need for an in-person visit.

Remote consultations are appropriate for conducting various tests and evaluations at home, including the use of questionnaires.

Greenhalgh et al. proposed a guideline for evaluating dyspnoea in patients during virtual consultations, which includes questions to help differentiate severely ill from mild patients. These questions are: "What didn't make you breathless yesterday, what is causing you to be breathless now?" (change in symptoms), "Are you so short of breath that you can't speak more than a few words?" (limitation of function) and "Do you have any associated symptoms or signs such as chest pain, audible wheezing, cyanosis, chills, clammy or confused feeling?" (associated symptoms and signs). They also recommend asking about any comorbidities such as asthma or cardiovascular disease [9].

Judson et al. have suggested the use of an online self-triage tool for patients with suspected COVID-19 and presenting with dyspnoea. The tool categorizes patients as "urgent" if they report symptoms such as "chest pain, severe shortness of breath, bluish lips or confusion" related to their dyspnoea complaint [10].

Kim et al. have implemented a telephone severity scoring system in patients with comorbidities like active cancer, end-stage renal disease, COPD, congestive heart failure or iatrogenic immunosuppression to recommend hospitalization [11].

Assessing dyspnoea in patients with varying degrees of severity is crucial for PC practitioners who need to make prompt and precise decisions. However, interpretation of the results should be done carefully. Most of the available tools need to be tailored to the specific population they are intended for, limiting their use in different healthcare settings. Developing a reliable and validated remote triage tool for acute respiratory disorders is essential, and more research is required in this area. The availability of an evidence-based tool for dyspnoea assessment through telemedicine will be critical in managing healthcare demand [12].

Regarding remote physical examination for cardiovascular dyspnoea, performing a physical examination by phone is nearly impossible, and it can be challenging even during a video consultation. Therefore, compromises need to be made.

During a remote consultation with video for dyspnoea in cardiovascular disease, the healthcare provider may perform a physical examination virtually by asking the patient to perform certain tasks and observing their responses. Some physical examination characteristics may be assessed during a remote consultation for dyspnoea in cardiovascular disease. This may involve inspection and asking the patient to take readings from instruments they have at home such as temperature, pulse, blood pressure (BP), blood glucose, peak expiratory flow rate and oxygen saturation [8].

During a video consultation, the healthcare provider should assess the patient's demeanour, including whether they are lying in bed or up and moving around. The provider should also observe the patient's skin features, such as flushing, pallor or cyanosis. However, it is important to note that assessing these features can be difficult if lighting is suboptimal [8].

The provider may observe the patient's breathing pattern, rate and effort. The healthcare provider can assess for any abnormal lung sounds, such as crackles or wheezing, by asking the patient to take deep breaths and cough. This can provide important information for diagnosing and managing respiratory conditions [13].

The provider may ask the patient to use a pulse oximeter to measure their oxygen saturation level. Occasionally, patients may have a home oximeter that can measure their oxygen saturation. If a healthcare professional records a reading made by the patient using such a device, it is important to note their confidence in its accuracy, particularly if the reading seems to be inconsistent with their overall assessment. By keeping accurate records of what they can and cannot see during the assessment, as well as the results of any readings taken, healthcare professionals can better monitor their patients and make informed decisions about their care [8].

A remote pulse oximeter also can be used by patients at home and data can be transmitted remotely to HCP for monitoring. This type of technology is particularly useful for patients with respiratory conditions or other illnesses that affect oxygen saturation levels in the blood. Remote pulse oximeters can help healthcare providers to monitor patients' conditions from a distance and make timely interventions if necessary [14].

Heart rate evaluation remotely can be done using various technologies such as wearable devices or smartphone applications. Wearable devices such as smartwatches can continuously monitor a patient's heart rate and send data to HCP for remote monitoring. Smartphone applications with built-in sensors can also measure heart rate by detecting changes in the colour of the patient's fingertip as blood flow changes. These technologies are particularly useful for patients with cardiovascular conditions or those at risk for heart-related issues [14].

BP monitors allow patients to monitor their BP levels at home. These devices can be used for self-monitoring and can provide valuable information for patients with hypertension or other cardiovascular conditions. Home BP monitors are available in various forms, including automatic arm cuffs, wrist cuffs and finger cuffs. The most commonly used type of home BP monitor is the automatic arm cuff, which measures BP in the upper arm [15]. Patients can take their BP readings at home and share the data with their HCP for remote monitoring. Home BP monitors are typically reliable and accurate when used correctly and can help patients to manage their BP levels effectively [15]. Some BP monitors are compatible with smart devices, allowing the device to transfer the blood pressure measurements to a computer or smartphone. These monitors offer a convenient way for patients to monitor their BP regularly, and the data can be easily shared with HCP electronically.

Smart devices for BP are wearable devices or smartphone applications that can measure and track BP readings. These devices often utilize Bluetooth or Wi-Fi technology to connect to a smartphone or other mobile device, allowing patients to track their BP readings over time and share the data with their HCP. Some of these devices can also provide additional features, such as heart rate monitoring and activity tracking. Smart devices for BP are convenient for patients who need to monitor their BP regularly, as they can provide accurate and reliable readings from the comfort of their own homes. However, it is important to note that not all smart devices for BP have been validated for accuracy and should be used with caution [16]. It is important to ensure that patients are using these devices correctly and to check their proper usage. In situations where the patient is unsure of how to use their equipment, it may be necessary to bring the physician's own device into camera view and demonstrate how it is used [8].

Moreover, new and potentially disruptive tools may play an increasingly important role in advanced cardiovascular consultations by providing remote access to real-time, high-quality patient data. These tools allow for the collection of critical metrics such as heart rate, BP and respiratory sounds, which can be reviewed by specialists even if the patient is not physically present. This ability to conduct remote examinations means patients can receive timely, accurate cardiovascular assessments from the comfort of their homes, improving access to care, reducing delays and enabling ongoing monitoring for at-risk individuals. As part of a broader telehealth ecosystem, such tools contribute to more efficient, preventive and personalized cardiovascular care.

14.2.3 Tachycardia

Monitoring of tachycardia and its treatment can be very difficult, especially in areas where there is no access to cardiology specialists. In addition, private cardiologists usually work in cities and can be expensive, including the movement of patients to these consultations. Moreover, once the diagnosis is made, follow-up is mandatory to ensure long term beneficial effects.

Faced with these problems, telemedicine is a tool that can be useful in this situation. The discussion of tachycardia and its classification is beyond the scope of this chapter, but we will discuss how telemedicine could help in the diagnosis, management and follow-up of this condition.

14.2.3.1 Emergency Management of Tachycardia

The use of a telemedicine program, especially in case of urgent patients and emergencies, must be in a structured and regulated project allowing to establish when and how to use it. Moreover, a training plan is mandatory for all the providers involved in the project to educate all the actors in play to act properly. This allows a correct diagnosis in proper time, and then correct therapeutic instructions could be provided to the correct management. In this way, the remote emergency doctor is intended as a supplement and a potentiation to the peripherical emergency doctor system and as a further structural element of the rescue service. However, it is not a substitute for the emergency doctor.

The successful application of telemedicine has been proven in many studies [17] to allow communication in rural areas where a specialist could not be found; in the case described above, patient's data, such as vital parameters, blood tests and ECGs, as well as live video of the patient can be sent to the specialist doctor so that he can think about the patient knowing almost complete amount of data and can thus decide the most appropriate treatment to follow (technical advantage).

Telemedicine is useful also in situations in which emergency systems could not reach the patients quickly. In a case report of a 33-year-old female patient who presented palpitations, chest pain and dizziness while on an international flight, the digital transmission of her vital signs and ECGs by an on-board device (Tempus IC) allowed the proper diagnosis of 220 bpm supraventricular tachycardia, which was confirmed by a doctor at the telemedicine centre. This allowed to promptly start vagal manoeuvres, placement of an intravenous line by a medical doctor on the flight and start of pharmacological chest pain management [18].

14.2.3.2 Tachycardia Monitoring at Home

Nowadays, new devices have been designed to monitor heart beats; some devices are based on electrocardiographic sensors, while others use photoplethysmography (PPG); these kinds of technique, often incorporated in smartwatches or sports bands, use an LED light emitter to enlighten the blood capillaries and calculate heart rate by measuring blood flow.

PPG-based devices allow to monitor the patient's pulse both during rest and during daily activities; moreover, proprietary algorithm allows to recognize an irregular beat that could be a surrogate for atrial fibrillation that needs to be confirmed by the ECG.

Furthermore, if it detects a change in the pulse, it could immediately notify the patient (and in some cases even to the doctor, depending on the system and the application); this could allow to inform asymptomatic patients about arrhythmic events that, when paroxysmal, could not be slipped by conventional ECG and cardiological visits. Some smartwatches may have good diagnostical detection, for example, a study shows that the Apple watch can detect the presence of atrial tachyarrhythmia in 93% of cases (showing high sensitivity and specificity) [19]. It can also adequately detect cases of atrial fibrillation, although with problems depending on where the system is placed. However, the role of asymptomatic atrial fibrillation events detected by these devices is still under debate and more studies are needed.

There are even some studies that have shown a reduction in medical visits by patients with chronic heart conditions. For example, the ALTITUDE study showed that patients with ICDs who had remote controls (based on telemedicine) had better survival rates compared with those who had hospital visits (physical) [20]. The MERLIN study also confirmed that remote controls were associated with increased survival, probably due to a better level of adherence [21].

14.2.3.3 Telemedicine in Tachycardia for Primary Care—Hospital Cardiology Service

In PC the use of telecardiology tools increases the quality and safety of work in the management of patients with cardiovascular diseases, including tachycardia. The use of telemedicine services that make it possible to perform ECGs at home is always more widely employed and appreciated [22]. Despite spending on digital monitoring tools, money is saved and the gap between primary and hospital care is reduced [23] .

Öner et al., in a study carried out in Germany, showed that telemedicine in the cardiovascular field is not better than standard-of-care, but that it did lead to a reduction in mortality, stroke, myocardial infarction and cardiac decompensation [24]. Other studies show that post-hospital telecardiology improves outcomes and reduces re-admissions or outpatient contacts in patients with heart failure, arrhythmias or implantable devices [25].

In addition, the shared use of PC and cardiology telemedicine can help to have early diagnoses not only in tachycardia but also in other cardiovascular pathologies, reducing costs and increasing the quality of life and patient satisfaction [26].

In monitoring patients in the home environment, wearable tools that document data to be evaluated by healthcare professionals are mandatory; tools such as smartwatches or pocket-ECG are even useful in the diagnosis of palpitations and tachycardia, where it has even been possible to find asymptomatic arrhythmias [27].

Telemedicine in cases of arrhythmia and tachycardia should be oriented towards diagnosis, ECG monitoring and treatment changes including emergency calls in life-threatening situations such as ventricular tachycardia or debilitating conditions like atrial fibrillation [28].

14.2.4 Syncope

14.2.4.1 Definition and Epidemiology

Syncope is a temporary loss of consciousness due to insufficient blood flow to the brain, often with spontaneous recovery. Episodes may or may not be preceded by warning signs, such as dizziness or nausea, known as prodromal symptoms. Presyncope refers to the sensations that suggest an impending syncope episode. It is a frequent concern in emergency care, accounting for approximately 6% of hospital admissions, according to surveys (72). Prevalence varies widely, affecting 15% of children and up to 23% of adults over 70 [29], particularly those with cardiovascular conditions or residing in the institutional care setting [30]. Patients with syncope are often admitted to hospital and undergo expensive investigations, many of which do not provide a definite diagnosis [31]. Although most causes of syncope are benign and require no further evaluation, there is a small subset of patients for whom a syncopal episode may herald a potentially life-threatening condition [32].

14.2.4.2 Remote Clinical Evaluation

In PC, remote assessment via telemedicine can be invaluable for initial evaluation. Collecting a comprehensive patient history—through telephonic or virtual consultation—enables clinicians to differentiate true syncope from other causes of transient loss of consciousness (TLOC). In cases where patients or witnesses can report symptoms accurately, remote consultations provide critical diagnostic insights and reduce unnecessary hospital visits. Frequent episodes within a short timeframe (days to weeks) may signal serious conditions like cardiac arrhythmias, whereas isolated events over years are typically benign. Recurrent episodes often require more in-depth evaluation, especially if multiple episodes occur in a single day, which may suggest psychogenic origins. Long-standing episodes without significant comorbidities often indicate a lower risk profile. However, recent episodes in young patients (<35 years) with structural heart concerns may warrant further investigation [33].

True syncope of any aetiology is usually brief since the loss of postural tone (and the subsequent gravitationally neutral position) generally restores brain blood flow. Longer periods of real or apparent loss of consciousness (especially if >5 minutes) suggest that the event is not syncope or is not syncope alone. A prolonged event could be syncope resulting in a fall complicated by head injury (concussion may prolong TLOC), a seizure or psychogenic pseudo-syncope (a collapse deemed secondary to a conversion reaction or dissociative episode [34]. It is important to remind also that familial associations have been observed for reflex syncope and for chronic cardiac conditions such as cardiomyopathy and channelopathy [35].

Reflex syncope can be triggered by emotional stress, pain or environmental factors. Situational syncope, which occurs after urination, coughing or eating, may indicate specific reflex syncope types, whereas syncope linked to neck movement could suggest carotid sinus syndrome, especially in older adults.

The position in which the syncope occurs is another relevant factor that must be considered: a syncope while standing or sitting often points to reflex syncope, whereas syncope occurring while supine suggests cardiac arrhythmia, necessitating urgent assessment.

Episodes occurring during exercise are especially concerning and may indicate serious heart conditions.

Warning signs such as light-headedness, nausea or visual changes often precede reflex syncope, while sudden TLOC without warning could indicate cardiac issues. Collecting details of these sensations remotely can guide the diagnostic pathway and help define time to treat and point of care. Clinical risk scores [36, 37] and clinical decision rules [38] have been developed to identify the population at the highest risk for adverse events, though those are not validated for remote assessment.

Telecardiology enables remote ECG monitoring, offering patients a convenient way to undergo assessment at home or a local clinic. Portable devices, including single-lead ECG watches, allow patients to record their heart rhythm and transmit the data to specialists for analysis. Such technology can detect serious arrhythmias and reduce diagnostic delays, improving outcomes for those at risk.

14.2.4.3 Implantable Loop Recorders

In cases of recurrent or unexplained syncope, an implantable loop recorder (ILR) may be recommended. ILRs provide continuous monitoring and enable long-term tracking, which is particularly useful for patients with infrequent but severe episodes. These devices communicate with remote monitoring systems to send alerts and detailed reports, allowing PC providers to adjust treatment plans promptly [39, 40].

14.3 Issues to Keep in Mind When Performing Telehealth for Cardiovascular Care in Primary Care

There are a range of issues that need to be kept in mind when performing virtual health encounters. The specificities of the various clinical situations that may arise in cardiovascular care are described in more detail in the sections below. However, the more general issues will be of importance in all encounters.

In terms of regulatory issues, the current regulatory landscape is sparse and disparate; there is no international consensus regarding the core features of telehealth encounters and how these may be assessed for quality. There is a lack of standardization regarding the complaints that are suitable for evaluation by telemedicine, and the data that should be collected during encounters. Data privacy must be adequately protected, and certain practitioners may need to ensure compliance with the requirements of the Health Insurance Portability and Accountability Act (HIPAA), a US law introduced in 1996 relating to the protection of sensitive patient health information against disclosure. There may also be licensing issues, which will vary between countries, and it is incumbent on every practitioner wishing to use, or already providing telehealth services to be aware of local legislation regarding the level of service, and the declaration and reimbursement of those activities. Indeed, establishing written protocols for best practices, or using available national guidelines is recommended to minimize any liability for missed or wrong diagnosis [41–43]. Different health systems will have different requirements regarding the appropriate tests or examinations to be recommended for each clinical situation in the absence of a physical examination, as in the case with virtual health encounters. Finally, provision of services to patients who are physically located overseas may be problematic in terms of jurisdiction, prescribing and reimbursement.

In terms of responsibility of the physician providing the telehealth services, it is important to be attentive to the follow-up of patients, since there is a risk of fragmentation of healthcare with telemedicine. Therefore, it is important to follow-up after a teleconsultation to ensure that the examinations prescribed were actually carried out, and the results transmitted to the appropriate HCP—either the GP who did the teleconsultation, or a relevant specialist, if required. This integrated patient flow is easier to accomplish when the patient is already known to the GP, but many consultations may be with patients who are unknown to the HCP, and there may be no immediate access available to prior health records for that patient. Building rapport is essential, especially with patients who were not previously known, and although this can consume precious time during a time-limited teleconsultation, it is nonetheless of key importance. Failure to establish rapport and trust may stymie communication and prevent accurate assessment, increasing the risk of missing a diagnosis, or misdiagnosis. The use of consumer-grade video-conferencing services like Skype or Zoom may reduce the diagnostic capabilities of the physician, since these services do not include technological enhancements designed for medical encounters, such as electronic heart monitoring. The reliability of visual inspection may also be affected by poor image quality. Physicians should also be attentive to unscrupulous patients who may be exploiting the current surge in telehealth to support drug overuse by obtaining multiple prescriptions for multiple providers. Finally, it is important to obtain confirmation of the patient's physical address, in case sudden escalation of care becomes necessary and emergency services have to be dispatched to the patient's location. This can be of particular relevant in cardiac disease.

14.4 Conclusions

Telemedicine can be particularly useful in patients with cardiovascular diseases, because of the chronic nature of many forms of cardiovascular disease, enabling long-term follow-up and monitoring. Many patients who suffer from chronic cardiac disease, such as heart failure, or arrhythmias, will be equipped with smart devices, such as home BP monitors, connected scales or watches, which can enable transmission of vital data to HCP, thus facilitating telehealth encounters. Telehealth can also enable forward triage of cardiovascular patients, enabling identification of acute, life-threatening symptoms of cardiovascular disease that requires urgent transfer to the nearest emergency department or cardiac care unit, also possibly enabling pre-activation of the catheterization laboratory, for acute ST elevation myocardial infarction, for example. Conversely, certain cardiovascular events may be more difficult to evaluate and accurately diagnose during a teleconsultation. The scenarios reviewed here, namely chest pain, dyspnoea, tachycardia and syncope, all have various possible aetiologies that it may not be possible to identify in a telehealth encounter. Accurate anamnesis and close observation of the patient's demeanour can allow the PC physician to assess the urgency of the situation, with a view to transfer if required, but may not always provide sufficient information to allow accurate etiological diagnosis. The use of clinical risk scores combined with clinical judgement can help PC physicians to make the best assessment possible with the available information. For patients with connected devices, additional clinical information may be available, if the PC physician has the necessary equipment to receive the data in a timely and secure manner.

While the remote delivery of healthcare eliminates time and costs associated with transport, is associated with increased patient satisfaction [41, 44, 45] and can give access to healthcare to people in areas that are otherwise underserved by medical facilities [41], there nonetheless remains a pressing need to define international standardization for the performance of virtual health encounters, to avoid variations in quality of care, and the effects of telehealth provision need to be documented to inform best practice.

References

1. Scalvini S, Zanelli E, Conti C, Volterrani M, Pollina R, Giordano A, et al. Assessment of pre-hospital chest pain using telecardiology. J Telemed Telecare. 2002;8(4):231–6.
2. Lin MH, Yuan WL, Huang TC, Zhang HF, Mai JT, Wang JF. Clinical effectiveness of telemedicine for chronic heart failure: a systematic review and meta-analysis. J Investig Med. 2017;65(5):899–911.
3. Jaén-Extremera J, Afanador-Restrepo DF, Rivas-Campo Y, Gómez-Rodas A, Aibar-Almazán A, Hita-Contreras F, et al. Effectiveness of telemedicine for reducing cardiovascular risk: a systematic review and meta-analysis. J Clin Med [Internet]. 2023 Jan 20 [cited 2024 Nov 28];12(3). Available from: http://www.ncbi.nlm.nih.gov/pubmed/36769487
4. Thygesen K, Alpert JS, Jaffe AS, Chaitman BR, Bax JJ, Morrow DA, et al. Fourth universal definition of myocardial infarction (2018). Eur Heart J. 2019;40(3):237–69.
5. Gencer B, Vaucher P, Herzig L, Verdon F, Ruffieux C, Bösner S, et al. Ruling out coronary heart disease in primary care patients with chest pain: a clinical prediction score. BMC Med. 2010;8:9.
6. Bösner S, Haasenritter J, Becker A, Karatolios K, Vaucher P, Gencer B, et al. Ruling out coronary artery disease in primary care: development and validation of a simple prediction rule. CMAJ. 2010;182(12):1295–300.
7. Chorin E, Padegimas A, Havakuk O, Birati EY, Shacham Y, Milman A, et al. Assessment of respiratory distress by the Roth score. Clin Cardiol. 2016;39(11):636–9.
8. Greenhalgh T, Koh GCH, Car J. Covid-19: a remote assessment in primary care. BMJ. 2020;368:m1182.
9. Greenhalgh T, Wherton J, Shaw S, Morrison C. Video consultations for covid-19. BMJ. 2020;368:m998.
10. Judson TJ, Odisho AY, Neinstein AB, Chao J, Williams A, Miller C, et al. Rapid design and implementation of an integrated patient self-triage and self-scheduling tool for COVID-19. J Am Med Inform Assoc. 2020;27(6):860–6.
11. Kim SW, Lee KS, Kim K, Lee JJ, Kim JY. A brief telephone severity scoring system and therapeutic living centers solved acute hospital-bed shortage during the COVID-19 outbreak in Daegu, Korea. J Korean Med Sci. 2020;35(15):e152.
12. Zheng Z, Peng F, Xu B, Zhao J, Liu H, Peng J, et al. Risk factors of critical & mortal COVID-19 cases: a systematic literature review and meta-analysis. J Infect. 2020;81(2):e16–25.
13. Braun SR. Respiratory rate and pattern. Clinical methods: the history, physical, and laboratory examinations [Internet]. 1990 [cited 2024 Nov 28]; Available from: http://www.ncbi.nlm.nih.gov/pubmed/21250206.

14. Alboksmaty A, Beaney T, Elkin S, Clarke JM, Darzi A, Aylin P, et al. Effectiveness and safety of pulse oximetry in remote patient monitoring of patients with COVID-19: a systematic review. Lancet Digit Health. 2022;4(4):e279–89.
15. Ringrose JS, Polley G, McLean D, Thompson A, Morales F, Padwal R. An assessment of the accuracy of home blood pressure monitors when used in device owners. Am J Hypertens. 2017;30(7):683–9.
16. Falter M, Scherrenberg M, Driesen K, Pieters Z, Kaihara T, Xu L, et al. Smartwatch-based blood pressure measurement demonstrates insufficient accuracy. Front Cardiovasc Med [Internet]. 2022 Jul 11 [cited 2024 Nov 28];9:958212. Available from: http://www.ncbi.nlm.nih.gov/pubmed/35898281
17. du Toit M, Malau-Aduli B, Vangaveti V, Sabesan S, Ray RA. Use of telehealth in the management of non-critical emergencies in rural or remote emergency departments: a systematic review. J Telemed Telecare. 2019;25(1):3–16.
18. Voerman JJ, Hoffe ME, Surka S, Alves PM. In-flight management of a supraventricular tachycardia using telemedicine. Aerosp Med Hum Perform. 2018;89(7):657–60.
19. Perez M V., Mahaffey KW, Hedlin H, Rumsfeld JS, Garcia A, Ferris T, et al. Large-scale assessment of a Smartwatch to identify atrial fibrillation. N Engl J Med [Internet]. 2019 [cited 2024 Nov 28];381(20):1909–1917. Available from: https://www.nejm.org/doi/full/10.1056/NEJMoa1901183
20. Saxon LA, Hayes DL, Gilliam FR, Heidenreich PA, Day J, Seth M, et al. Long-term outcome after ICD and CRT implantation and influence of remote device follow-up: the ALTITUDE survival study. Circulation [Internet]. 2010 [cited 2024 Nov 28];122(23):2359–2367. Available from: https://pubmed.ncbi.nlm.nih.gov/21098452/
21. Mittal S, Piccini JP, Snell J, Prillinger JB, Dalal N, Varma N. Improved survival in patients enrolled promptly into remote monitoring following cardiac implantable electronic device implantation. J Interv Card Electrophysiol [Internet]. 2016 [cited 2024 Nov 28];46(2):129. Available from: https://pmc.ncbi.nlm.nih.gov/articles/PMC4923102/
22. Vermunicht P, Grecu M, Deharo JC, Buckley CM, Palà E, Mairesse GH, et al. General practitioners' perceptions on opportunistic single-time point screening for atrial fibrillation: a European quantitative survey. Front Cardiovasc Med [Internet]. 2023 [cited 2024 Nov 28];10:1112561. Available from: http://www.ncbi.nlm.nih.gov/pubmed/36873407
23. Vodička S, Naji HF, Zelko E. The role of telecardiology in dealing with patients with cardiac rhythm disorders in family medicine – systematic review. Zdr Varst [Internet]. 2020 [cited 2024 Nov 28];59(2):108–16. Available from: http://www.ncbi.nlm.nih.gov/pubmed/32952710
24. Öner A, Dittrich H, Arslan F, Hintz S, Ortak J, Brandewiede B, et al. Comparison of telemonitoring combined with intensive patient support with standard care in patients with chronic cardiovascular disease – a randomized clinical trial. Eur J Med Res. 2023;28(1):22.
25. Molinari G, Molinari M, Di Biase M, Brunetti ND. Telecardiology and its settings of application: an update. J Telemed Telecare. 2018;24(5):373–81.
26. Mohammadzadeh N, Rezayi S, Tanhapour M, Saeedi S. Telecardiology interventions for patients with cardiovascular disease: a systematic review on characteristics and effects. Int J Med Inform. 2022:158, 104663.
27. Bieganowska K, Miszczak-Knecht M, Brzezińska M, Posadowska M, Pręgowska K, Kaszuba A, et al. Usefulness of long-term telemetric electrocardiogram monitoring in the diagnosis of tachycardia in children with a medical history of palpitations. Kardiol Pol. 2021;79(2):129–38.
28. Ghilencea LN, Chiru MR, Stolcova M, Spiridon G, Manea LM, Stănescu AMA, et al. Telemedicine: benefits for cardiovascular patients in the COVID-19 era. Front Cardiovasc Med [Internet]. 2022 [cited 2024 Nov 28];9:868635. Available from: http://www.ncbi.nlm.nih.gov/pubmed/35935629
29. Sarasin FP, Louis-Simonet M, Carballo D, Slama S, Rajeswaran A, Metzger JT, et al. Prospective evaluation of patients with syncope: a population-based study. Am J Med [Internet] 2001 [cited 2024 Nov 28];111(3):177–184. Available from: https://pubmed.ncbi.nlm.nih.gov/11530027/
30. Lipsitz LA, Wei JY, Rowe JW. Syncope in an elderly, institutionalised population: prevalence, incidence, and associated risk. QJM. 1985;55(1):45–54.

31. Disertori M, Brignole M, Menozzi C, Raviele A, Rizzon P, Santini M, et al. Management of patients with syncope referred urgently to general hospitals. Europace. 2003;5(3):283–91.
32. Quinn J, McDermott D, Stiell I, Kohn M, Wells G. Prospective validation of the San Francisco syncope rule to predict patients with serious outcomes. Ann Emerg Med. 2006;47(5):448–54.
33. Albassam OT, Redelmeier RJ, Shadowitz S, Husain AM, Simel D, Etchells EE. Did this patient have cardiac syncope?: the rational clinical examination systematic review. JAMA. 2019;321(24):2448–57.
34. Furlan R, Alciati A. Psychogenic pseudosyncope and pseudoseizure: approach and treatment. Syncope [Internet]. 2020 [cited 2024 Nov 28];135–47. Available from: https://link.springer.com/chapter/10.1007/978-3-030-44507-2_11
35. Fedorowski A, Pirouzifard M, Sundquist J, Sundquist K, Sutton R, Zöller B. Risk factors for syncope associated with multigenerational relatives with a history of syncope. JAMA Netw Open. 2021;4(3):e212521.
36. Thiruganasambandamoorthy V, Sivilotti MLA, Le Sage N, Yan JW, Huang P, Hegdekar M, et al. Multicenter emergency department validation of the Canadian syncope risk score. JAMA Intern Med. 2020;180(5):737–44.
37. Sarasin FP, Hanusa BH, Perneger T, Louis-Simonet M, Rajeswaran A, Kapoor WN. A risk score to predict arrhythmias in patients with unexplained syncope. Acad Emerg Med [Internet]. 2003 [cited 2024 Nov 28];10(12):1312–7. Available from: https://pubmed.ncbi.nlm.nih.gov/14644781/
38. Quinn JV, Stiell IG, McDermott DA, Sellers KL, Kohn MA, Wells GA. Derivation of the San Francisco syncope rule to predict patients with short-term serious outcomes. Ann Emerg Med. 2004;43(2):224–32.
39. Cheung CC, Krahn AD. Loop recorders for syncope evaluation: what is the evidence? Expert Rev Med Devices. 2016;13(11):1021–7.
40. Krahn AD, Klein GJ, Yee R, Skanes AC. Randomized assessment of syncope trial: conventional diagnostic testing versus a prolonged monitoring strategy. Circulation. 2001;104(1):46–51.
41. Takahashi EA, Schwamm LH, Adeoye OM, Alabi O, Jahangir E, Misra S, et al. An overview of telehealth in the management of cardiovascular disease: a scientific statement from the American Heart Association. Circulation. 2022;146(25):E558–68.
42. Di Lenarda A, Casolo G, Gulizia MM, Aspromonte N, Scalvini S, Mortara A, et al. The future of telemedicine for the management of heart failure patients: a Consensus Document of the Italian Association of Hospital Cardiologists (A.N.M.C.O), the Italian Society of Cardiology (S.I.C.) and the Italian Society for Telemedicine and eHealth (Digital S.I.T.). Eur Heart J Suppl [Internet] 2017 [cited 2024 Nov 26];19(Suppl D):D113–29. Available from: http://www.ncbi.nlm.nih.gov/pubmed/28751839
43. Schwamm LH, Chumbler N, Brown E, Fonarow GC, Berube D, Nystrom K, et al. Recommendations for the implementation of telehealth in Cardiovascular and stroke care: a policy statement from the American Heart Association. Circulation. 2017;135(7):e24–44.
44. Russo JE, McCool RR, Davies L. VA telemedicine: an analysis of cost and time savings. Telemed J E Health. 2016;22(3):209–15.
45. Xu T, Pujara S, Sutton S, Rhee M. Telemedicine in the management of type 1 diabetes. Prev Chronic Dis. 2018;15(1):E13.

15 Remote Consultation for Skin Complaints

Sonia Guarguagli, Sofia Acciai, and Jacopo Demurtas

15.1 Introduction

Skin conditions are a prevalent reason for consultation in primary care, with estimates suggesting that up to 15% of general practitioner consultations involve dermatological issues [1–3]. The COVID-19 pandemic has accelerated the adoption of telemedicine for remote dermatological assessments, with both patients and providers reporting high satisfaction with the convenience and accessibility of remote consultations. However, the use of telemedicine for skin disorders poses unique challenges, as the quality of clinical photos submitted by patients is often insufficient for accurate diagnosis and assessment [4]. Clinicians require high-quality images that capture the key features of skin lesions, but patients frequently struggle to take adequate photos, leading to wasted time and inefficiency in the telemedicine workflow [4].

S. Guarguagli (✉)
Family Medicine Department, ASL Città di Torino, Turin, Italy

Member of the Solidarity Commission, Medical Association of Turin, Turin, Italy

Master of Science in Health Services Management, Turin, Italy

S. Acciai
Family Medicine Department, USL Toscana Sud-Est, Arezzo, Italy

J. Demurtas
Clinical and Experimental Medicine PhD Program, University of Modena and Reggio Emilia, Modena, Italy

Family Medicine Department, USL Toscana Sud-Est, Capalbio, Italy

J. Demurtas (ed.), *Remote Consultation in Primary Care*, TELe-Health,
https://doi.org/10.1007/978-3-031-89661-3_15

In this chapter, we will review the current state of remote consultations for dermatological care in primary care, highlighting the challenges and opportunities of this rapidly evolving field.

15.2 Telemedicine in Dermatology

Knowing if a rash or something on the skin of your patients is blanching or not may be vital and dramatically change the prognosis and the triaging of that patient [5]. Luckily, it can be done even on a remote telephone consultation.

Dermatology, nevertheless, heavily relies on visual diagnosis, and that is why, telemedicine holds a unique importance in this field compared with elsewhere in medicine, with teledermatology platforms and services spreading [6].

Skin conditions are often visible, making telemedicine an ideal platform for dermatologists to assess and diagnose many skin issues.

High-resolution images and videos can provide a wealth of visual information for accurate assessments. Moreover, as technology continues to advance, and telemedicine becomes more integrated into healthcare systems, its importance in dermatology is only expected to grow, ultimately benefiting patients and healthcare providers alike. It is obvious that with the advent of remote consultation, the diagnostic and investigative aspects of dermatology have become increasingly important and that remote consultation in primary care offers convenience and accessibility to patients, but it is also important to remember that it presents challenges in accurately diagnosing: using telemedicine for dermatological consultations requires careful planning and adherence to best practices to ensure effective and secure communication between patients and dermatologists.

Patients frequently struggle to capture high-quality images of their skin conditions, leading to wasted time for both the patient and the clinician as they work to obtain usable photos [7]. To address this, researchers have developed AI-powered tools to automatically evaluate the quality of telemedicine photos and provide guidance to patients on how to improve their submissions [7]. For example, a study on an AI-based tool called "TrueImage" found that it was able to accurately assess photo quality and provide tailored feedback to patients, leading to significant improvements in subsequent photo submissions [7].

Beyond photo quality, the regulatory and legal landscape for telemedicine in dermatology varies widely between countries, with differing rules and requirements for remote consultations. Some jurisdictions have implemented new policies to facilitate the expanded use of telemedicine during the pandemic, while others maintain more restrictive guidelines [8].

A comprehensive approach to remote dermatological investigation is pivotal to ensure that patients receive accurate diagnoses and appropriate management: this short chapter of the book aims at explaining good practices and at giving suggestions that we hope can help the reader when performing a dermatological teleconsultation.

15.3 History

In addition to visual cues, obtaining a comprehensive medical history from the patient is crucial for an accurate diagnosis. Questions about the onset, progression, associated symptoms, and exposure to potential triggers can provide valuable insights. Ideally, the clinician should guide the patient through a structured interview, similar to an in-person consultation. Moreover, traditionally, telemedicine in dermatology has relied on asynchronous consultations, where the patient submits images and a medical history, and the clinician provides a diagnosis and treatment plan at a later time. However, the reliance on visual information in dermatology means that the quality and adequacy of patient-submitted images are paramount.

15.4 Take a Picture!

Photos and videos of skin lesions play a critical role in the diagnostic and assessment process for remote dermatological consultations. These visual aids can be obtained in various ways, such as during the consultation by a healthcare professional, or by the patient or a caregiver either in real time or asynchronously [5]. Capturing high-quality images and submitting them to the dermatologist or primary care provider can significantly facilitate the diagnosis and prognosis of skin lesions or rashes. To improve the efficacy of remote assessments, patients may be guided on how to capture high-quality photos of their skin condition [5].

Teledermatology platforms that incorporate AI-powered tools to automatically evaluate photo quality and provide tailored feedback to patients have demonstrated the potential to enhance the diagnostic process [7, 9].

Whether we are AI powered or not, we have to evaluate:

Features (visual, palpatory)
Distribution
Symmetry
Measures of the lesion/lesions
Blanching

It is important to obtain close-up pictures of the lesion and pictures that help identify the zone where the lesion is. Moreover, pictures should be taken in more dimension, and distant photo to help clinicians define the symmetry and distribution [5].

When evaluating a dermatological presentation or lesion, rely on pictures taken from different angles, to have an idea of it in all three dimensions: pictures taken from above may help you identifying the core features of the lesion, its symmetry, colour, and shape; pictures taken from the side, even if more difficult to take, make possible an evaluation of the height or projection of the lesion examined [5]. If possible, try to guide the patient in the assessment using landmarks rather than direction [5]. For instance, asking the patient to move the camera toward a certain part of the body may be better than just saying to move further up, right, left, and down [5].

Patients may help themselves by using objects of reference like a ruler, a coin or a pen to help visualize the size of the lesion.

15.5 Main Dermatological Scenarios

15.5.1 Rashes

To begin with, we have to say that a rash is a broad term used to describe any noticeable change in colour, texture, or appearance of skin. Rashes can manifest as redness, bumps, blisters, pustules, scaling, itching, or other alterations of the skin normal condition. They can occur for a wide range of reasons, including infections, allergies, autoimmune disorders, and irritants.

Rashes can vary greatly in appearance and severity, and they may affect different parts of the body or be localized to a specific area.

Common types of rashes seen in dermatology include contact dermatitis, atopic dermatitis (eczema), psoriasis, hives (urticaria), impetigo, ringworm (tinea), and many others, each with its own distinctive characteristics and causes.

Rashes are a common cause of dermatological consultation. The part of the body involved, the primary lesion of the dermatosis, the onset, and the spreading, even the timing of the disease, are culprits for diagnosis.

The first question is to know where the rash is: if it involves the whole body, or just an area. If it's with sharp borders, or if it fades in the healthy skin. If it's itchy or painful, or if it's not symptomatic. How it started, and how is going. If the lesion changed in time. There must be a very detailed drug and ointment use history: previous or subsequent self-administration of drugs can change the appearance of the dermatosis.

15.5.2 Allergic Rashes

The most common rashes are the allergic ones: Often there is an history of previous flare-ups or allergic-related diseases (allergic rhinitis, asthma, allergic conjunctivitis, etc.). Sometimes, the first steps go unnoticed, so it's useful to ask about frequent and subsequent sneezing episodes, or the presence of recurrent cradle cap in infancy. Usually the allergic rashes are very itchy, so we have to ask if there are secondary sleeping disorders. They start in a place to spread even to the whole body. If the whole body is affected, usually the thinnest skin is more compromised, like the eye lids and the lips. In chronic disease, there can be an elderly look even in young people, due to the presence of Dennie Morgan sign, a wrinkle of the lower eyelid due to chronic inflammation and oedema. The eczema can arise from a systemic exposure, as the ingestion of something responsible for the flare-up (e.g. nickel), as a sign of a distant infection (e.g. tinea pedis) or after direct contact with substances. The eczema appears differently as the time passes by: start as erythema with fragile blisters, usually broken, leaving a wet surface from exudate. After a few days, it became scaly, with a honey and wax appearance, often the sign of a bacterial infection (*Staphylococcus aureus*). In the later stages, the skin thickens, and the skin texture appears magnified, as elephant skin, sometimes with brown/grey discoloration. The improvement during the weekend or after the abstention from work is a sign of a work-related disease (e.g. contact dermatitis from hair colour in hair stylists). The main suggestion is to avoid contact with the suspected agent, start antihistaminic drugs, steroid, or calcineurin ointments, and use gentle cleanser followed by abundant balms. A distinctive allergic rash may develop following the use of certain drugs; among the most common is a measleslike eruption that can occur after betalactam antibiotic administration in the context of mononucleosis infection. Adverse drug reactions often involve the palms and the soles; a sign of worsening can be the involvement of mucosa (oral, conjunctiva, etc.) and can arise after the first (uncommon) or after several contacts with the drug. Always stop the drug, start steroids and antihistaminic drugs, and follow up carefully.

15.5.3 Urticaria

The onset of urticaria is typically rapid, and the resolution of the lesions is a key diagnostic feature. When a patient seeks medical attention for urticaria, the rash may have already resolved or migrated by the time the clinician examines the patient, leaving the individual feeling frustrated [10]. Urticaria is characterized by intensely pruritic lesions that resemble mosquito bites, but fade without leaving any trace. It often develops within 2 weeks following a viral infection, which may go unnoticed. The rash can be triggered by various physical stimuli, such as exercise, temperature extremes, pressure, contact with ice or water, as well as the use of certain medications or the ingestion of histamine-rich or histamine-releasing foods and beverages, or even emotional factors [11]. Urticaria usually resolves spontaneously within 3 weeks, and extensive investigation for underlying organic diseases is not recommended unless the condition is chronic. The mainstay of treatment involves antihistamine medications, and the use of systemic corticosteroids should be avoided in the absence of signs of systemic involvement. If the urticaria persists for more than 6 weeks, a search for potential aetiologies may be warranted, but often leads to inconclusive findings. In the majority of cases, urticaria resolves spontaneously within 5 years [11, 12].

15.5.4 Parasitic Rashes

In parasitic diseases like scabies, the rash can appear as papules or single lesions, and may sometimes resemble eczema, often with a bacterial infection present [13]. The rash typically avoids the scalp and face in adults, instead preferring the hands, feet, and other areas such as the spaces between fingers, the nipples, armpits, and buttocks. The lesions may appear as papules, and if highly inflamed, the mite's path can fill with pus, resulting in a characteristic linear, curved pustule that is very suggestive of the condition.

Proper diagnosis and treatment with topical creams or oral ivermectin are essential, as these conditions can be highly contagious.

The condition is highly itchy and often affects multiple family members. In the case of Norwegian scabies, the skin has a scaly appearance. Ask if there is worsening of prurigo (itchy skin rash) at night, and if antihistamine medications are ineffective, as these are common signs of a parasitic infestation. There is an incubation period of about 30 days, so it is important that everyone in the family is treated simultaneously, even if they are not yet symptomatic. Therapy involves using permethrin lotions, ivermectin pills for Norwegian scabies, thoroughly cleaning the domestic environment to address the parasite's life cycle, repeating the treatment every 2 weeks to kill newly hatched parasites, and tracking all cases to prevent a small-scale outbreak [14]. Prurigo can persist for weeks as a neurological response even after the condition has healed.

15.5.5 Viral Rashes

Among the possible rashes that may be assessed remotely and have a viral aetiology, we will describe measles, chickenpox, coxsackie, and erythema infectiosum (parvovirus B19) infection, scarlet fever, and rubella.

15.5.5.1 Measles

Although the onset of measles-like rashes is now uncommon due to widespread vaccination, the condition can still occur. The rash appears as small red macules that start on the head and spread to the entire body. Measles in adults is associated with high fever, tender lymph nodes, profound fatigue, sore throat, cough, photophobia, and a rash that involves the whole body, beginning with a mucosal enanthema. If the lesions are pressed with a glass, they disappear, and they heal without scarring. It is important to inquire about the patient's vaccination status and be prepared for hospitalization if diarrhoea or altered consciousness develops [15].

15.5.5.2 Chickenpox

Chickenpox is caused by the varicella-zoster virus, for which a vaccine is available. The onset is usually marked by high fever, with small macules appearing on the head that evolve into small blisters, often on the scalp. New lesions of varying size then spread throughout the body before the older ones heal. The itching is intense, and scratching can lead to permanent scarring, so antihistamines and topical antibiotics to cover facial lesions are important. Chickenpox typically resolves within 2 weeks but remains highly contagious until all lesions have healed. Contagion can also occur from herpes zoster, so it is important to ask if the patient has had contact with someone with shingles in the 15 days preceding the dermatosis onset [16].

15.5.5.3 Coxsackie Virus and Parvovirus B19

Coxsackie virus and parvovirus B19 can lead to viral rashes, usually in children, with pink-red macules, which tend to be confluent on cheeks, like after a mild trauma, but can involve the whole skin, even palm and soles sometimes with purpuric aspect (socks and gloves syndrome), so if you put the glass on the lesions, they still appear, because of the blood under the skin. They start usually with mild fever, asthenia, and resolve without therapy. It's contagious, but not everyone seems to have the rash; it only occurs in genetically predisposed.

15.5.5.4 Scarlet Fever

Scarlet fever is typically caused by a streptococcal infection, so it is important to inquire about the presence of a sore throat, high fever, tender lymph nodes, or recent contact with someone who had a sore throat [17]. The rash usually begins on the face, often sparing the area around the mouth, and is accompanied by a strawberry-like appearance of the tongue. The rash then spreads to the arms and legs, from the axillary and inguinal regions towards the limbs. When examining the rash, it may have a sandpaper-like texture, with small, firm, reddish lesions [18]. Treatment involves antibiotics, and it is recommended to repeat a throat swab approximately 10 days after the initial treatment to ensure clearance of the infection and prevent recurrences. If there are more than two failed treatments, long-term monthly intramuscular penicillin administration should be considered.

15.5.5.5 Rubella

Rubella is a viral infection that was once common but is now rare due to widespread vaccination [19]. It typically begins with flu-like symptoms, followed by the appearance of macular rashes that start on the face and then spread throughout the body.

15.5.6 Secondary Syphilis

Secondary syphilis is considered the "great pretender" because it can mimic a variety of different dermatological conditions [20]. Typically, the patient is asymptomatic, with the only complaint being the presence of maculopapular lesions that can be difficult to identify. The key distinguishing feature is the involvement of the palms and soles, which are usually spared in other dermatoses. Diagnosis is made through blood tests [21]. It is useful to inquire about the presence of swollen lymph nodes, fever, and bone pain. Accurate diagnosis is crucial to prevent the development of irreversible late-stage lesions. The treatment involves high-dose antibiotics, starting at a lower dose to avoid a severe reaction from the destruction of the bacteria.

15.5.7 Pityriasis Rosea of Gibert

Pityriasis rosea is a common and benign skin condition that can be visually alarming due to the presence of an initial large, round lesion that may resemble other dermatological conditions, such as fungal infections. The condition typically begins with the appearance of this primary lesion, the herald patch [22] approximately 2 weeks after a mild, often unnoticed, viral illness. The initial lesion then heals within 2 weeks, followed by the emergence of smaller secondary lesions that spread in waves across the body, frequently affecting the back while typically sparing the face [23]. The diagnostic hallmarks of pityriasis rosea include the absence of fever or other systemic symptoms, the presence of slight scaling with the scales pointing towards the centre of the lesions (rather than being peripheral as in fungal infections), and the tendency for the lesions to align with the skin's tension lines, creating a characteristic "Christmas tree" pattern [24]. While the condition can last for several months, it typically resolves without the need for specific treatment. In cases of concurrent atopic dermatitis, the use of antihistamines or topical corticosteroids may be helpful in reducing the visibility of the most prominent lesions.

15.5.8 Kawasaki Disease

Kawasaki disease is often a great mimic of scarlet fever. The cause is unknown, but it can occur following COVID-19 infection as well.

The key features include a strawberry-red tongue, red eyes, enlarged and tender lymph nodes, sore throat, irritability, and a high fever lasting more than 5 days. The rash is maculopapular and covers the entire body, including the palms and soles, which are also swollen and very painful. The diagnostic clue is the fever, which is unresponsive to common medications like ibuprofen or acetaminophen, along with the involvement of the palms and soles [25, 26].

Diagnosis is crucial, as untreated Kawasaki disease can lead to coronary artery dilation or even aneurysm formation [27]. Therefore, a cardiologic evaluation and blood tests are essential. The treatment involves aspirin and intravenous immunoglobulin. The condition resolves with desquamation, characterized by large-scale peeling of the palms and soles, which can persist for years [25].

15.5.9 Rheumatologic Diseases

Lupus can present with a characteristic butterfly rash that involves the cheekbones and nose, which is highly suggestive of the condition. However, this must be considered as part of the overall clinical picture, as the presence of erythema alone may indicate rosacea instead. Therefore, it is important to inquire about signs of arthritis, such as morning stiffness lasting more than 30 min, joint pain, and pain persisting during rest. The diagnosis is made clinically, supported by blood tests. The treatment involves sun avoidance and using high sun protection creams.

Dermatomyositis can also present with a rash similar to lupus, but the presence of Gottron's papules is a key distinguishing feature. These are red-violaceous papules that appear over the small joints of the hands and are often worsened by sun exposure. The rash frequently involves sun-exposed areas, adopting a shawl-like distribution. Dermatomyositis can also affect the muscles and may be associated with an underlying malignancy.

Proper diagnosis requires a comprehensive medical history, thorough physical examination, and sometimes additional tests such as skin biopsies or allergy evaluations. As mentioned previously, the aim of this chapter is not to explore all types of rashes and their differential diagnoses in depth. This is not a dermatological essay, but rather, it emphasizes the importance of accurate diagnosis, timely assessment, and appropriate treatment to ensure optimal skin health and overall patient well-being in the context of telemedicine.

Many rashes are visually diagnosable. Dermatologists can examine images or live video during a telemedicine consultation, often leading to treatment recommendations.

Other than that, telemedicine facilitates easy follow-up appointments, enabling GPs and dermatologists to monitor the progress of treatment and adjust recommendations as necessary in longitudinal continuity.

15.5.10 Vasculitis

Purpuric lesions can appear after viral infection (coxsackie, echo), after bacterial infection, after rheumatic diseases, and after blood diseases. The culprit is the presence of blood under the skin, and it can be very easy to spot: just push gently a transparent surface on the skin (plastic, glass) and if the lesion fades away, it means that the red colour is due to vasodilatation, and it's not purpura. If it stays, it means the red is due to blood leaked from damaged vessels, so the problem is systemic. In the best of situation, the problem arises after scratching due to senile skin in patient using antithrombotic or antiplatelet drugs, so the purpura is linear or in single maculae and is usually in the upper part of legs, or in the area with minor trauma as hands and arms. Signs of danger are the presence of lesions in the lower part of the body, symmetric lesions, which means that there is gravity-related vascular damage, as in rheumatic and septic diseases. Blood test is mandatory, to check on platelets, autoimmune diseases, sepsis, so the referral to hospital is often the only solution.

15.5.11 Shingles

Shingles, also known as herpes zoster, results from the reactivation of the varicella-zoster virus, which also causes chickenpox [28]. The initial symptom is often a burning or tingling sensation in a specific dermatome, followed by the development of a unilateral, painful, blistering rash in a dermatomal distribution.

The rash typically begins as erythematous macules that progress to papules, vesicles, and ultimately crusted lesions. The diagnosis is often clinical, but distinguishing shingles from other rashes can be challenging, especially in the early stages.

15.5.12 Psoriasis

Psoriasis is a chronic inflammatory skin condition characterized by well-demarcated, erythematous, scaly plaques. Its diagnosis may be assessed or at least suspected based on the dermatological involvement and medical history. In some cases, psoriasis may be triggered or exacerbated by infections, medications, stress, or other factors. The Koebner phenomenon may be present, which is the appearance of new lesions at sites of trauma.

Psoriasis affects approximately 2–3% of the population and can have a significant impact on quality of life. Treatment typically involves topical therapies, such as corticosteroids and vitamin D analogues, as well as systemic medications for more severe cases. Its monitoring and management can be effectively conducted through telemedicine.

15.6 Remote Assessment of Malignant Skin Lesions

While most skin conditions discussed thus far can be adequately managed through telemedicine, there are certain malignant skin lesions that require more specialized evaluation and in-person assessment [29]. Melanomas, basal cell carcinomas, and squamous cell carcinomas can often be visually identified, but a definitive diagnosis requires a skin biopsy. We can roughly divide or suspect skin lesion to be malignant based on the ABCDE criteria and distinguish among melanotic and not melanotic skin lesions.

15.7 Top Tips

Using high-resolution images and videos can help visualize the rash/lesion and its characteristics, such as color, distribution, and morphology [30]. Patients can be guided to capture images using smartphones or cameras, ensuring proper lighting and focus [5]. Many dermatological conditions can be effectively assessed through remote consultations, provided that the patient can adequately display the lesion and describe aspects that are challenging to perceive on camera, such as dryness and texture. The following seven techniques can optimize your ability to evaluate your patients' skin: (1) Lighting: To thoroughly examine the skin, ensure adequate lighting. Natural light from windows is superior to artificial sources, so consider suggesting that patients position themselves closer to a window to enhance visibility [5]. (2) Double-check: Confirming with patients whether the on-screen image accurately represents the rash as they see it in person can provide confidence in your assessment or prompt you to seek a more representative view. (3) Measurement: Gauging the size of skin anomalies through a webcam can be challenging. Request that the patient uses a ruler or another reproducible object, like a coin, for scale reference. (4) Exposure: Do not hesitate to ask patients to remove clothing to expose broader areas of the body when dealing with widespread rashes. (5) Angles: Obtain a comprehensive understanding of any lesion in three dimensions. Request multiple views, both from above and from the side, to assess the lesion's projection or height. Use landmarks, such as "move towards your elbow," when directing camera adjustments for clarity. (6) Palpation: Encourage patients to run a hand over the lesion. Most patients can effectively convey characteristics such as heat, texture, tenderness, and moisture. (7) Glass test: Non-blanching rashes should raise concerns whether in remote or face-to-face examinations. Ask the patient to use a wide glass and roll it over the rash. If the rash does not fade, treat it as a medical emergency. This applies to both petechiae and purpura.

These techniques are just a few examples that can empower dermatologists and healthcare providers to conduct thorough assessments of skin conditions via remote consultations, ensuring the best possible care for patients.

15.8 Red Flags

Although telemedicine in dermatology presents numerous benefits, it is important to recognize that it may not be appropriate for all clinical scenarios. Situations that necessitate physical examinations, biopsies, or more intricate procedures still warrant in-person visits. During a remote dermatological consultation, it is paramount for both dermatologists and general practitioners to remain vigilant for red flags or indicators that may suggest a more severe or complex skin condition, which would require further assessment or an in-person evaluation.

Here are some common red flags to be aware of:

Rapid changes: If the patient reports rapid changes in the appearance of a skin lesion, such as sudden growth, significant colour changes, or the development of new symptoms, this could be a sign of a potentially serious condition.

Suspected cancer: Any skin lesion that raises suspicion of skin cancer should be considered a red flag. Look for irregular borders, asymmetry, variegated colour, or a lesion that is evolving (the ABCDE criteria) [31].

Non-healing sores: Ulcers, sores, or wounds that do not heal or continue to worsen over time may indicate a chronic or infectious skin condition, which requires prompt attention.

Severe pain or discomfort: If the patient reports severe pain, itching, or discomfort associated with a skin condition, this could be indicative of a more serious problem that requires immediate evaluation.

Systemic symptoms: Fever, chills, or other systemic symptoms accompanying a skin issue may suggest an underlying infection or inflammatory condition requiring further investigation.

Bleeding or oozing: Skin lesions that bleed, ooze, or have an unusual discharge should raise concerns, especially if they persist or worsen.

Non-responsive to treatment: If a patient has been following a prescribed treatment regimen for an extended period without improvement, it suggests the need for re-evaluation and potentially a change in treatment.

Persistent rash or eczema: Chronic or recurrent rashes or eczema that do not respond to standard treatments may require a more in-depth assessment.

Pay particular attention to immunocompromised patients—because they may be at higher risk of severe skin infections or complications—and to patients with history (or family history) of skin cancer—they may have an increased risk and should be evaluated thoroughly.

Special attention should also be paid to paediatric patients, as some skin conditions in children may be indicative of underlying systemic diseases.

Whenever a red flag is identified during teleconsultation, it is essential to communicate the need for further evaluation or in-person assessment to the patient.

15.9 Conclusion

One of the primary challenges of remote consultations is the inability to perform hands-on physical examinations. Dermatologists often rely on touch, texture, and palpation to assess skin condition, which cannot be replicated in a remote setting; even with high-quality images, certain aspects of a rash might be difficult to detect, such as depth, subtle variations in color, and three-dimensional characteristics.

Despite these challenges, telemedicine technology has the potential to revolutionize dermatological investigations by improving access, accuracy, and convenience. With the appropriate guidance and techniques, such as using proper lighting, angles, scale references, and interactivity with the patient, healthcare providers can conduct comprehensive remote evaluations and provide high-quality care to patients.

However, by leveraging strategies such as lighting optimization, use of visual scales and landmarks, verbal description, and virtual palpation, dermatologists can still gather essential diagnostic information to guide patient care. Furthermore, the flexibility and increased accessibility of teledermatology have the potential to improve timely diagnosis and treatment in many cases, ultimately benefiting patients [4, 6].

As technology continues to advance, telemedicine will likely play an increasingly important role in the field of dermatology, benefiting both patients and healthcare providers.

References

1. Kerr O, Tidman MJ, Walker JE, Aldridge RD, Benton EC. The profile of dermatological problems in primary care. Clin Exp Dermatol. Oxford University Press. 2010;35(4):380–3. https://doi.org/10.1111/j.1365-2230.2009.03586.x.
2. Lowell B, Froelich CW, Federman DG, Kirsner RS. Dermatology in primary care: prevalence and patient disposition. J Am Acad Dermatol. Elsevier BV. 2001;45(2):250–5. https://doi.org/10.1067/mjd.2001.114598.
3. Schofield J, Fleming DM, Grindlay DJC, Williams HC. Skin conditions are the commonest new reason people present to general practitioners in England and Wales. Br J Dermatol. Oxford University Press. 2011;165(5):1044–50. https://doi.org/10.1111/j.1365-2133.2011.10464.x.

4. Vodrahalli K, Ko J, Chiou AS, Novoa RA, Abid A, Phung M, Yekrang K, Petrone P, Zou J, Daneshjou R. Development and clinical evaluation of an AI support tool for improving telemedicine photo quality. Cornell University; 2022. https://doi.org/10.48550/arxiv.2209.09105.
5. Abbs AD. Remote consultations handbook: strategies to ensure a safe and effective consultation via video or telephone; 2022.
6. Pala P, Bergler-Czop B, Gwiżdż J. Teledermatology: idea, benefits and risks of modern age – a systematic review based on melanoma. Postepy Dermatol Alergol. Termedia Publishing House. 2020;37(2):159–67. https://doi.org/10.5114/ada.2020.94834.
7. Vodrahalli K, Daneshjou R, Novoa RA, Chiou AS, Ko J, Zou J. TrueImage: a machine learning algorithm to improve the quality of telehealth photos. Cornell University; 2020. https://doi.org/10.48550/arxiv.2010.02086.
8. Araujo KM, Denadai R. Digital clinician–patient consultation for dermatology care in stressful COVID-19 environment. J Patient Exp. SAGE Publishing. 2020;7(4):426–7. https://doi.org/10.1177/2374373520942376.
9. Xiong M, Pfau J, Young AT, Wei ML. Artificial intelligence in teledermatology. Curr Dermatol Rep. Springer Science+Business Media. 2019;8(3):85–90. https://doi.org/10.1007/s13671-019-0259-8.
10. Bernstein JA, Lang DM, Khan DA, Craig T, Dreyfus DH, Hsieh FH, Sheikh J, Weldon D, Zuraw BL, Bernstein DI, Blessing-Moore J, Cox L, Nicklas RA, Casale TB, Portnoy JM, Randolph C, Schuller DE, Spector SL, Tilles SA, Wallace D. The diagnosis and management of acute and chronic urticaria: 2014 update. J Allergy Clin Immunol. Elsevier BV. 2014;133(5):1270–1277.e66. https://doi.org/10.1016/j.jaci.2014.02.036.
11. Kaplan AP. Diagnosis, pathogenesis, and treatment of chronic spontaneous urticaria. Allergy Asthma Proc. OceanSide Publications, Inc. 2018;39(3):184–90. https://doi.org/10.2500/aap.2018.39.4121.
12. Guha K, Youngberg G. Acute and chronic urticaria. 2016. https://www.tandfonline.com/doi/full/10.3810/pgm.2001.02.861.
13. Johnston G, Sladden M. Scabies: diagnosis and treatment. BMJ. 2005;331(7517):619–22. https://doi.org/10.1136/bmj.331.7517.619.
14. Amato E, Dansie L, Grøneng G, Blix HS, Bentele H, Veneti L, Stefanoff P, Macdonald E, Blystad H, Soleng A. Increase of scabies infestations, Norway, 2006 to 2018. Eurosurveillance. 2019;24(23):190020. https://doi.org/10.2807/1560-7917.es.2019.24.23.190020.
15. Gould D. Measles: symptoms, diagnosis, management and prevention. Prim Health Care. Royal College of Nursing. 2015;25(1):34–40. https://doi.org/10.7748/phc.25.1.34.e908.
16. Chickenpox Clinical Presentation. 2022. https://emedicine.medscape.com/article/1131785-clinical.
17. Basetti S, Hodgson JA, Rawson TM, Majeed A. Scarlet fever: a guide for general practitioners. Lond J Prim Care. Taylor & Francis. 2017;9(5):77–9. https://doi.org/10.1080/17571472.2017.1365677.
18. Alotaibi A, Binsaqr MA, Mutlaq MR, Khojah AA, Khojah SA, Mohamed HA. Atypical presentation of scarlet fever. Cureus. 2022;14:e33142. https://doi.org/10.7759/cureus.33142.
19. Plotkin SA. The history of rubella and rubella vaccination leading to elimination. Clin Infect Dis. Oxford University Press. 2006;43(Supplement_3):S164–8. https://doi.org/10.1086/505950.
20. Tang MBY, Yosipovitch G, Tan S. Secondary syphilis presenting as a lichen planus-like rash. J Eur Acad Dermatol Venereol. Wiley. 2004;18(2):185–7. https://doi.org/10.1111/j.1468-3083.2004.00859.x.
21. Mansouri S, Mai S, Senouci K, Hassam B. Secondary syphilis resembling erythema annulare centrifugum. BMJ. 2019;12(5):–e230301. https://doi.org/10.1136/bcr-2019-230301.
22. McLeod RP. Lumps, bumps, and things that go itch in your office! J Sch Nurs. SAGE Publishing. 2004;20(3):185–6. https://doi.org/10.1177/10598405040200031001.
23. González LM, Allen RE, Jänniger CK, Schwartz RA. Pityriasis rosea: an important papulosquamous disorder. Int J Dermatol. Wiley. 2005;44(9):757–64. https://doi.org/10.1111/j.1365-4632.2005.02635.x.

24. Saravanan N, Ramasamy S, Murugan S, Sridhar V, Vanathi T, Sarathchandran B, Rekha GP. An analytical study of clinical features in 100 cases of Pityriasis rosea. J Evol Med Dent Sci. 2017;6(26):2142–8. https://doi.org/10.14260/jemds/2017/465.
25. Burns JC, Glodé MP. Kawasaki syndrome. Lancet. Elsevier BV. 2004;364(9433):533–44. https://doi.org/10.1016/s0140-6736(04)16814-1.
26. Leung DY, Meissner HC. The many faces of Kawasaki syndrome. Hosp Pract. Taylor & Francis. 2000;35(1):77–94. https://doi.org/10.3810/hp.2000.01.182.
27. Belay E. Kawasaki disease. 2020. https://link.springer.com/content/pdf/10.1007/978-1-84628-715-2_44.pdf.
28. Peate I. Preventing shingles: symptoms, treatment and management. Br J Health Care Manag. Mark Allen Group. 2010;4(3):120–3. https://doi.org/10.12968/bjha.2010.4.3.47061.
29. Finnane A, Curiel-Lewandrowski C, Wimberley G, Caffery LJ, Katragadda C, Halpern AC, Marghoob AA, Malvehy J, Kittler H, Hofmann-Wellenhof R, Abraham I, Soyer HP. Proposed technical guidelines for the acquisition of clinical images of skin-related conditions. JAMA Dermatol. American Medical Association. 2017;153(5):453. https://doi.org/10.1001/jamadermatol.2016.6214.
30. Witmer WK, Lebovitz PJ. Clinical photography in the dermatology practice. Semin Cutan Med Surg. 2012;31(3):191–9. https://doi.org/10.1016/j.sder.2012.06.004.
31. Signs and Symptoms of Skin Cancer. 2014. https://www.ncbi.nlm.nih.gov/books/NBK247171/.

Remote Consultation in Neurology 16

Simone Quintana, Raquel Gomez Bravo, Ogulcan Come, and Vildan Mevsim

16.1 Remote Consultation in Neurology Clinical Practice

The advent of telemedicine and virtual consultations has revolutionized how healthcare providers approach the assessment and management of neurological conditions in primary care. Traditionally, neurological examinations and diagnoses have relied heavily on in-person interactions, with clinicians using physical examinations and hands-on assessments to evaluate patients. However, the COVID-19 pandemic has accelerated the adoption of remote healthcare, necessitating the development of novel approaches to neurological assessments that can be conducted virtually [1].

One key consideration in the remote assessment of neurological scenarios is the emphasis on effective verbal communication skills. As patients and providers interact through video or telephone consultations, there is a greater reliance on verbal cues and the ability to convey and interpret information effectively. Telemedicine and remote medical consultation have found positive applications in the field of neurology. Like other branches of medicine, the neurological clinic serves a large population of patients with chronic diseases who can benefit from a teleconsultation or a televisit to update their own doctor on the progress of their diagnosed and

S. Quintana (✉)
Headache Centre, Neurology Unit, Neuromotor and Rehabilitation Department, Azienda USL-IRCCS di Reggio Emilia, Reggio Emilia, Italy
e-mail: simone.quintana@ausl.re.it

R. G. Bravo
Centre Hospitalier Neuro-psychiatrique (CHNP), Rehaklinik, Ettelbruck, Luxembourg

Department of Behavioural and Cognitive Sciences, University of Luxembourg, Esch-sur-Alzette, Luxembourg

O. Come · V. Mevsim
Dokuz Eylul University, Faculty of Medicine, Department of Family Medicine, Izmir, Turkey
e-mail: ogulcan.come@deu.edu.tr; vildan.mevsim@deu.edu.tr

J. Demurtas (ed.), *Remote Consultation in Primary Care*, TELe-Health, https://doi.org/10.1007/978-3-031-89661-3_16

treated clinical condition. Telemedicine allows for the real-time monitoring of the progress of pathologies such as neurodegenerative disorders, chronic headache, epilepsy, and other neurological conditions [2].

Telemedicine has been widely embraced in the field of neurology to bridge gaps in access to care. One notable example is telestroke, which gained prominence in stroke centres during the mid-2000s following the success of the STRokE DOC2 trial, which demonstrated the diagnostic accuracy of telemedicine in acute stroke care [3]. In the outpatient setting, teleneurology serves as an alternative for patients with chronic conditions and disabilities that hinder their ability to visit subspecialty clinics in person. The Telemedicine Work Group's recent update provides a comprehensive overview of teleneurology support for outpatient neurology care. The review emphasizes the positive impact of teleneurology on patient satisfaction, associated costs, and caregiver burden, all while maintaining high-quality care standards [4]. Robust literature data on the safety and efficacy of telemedicine are now available for three types of neurological patients: patients with Parkinson's disease [5], patients with epilepsy [6], and patients with headache [7].

The teleconsultation tools in the doctor-patient relationship make it possible to monitor the progress of the pathology, the response to the proposed treatments, and the detection of the patient's and family unit's assistance needs. In advanced care models, the possibility of having an interaction between healthcare professionals has also been activated: this possibility allows in some rural areas to be able to promptly submit the patients in charge to the general practitioner or any other specialists to time-dependent therapies, for example fibrinolytic therapy in the ischemic stroke [8].

16.2 Strengths and Limitations of Telemedicine Applications in Neurology

Telemedicine presents numerous advantages for patients and healthcare providers [9]:

· Improved comfort, convenience, and safety: Particularly beneficial for patients with limited mobility or those requiring home medical support equipment, telehealth enables medical consultations and support from the safety and convenience of their own homes, reducing the need for travel and minimizing the risk of accidents or infections associated with hospital visits.

- Decreased travel time and costs: By eliminating the necessity for patients to travel long distances, telehealth saves time and money, eliminating expenses related to transportation, accommodation, and other associated costs.
- Minimized disruption to daily life: Telehealth reduces the need for extensive travel and waiting times, enabling patients to spend less time away from work or other essential activities. This reduces the impact on their daily routines and responsibilities.

- Reduced stress for caregivers: Telehealth eases the burden on caregivers by providing remote access to healthcare providers, allowing them to discuss concerns and receive guidance. This helps reduce the stress and challenges associated with coordinating and attending in-person appointments.
- Increased involvement during visits: Telehealth promotes greater participation from care partners and providers during medical consultations. Care partners can actively engage in discussions, ask questions, and contribute valuable input, resulting in a more comprehensive and collaborative approach to patient care.
- Improved assessment of social determinants of health: Telehealth enables healthcare providers to gain a better understanding of the patient's home environment and other social factors influencing their health. This information can inform treatment plans and interventions to address specific patient needs.
- Early intervention based on continuous assessment: Through continuous monitoring and evaluation of neurologic disease progression and treatment effectiveness, telehealth enables early identification of warning signs or changes in a patient's condition. This facilitates timely interventions and adjustments to treatment plans.
- Protection against infectious diseases: Telehealth reduces the risk of infectious disease transmission for both patients and providers by minimizing the need for in-person visits. This helps conserve personal protective equipment (PPE) for situations requiring direct physical contact.
- Supported by evidence: Multiple studies have provided evidence supporting the effectiveness of telehealth in various neurologic subspecialties, both in inpatient and outpatient settings. This evidence supports its use for acute evaluations, routine assessments, and ongoing management of neurologic conditions.

Evidence supports the effectiveness of telehealth in inpatient and outpatient settings, for acute evaluation and routine assessment and for neurological condition. There are of course limitations to the use of telemedicine tools in neurology [10, 11]:

- Limited physical examination: Patients with advanced neurodegenerative pathology, patients with severe impairment of autonomies due to the underlying pathology such as amyotrophic lateral sclerosis, severe muscular dystrophies, multiple sclerosis in an advanced state, patients with neuro-oncological pathology: in these conditions, it is challenging to evaluate accurately the patient and the traditional visit becomes indispensable both specialists, neurologist and general practitioner. The lack of physical contact can hinder the doctor's ability to make precise diagnoses and treatment decisions.
- Technological constraints: Stable Internet connections, high-quality video/audio transmission, and reliable platforms are crucial for telemedicine to maintaining data security and patient privacy remotely. In some rural areas, this Internet infrastructure may be limited and influence the effectiveness of the online consultations.
- Limited access to diagnostic tests and physical procedures: The procedures such as EEG (electroencephalography), EMG (electromyography), or neuroimaging (MRI, CT scans), which are typically performed in a clinical setting with special-

ized equipment, may restrict the ability to make accurate diagnoses and treatment decisions. The same situation applies to hands-on procedures such as lumbar punctures, nerve blocks, or botulinum toxin injections that need in-person consultation.
- Incomplete patient assessment.
- Patients' varying levels of digital literacy can affect their ability to engage in teleconsultations effectively.
- Patients' preferences.

16.3 Role of Remote Consultation Teaching to Physicians

As telemedicine becomes more widespread, it is starting to be incorporated into medical curricula. Studies have outlined specific competencies related to teleneurology that are recommended for inclusion in medical curricula. These competencies aim to prepare medical students and healthcare professionals for effectively practicing teleneurology [12]. Competencies are as follows.

16.3.1 Setting

- Background: minimal complexity and movement to preserve video quality; avoid fans; prefer a plain wall and a smaller room
- Lighting: bright light in front of doctor's face; avoid backlighting
- Sound: headset ideal to prevent feedback; if you get feedback, turn down the speaker volume; avoid moving the microphone farther away, which will worsen feedback
- Ask the patient to minimize number of people to 1–2, and to minimize movement; ideally, rest device on firm surface rather than hand-held
- Recommend a quiet well-lit room away from pets, children, nonessential staff; encourage participants to speak one at a time
- Ask scheduler to coordinate availability with home health if possible

16.3.2 Telepresence

- Note delta angle between camera and patient image on screen; to maintain eye contact, practice looking counterintuitively at camera, not the screen, when speaking to the patient.
- When multitasking, documenting in the electronic record, or reviewing films and laboratory studies, be explicit what you are doing so it does not seem that you are not paying attention.
- Start encounter by obtaining all participant names; use names (instead of body language) to direct questions and get attention.

- Ask those speaking to come into view of the camera, both to get your attention and optimize use of directional microphones.
- At visit conclusion, explicitly address the future nature of your relationship including follow-up and modality.

16.3.3 Teleneurologic Examination

- Conduct the neurologic examination in order to minimize need to reposition cameras.
- Use examination demonstration and mimicking, particularly in the absence of an assistant.
- Mental status: mostly observational; mini-cognitive examination possible; with a trained assistant, more complex cognitive tests are possible.
- Cranial nerves: zoom in for eye movements, face, tongue; may rely largely on voluntary saccades to each direction; zoom out for everything else; visual fields can be checked with patient's hands extended in front of the field of view or more formally if an assistant is present.
- Zoom out slightly: pronator drift, satellite sign, digiti minimi sign, finger escape sign; more formal strength testing is possible with an assistant; test coordination with nose-full extension-nose, or finger-nose-finger if an assistant is present.
- Zoom out more: leg drift, heel-knee-shin, sensation of face/arms/legs, gait.
- May be able to test more detailed strength, tone, reflexes, sensation if an assistant is present.

16.4 Neurological Examination

Our purpose is to provide essential elements for conducting a complete neurological tele-evaluation, with elements of semiotics that are easy to perform for the patient and highly informative for the doctor. After the clinical evaluation section, some neurological pathology scenarios and the most suitable approach to put into practice with remote consultation will be examined.

The practical neurological evaluation involves three main steps:

1. The evaluation of the higher functions, i.e. the aspects of language, understanding, memory, attention, and all that more generally is called neuropsychological evaluation
2. The second part involves a careful assessment of cranial nerve function.
3. The third part provides for the evaluation of motion, sensitivity, and coordination functions at the level of the upper and lower limbs.

16.4.1 Essential Assessment of Higher Cognitive Functions

Assess Patient's

Space-time orientation: ask for the date, complete with day-month-year. Ask where the patient is located.

Alterations to these types of questions are typical of patients with dementia or patients with an acute confusional state.

Language

To evaluate the presence of complete or partial aphasic disorders, it is advisable to listen to some complete sentences pronounced by the patient in relation to circumstantial questions (for example questions about his health condition or family activities).

The function of language is generally impoverished during physiological ageing. Sudden worsening can be attributable to neurodegenerative diseases or cerebral ischemic events.

Praxia

The patient may be asked to perform simple commands, such as lifting a specific limb or picking up an object and showing it to the doctor. Apraxias, divided into ideational, motor, or ideo-motor, are usually secondary to neurodegenerative processes. The degree of impairment of the praxic functions is correlated to the degree of residual autonomy of the patient.

16.4.2 Essential Assessment of Cranial Nerves

Cranial nerves can be assessed with good approximation from remote as follows:

I Olfactory

Ask the patient if they've lost their sense of smell

Progressive loss of smell is a common early symptom of Parkinson's disease, occurring during the premotor phase, and can also indicate space-occupying lesions in the anterior cranial fossa. Patients can be asked to smell a selected scent and report whether they are able to identify it.

II Optic

The patient is asked if he has subjectively lost visual acuity, he can be asked to read a book or a newspaper.

Optic nerve disorders may be secondary to damage to the optic nerve, chiasm, retrochiasmatic tracts, or primary visual cortex. The association between visual loss and pain on eye movements is typical of retrobulbar optic neuritis, often the presenting symptom of multiple sclerosis.

III, IV, and VI Oculomotor, Trochlear, and Abducens

The patient is asked to voluntarily move the eyes through the six gaze directions while the doctor visually monitors the symmetry and timing of the ocular movements.

The doctor can also ask the patient to follow the movement of a pen or of their own fingers.

Ask the patient to keep their head still and move their eyes slow from left to right and then up and down. Observe the position of the pupil of both eyes. It should be parallel, wherever the eyes look. If there is asymmetry, there is a likely deficit. Also observe for nystagmus.

Eye motion disorders have many possible etiologies. A relevant form is horizontal gaze palsy due to cranial nerve VI deficiency, typical of diabetic mononeuropathy.

V Trigeminal

For the sensory function, ask the patient to pass some cotton or gauze first over the forehead, then at the level of the cheekbone and then at the level of the jaw, first on the right and then on the left to compare it.

For motor function, make the mouth open and close; with your mouth closed, ask to grit your teeth and observe the masseters.

Selective changes in the trigeminal territory may be the result of an exacerbation of the varicella-zoster virus. In trigeminal neuralgia, attacks of acute neuropathic pain may be elicited during the sensory assessment phase.

VII Facial

Possible anomalies can already be observed in the rest condition. Subsequently the patient is asked to open and close his eyes, smile, puff out his cheeks. Asymmetries and hypofunctions are relevant.

Acute complete deficit of a facial nerve in the absence of other neurologic deficits is typical of Bell's palsy; acute unilateral lower facial deficit is typical of stroke.

VIII Vestibulocochlear

Ask the patient to rub their fingers next to the ear, first on one side and then on the other. Asymmetries and hypofunctions are relevant. Vestibular function can be assessed by asking the patient if they have experienced dizziness or dizziness.

Presbycusis is typically a progressive, bilateral, symmetrical hearing loss that occurs in old age. Significant hearing asymmetries require further neuroimaging.

IX, X, XII Glossopharyngeal, Vagus, and Hypoglassal Nerves

The reflex functions of these two important nerves are evaluated by asking the patient to cough and swallow.

Progressive neurodegenerative disorders such as amyotrophic lateral sclerosis and corticobasal degeneration lead to progressive dysphagia, dysarthria, and hoarseness.

XI Accessory of Vagus

Ask the patient to raise the shoulders, either one at a time or both at the same time to assess for asymmetries. Ask the patient to rotate his head, during the movements observe the state of trophism of the sternocleidomastoid muscle. Pathologies of the eleventh cranial nerve are usually accompanied by alterations of the ninth and tenth.

XII Hypoglossal

Ask the patient to stick their tongue out in order to assess for asymmetry, fasciculations, or wasting of the tongue.

Neuromuscular disorders can selectively affect the cranial nerves or involve them first in the evolution of the pathology (amyotrophic lateral sclerosis).

16.4.3 Essential Assessment of Motion, Sensation, and Coordination

Once the patient's collaboration and the function of the cranial nerves have been evaluated, the remaining somatic objectivity can be evaluated. It is advisable to evaluate the upper limbs separately from the lower limbs with dedicated tests.

Upper limbs:

- Evaluate the strength against gravity by asking the patient to lift his limbs in front of him and hold the position for a few tens of seconds. The evaluation can be enriched by asking the patient to perform selective joint movements, both free-body and by moving a small weight (1 kg dumbbell, bottle of water).
- The evaluation of sensitivity can be made use of a tactile stimulus applied by the patient on the parts of the upper limb, to be evaluated in comparison with the contralateral part. The data reported are of a subjective nature and therefore to be evaluated critically.
- For the upper limbs, coordination is assessed with the index-nose test to be performed by the patient in a suitable environment, in an initial sequence with eyes open and then with eyes closed. Asymmetries, dyssynergies, and dissymmetries should be noted.

Lower limbs:

- Strength can be assessed by asking the patient to stand up, stand, and then stand on one limb at a time. Segmental strength can be assessed by asking the patient to sit up using a single lower limb.
- Sensitivity can be evaluated as for the upper limbs, by applying a tactile stimulus on symmetrical parts of the limbs.
- Coordination can be assessed with the patient sitting down and asking him to reach his contralateral knee with his heel, first with his eyes open and then with his eyes closed, always evaluating dyssynergies and dissymmetries.

The evaluation of the upright position and the gait, complex functions that bring into play the sharing of everything previously examined, complete the evaluation of the neurological objectivity: one side dragging gears, stepping gears, unstable or asymmetrical gears should be noted.

16.5 Clinical Scenarios: Elements of Neurological Teleconsultation

16.5.1 Headache

The area of diagnosis and treatment of headaches is a challenging area for general practitioners and neurologists. There are some essential elements that every doctor-patient consultation must take into consideration: every headache must be highly characterized by the doctor by asking the patient detailed questions in the anamnestic collection, the fundamental distinction between primary headaches (basically benign) and secondary (possibly life-threatening) headaches.

To best characterize a headache, the patient should be asked for a series of characteristics:

- Site of the headache
- Quality and intensity of pain
- Associated neurovegetative symptoms such as nausea, vomiting, photophobia, phonophobia
- Associated trigeminal-autonomic signs such as eye redness, lacrimation, nasal congestion and rhinorrhea, palpebral edema
- Behavior of the patient during the headache
- Duration of the attacks
- Response to pain relief treatments

By collecting this information, it is possible to reach at least a first-level diagnosis with reference to the international classification of headaches [1]. It is then necessary to go in search of red flags, that is, those signs and symptoms that are most often associated with the presence of a structural organic cause at the base of the headache. If you identify the patient, he should be referred to a specialist or to the emergency-urgency service in a timely manner. The red flags are as follows:

Sudden onset severity, reaching maximal intensity within 5 min

This is the typical presentation of rupture of intracranial vascular malformations or bleeding lesions occupying space within the skull which, being inexpandable, suffers from the increase in pressure resulting from the increase in contents.

Change in neurological status, personality, or a new focal neurological deficit

This is the typical presentation of brain tumors that progressively extend to different brain areas by accumulating progressive deficits and increasing intracranial pressure

Aura lasting over 1 h that is atypical for the patient in conjunction with combined oral contraceptive use
This is the typical presentation of ischemic or hemorrhagic lesions
New-onset headache in immunosuppressed patients (AIDS, oncological therapy, immunosuppressed for chronic autoimmune diseases)
Headache in these cases may represent the first and only clinical element underlying neoplasms or intracranial infections
Headache associated with fever, vomiting, and other systemic symptoms
This condition can be sustained by meningitis or meningo-encephalitis, a condition that requires the prompt execution of laboratory tests and advanced treatments

16.5.2 Stroke and Transient Ischemic Attacks

Cerebrovascular disease represents a medical emergency; therefore, any patient with an acute onset of a neurological deficit should be referred to the emergency services because time-dependent treatments are available with proven efficacy in reducing mortality and disability. However, it is important to have the ability to grasp those transient clinical events that often precede major events such as ischemic or hemorrhagic strokes: these are transient ischemic attacks (TIAs). Typical TIAs (in which the likelihood of ischemia is relatively high) are characterized by transient, focal neurologic symptoms, generally with sudden onset, which can be localized to a single vascular territory within the brain, including one or more of the following:

- Transient monocular blindness or hemianopia
- Aphasia or dysarthria
- Hemiparesis and/or hemisensory loss

Other symptoms that are less likely to be due to a transient ischemic genesis are defined as atypical TIAs: gradual build-up of symptoms or march of symptoms from one body part to another, progression of symptoms from one type to another, isolated disturbance of vision in both eyes characterized by the occurrence of positive phenomena, isolated sensory symptoms with remarkably focal distribution, very brief spells lasting less than 30 s, identical spells occurring over a period of more than 1 year, isolated brainstem symptoms, such as dysarthria, diplopia, or hearing loss, amnesia, confusion, incoordination of limbs. In patients with a typical or atypical presentation of possible cerebral ischemic significance it is advisable to try to predict the risk of major events, to do this it is useful to use the score ABCD2 [2]:

Age
≥60 years
1 point
Blood pressure elevation when first assessed after TIA

Systolic ≥140 mmHg or
Diastolic ≥90 mmHg
1 point
Clinical features
Unilateral weakness
2 points
Isolated speech disturbance
1 point
Other
0 points
Duration of TIA symptoms
≥60 min
2 points
10–59 min
1 point
<10 min
0 points
Diabetes
Present
1 point

The ABCD2 score is designed to identify patients at high risk of ischemic stroke in the first 7 days after TIA occurs: 0–3 are at low risk, 4–5 are at moderate risk, 6–7 are at high risk. The predictive power of the ABCD2 score is generally higher in population-based setting compared with hospital settings.

16.6 Future Development Possibilities

The future of telemedicine in neurology holds promise for significant advancements, particularly through the integration of artificial intelligence and machine learning. These technologies could enhance diagnostic accuracy in remote settings by analyzing patient data and identifying patterns in neurological conditions that might otherwise be overlooked in virtual consultations. Additionally, wearable devices and mobile health applications offer opportunities for continuous monitoring of neurological symptoms, facilitating early intervention and personalized treatment plans. Expanding broadband Internet and telemedicine infrastructure, especially in underserved rural areas, is essential to improving the accessibility and effectiveness of remote neurological care. As these technologies evolve, collaborations between primary care providers and neurologists will become more seamless, enabling shared management of chronic and complex neurological conditions. Further development in VR- and AR-based telehealth could also support more comprehensive remote neurological examinations, bringing virtual assessments closer to the depth of in-person evaluations.

16.7 Conclusion

Remote neurology consultations represent a transformative shift in primary healthcare, offering new ways to effectively and conveniently manage chronic neurological conditions. Telemedicine has proven valuable in enhancing access to care, reducing travel burdens, and alleviating the strain on patients and caregivers. Despite limitations, such as challenges in performing physical examinations and the need for reliable technology, telemedicine has demonstrated positive outcomes in terms of patient satisfaction, cost efficiency, and care quality. As technological advances continue and telehealth training expands, remote neurology consultations will likely become a standard in both primary and specialized care. By embracing these innovations, healthcare systems can ensure more inclusive, efficient, and sustainable care models for patients with neurological needs.

References

1. Al-Hazmi A, Sheerah HA, Arafa A. Perspectives on telemedicine during the era of COVID-19; what can Saudi Arabia do? Int J Environ Res Public Health. Multidisciplinary Digital Publishing Institute. 2021;18(20):10617. https://doi.org/10.3390/ijerph182010617.
2. Martinelli M, Moroni D, Bastiani L, Mrakic-Sposta S, Giardini G, Pratali L. High-altitude mountain telemedicine. J Telemed Telecare. SAGE Publishing. 2020;28(2):135–45. https://doi.org/10.1177/1357633x20921020.
3. Meyer BC, Raman R, Hemmen T, Obler R, Zivin JA, Rao R, et al. Efficacy of site-independent telemedicine in the STRokE DOC trial: a randomised, blinded, prospective study. Lancet Neurol. 2008;7(9):787–95.
4. Hatcher-Martin JM, Adams JL, Anderson ER, Bove R, Burrus TM, Chehrenama M, et al. Telemedicine in neurology: telemedicine work group of the American Academy of Neurology update. Neurology. 2020;94(1):30–8.
5. Houston E, Kennedy AG, O'Malley D, Rabinowitz T, Rose GL, Boyd J. Telemedicine in neurology: a scoping review of key outcomes in movement disorders. Telemed J E Health. 2022;28(3):295–308.
6. Samia P, Sahu JK, Ali A, Caraballo RH, Chan J, Coan AC, et al. Telemedicine for individuals with epilepsy: recommendations from the international league against epilepsy telemedicine task force. Seizure-Eur J Epilep. 2023;106:85–91.
7. Noutsios CD, Boisvert-Plante V, Perez J, Hudon J, Ingelmo P. Telemedicine applications for the evaluation of patients with non-acute headache: a narrative review. J Pain Res. 2021;14:1533–42.
8. Wechsler LR, Tsao JW, Levine SR, Swain-Eng RJ, Adams RJ, Demaerschalk BM, et al. Teleneurology applications: report of the telemedicine work group of the American Academy of Neurology. Neurology. 2013;80(7):670–6.
9. Hatcher-Martin JM, Busis NA, Cohen BH, Wolf RA, Jones EC, Anderson ER, et al. American Academy of Neurology telehealth position statement. Neurology. 2021;97(7):334–9.
10. Timpano F, Bonanno L, Bramanti A, Pirrotta F, Spadaro L, Bramanti P, et al. Tele-health and neurology: what is possible? Neurol Sci. 2013;34(12):2263–70.
11. Wechsler LR. Advantages and limitations of teleneurology. JAMA Neurol. 2015;72(3):349–54.
12. Zha AM, Chung LS, Song SS, Majersik JJ, Jagolino-Cole AL. Training in neurology: adoption of resident teleneurology training in the wake of COVID-19: telemedicine crash course. Neurology. 2020;95(9):404–7.

Further Readings

1. Headache Classification Committee of the International Headache Society (IHS). The international classification of headache disorders, 3rd edition. Cephalalgia Int J Headache. 2018;38(1):1–211.
2. Johnston SC, Rothwell PM, Nguyen-Huynh MN, Giles MF, Elkins JS, Bernstein AL, et al. Validation and refinement of scores to predict very early stroke risk after transient ischaemic attack. Lancet Lond Engl. 2007;369(9558):283–92.

Telepsychiatry and Remote Assessment of Psychiatric Disorders in Primary Care

17

Alessandro Miola, Tommaso Boldrini, Marco De Toffol, Stefania Carpenzano, Gaetano Di Virgilio, Jacopo Demurtas, and Marco Solmi

A. Miola
Department of Neuroscience, University of Padova, Padua, Italy

T. Boldrini
Department of Psychology and Health Science, Pegaso University, Naples, Italy

M. De Toffol
Autism Service Center "Amici di Nico", Matino, Lecce, Italy

L'Adelfia Social Cooperative, Alessano, Lecce, Italy

S. Carpenzano
Private Psychology Practice, Padua, Italy

G. Di Virgilio
Psychology Department, University of Turin, Master Degree in Clinical Psychology Program, Turin, Italy

J. Demurtas
Clinical and Experimental Medicine PhD Program, University of Modena and Reggio Emilia, Modena, Italy

Family Medicine Department, USL Toscana Sud-Est, Capalbio, Italy

M. Solmi (✉)
Sciences Lab, Department of Psychiatry, University of Ottawa, Ottawa, ON, Canada

Department of Mental Health, The Ottawa Hospital, Ottawa, ON, Canada

Ottawa Hospital Research Institute (OHRI), Clinical Epidemiology Program, University of Ottawa, Ottawa, ON, Canada

School of Epidemiology and Public Health, Faculty of Medicine, University of Ottawa, Ottawa, ON, Canada

Department of Child and Adolescent Psychiatry, Charité Universitätsmedizin, Berlin, Germany

J. Demurtas (ed.), *Remote Consultation in Primary Care*, TELe-Health,
https://doi.org/10.1007/978-3-031-89661-3_17

17.1 Bridging Gaps in Mental Health: Global Burden, Mortality Disparities, and Differences in Access to Care

Mental health burden is a significant global concern, affecting individuals across various demographics and geographical locations [18]. According to the World Health Organization (WHO), mental health conditions contribute to a substantial portion of the global disease burden [46], with depression alone being the leading cause of disability worldwide [31]. This burden extends beyond individual suffering, impacting families, communities, and economies.

One striking aspect of mental health disparities is the stark difference in mortality rates between individuals with mental disorders and those without [50, 51]. Studies consistently show that individuals with severe mental illness have a significantly reduced life expectancy compared to the general population [9, 29]. This mortality gap is not solely attributable to suicide [24] but also to physical health conditions, such as cardiovascular disease, diabetes, and respiratory illnesses, which are often exacerbated by factors like inadequate healthcare access, socioeconomic disadvantage, and lifestyle factors. Furthermore, individuals with severe mental illness frequently receive lower-quality care for physical comorbidities due to various barriers related to patient, treatment, physician, and service [12, 43, 44].

While mental health conditions affect individuals worldwide, there are notable differences in the prevalence, presentation, and cultural perceptions of mental disorders across different regions. Factors such as socioeconomic status, cultural beliefs, access to healthcare, and stigma contribute to these variations [27]. For instance, high-income countries may have better resources for early detection and treatment, whereas low-income countries may face greater challenges due to limited mental health infrastructure, societal attitudes, and access to older medications [37].

The evolution of technology has revolutionized the field of mental healthcare delivery, particularly with the advent of telemedicine. However, there are disparities in access to technology and infrastructure across different regions, necessitating varied approaches to telepsychiatry implementation [8, 23, 48]. In high-income countries, where digital connectivity is widespread, telepsychiatry may be seamlessly integrated into existing healthcare systems [7]. In contrast, in low-income countries with limited internet access and technological resources, alternative strategies — such as mobile-based interventions or telepsychiatry via phone calls — may be more feasible [48]. The involvement of local stakeholders, community representatives, policymakers, and clinicians is crucial to ensure a co-designed integration of telepsychiatry [17, 21], in contrast to top-down solutions that risk low adoption by the target population.

17.2 Telepsychiatry

Telepsychiatry is a rapidly growing field that leverages technology to provide psychiatric care to patients remotely [11]. The COVID-19 pandemic has accelerated the adoption of telepsychiatry, with healthcare providers increasingly utilizing video conferencing, mobile apps, and other digital tools to assess and treat patients remotely [11].

One of the key benefits of telepsychiatry is its ability to address the maldistribution of mental health resources, particularly in underserved and rural areas [22]. By enabling remote consultations, telepsychiatry can improve access to specialized psychiatric care for patients who may have difficulty traveling to in-person appointments. Additionally, telepsychiatry can be a more convenient and accessible option for patients, potentially increasing engagement, and adherence to treatment [30].

On the other hand, assessments of depressive, anxiety, and psychotic symptoms, as well as suicidal risk, generally show good reliability in telepsychiatry when compared with face-to-face interviews [54]. Additionally, a previous review aimed at clarifying the evidence on telepsychiatry's effectiveness found that it was reliable for diagnosing common psychiatric disorders, with diagnostic accuracy comparable to face-to-face consultations, despite the wide variety of diagnostic measures used across different studies [38].

Of note, telepsychiatry can achieve a symptom improvement effect for various psychiatric disorders similar to that of face-to-face treatment [20, 38]. Interestingly, treatment via telemedicine interventions is beneficial for depressive symptoms and quality of life in individuals with depression [39]. Again, a comprehensive meta-analysis comparing telepsychiatry with face-to-face treatment for psychiatric disorders revealed that telepsychiatry was superior to face-to-face treatment regarding symptom improvement for depressive disorders [20]. In depression, telepsychiatry was also reported to improve medication adherence and quality-of-life scores, helping to prevent relapses and recurrences [38]. Regarding tolerability, measured by all-cause discontinuation rates, telepsychiatry showed similar results to face-to-face treatment, except for substance misuse, where in-person therapy led to fewer dropouts [20].

Thus, the main barrier to telepsychiatry is not a lack of evidence but rather clinicians' reluctance to incorporate it into their practice and the absence of consistent professional guidance [38]. Although both patients and clinicians are generally satisfied with telepsychiatry, concerns about establishing rapport, maintaining privacy, ensuring safety, and addressing technology limitations have hindered its broader acceptance [10].

17.3 Effective Communication Skills in Psychiatry and Telepsychiatry: Verbal, Nonverbal, and Virtual Interaction

Effective verbal communication is the cornerstone of psychiatric practice, especially in remote consultations where non-verbal cues may be limited (i.e., phone consults). Clinicians must employ clear, empathetic, and culturally sensitive language to build rapport, convey information, and facilitate therapeutic alliance [4, 16, 33]. Active listening, summarization, and validation of patient experiences are essential skills that promote engagement and trust [34]. With patient consent, communication should also include close family members—facilitators if needed to complete collateral information collection [15].

In remote consultations, nonverbal communication takes on new dimensions. Clinicians should be mindful of background noise, ensuring a quiet and private environment conducive to meaningful interaction [1]. Inviting or supporting patients to ensure privacy during online consultations can be highly beneficial, as the lack of private space at home has been identified as a significant barrier in virtual clinical settings [3]. The choice of setting, whether virtual or real, can also impact patient perception and engagement. Virtual backgrounds should be culturally safe, professional, and nondistracting, while real backgrounds should be tidy and devoid of potential distractions [41]. Clinicians may also consider encouraging patients to disable the self-view during video calls. This simple rule can help reduce distractions and alleviate anxiety related to one's appearance, as distress and intensified body dysmorphia may arise with frequent video call usage [35, 49]. More generally, the so-called "zoom fatigue" refers to exhaustion and stress experienced after prolonged video calls, arising from factors like distress from constantly seeing one's own image (i.e., mirror anxiety), the need to stay within the camera's frame (i.e., feeling physically trapped), the perception of continuous direct eye contact from participants (i.e., hyper gaze), and increased cognitive load (from both intentionally producing increased nonverbal cues and struggling to interpret others' cues accurately) [13, 36]. Clinicians may benefit to keep these factors in mind when delivering online consultations, both regarding the patient and for themselves—also to prevent professional burnout.

17.4 Digital Phenotyping for Psychiatric Assessment and Monitoring

The rise of digital technologies has opened new frontiers in psychiatric assessment and monitoring. Digital phenotyping, the passive collection and analysis of data from digital devices, holds promise for remote psychiatric evaluation. Objective data on sleep patterns, physical activity, social interactions, and other behavioral markers can offer valuable insights into a patient's mental health status, potentially complementing traditional clinical assessments [17].

As highlighted in Topol's Deep Medicine, artificial intelligence (AI)-powered digital phenotyping could enable continuous, real-time monitoring of mental health, alerting clinicians to potential exacerbations or relapses.

Furthermore, research suggests that digital phenotyping may be particularly useful for conditions like depression, where objective data on sleep, daily activity, and social engagement can inform treatment decisions [17]. Wearable technologies like wrist-worn biosensors have shown promise in detecting physiological signals, such as heart rate variability and electrodermal activity, which are linked to emotional regulation and can be used to predict adverse outcomes in vulnerable populations [53].

The parameters used to construct the digital phenotype are either active or passive. Various digital biomarkers leveraged in digital phenotyping include geolocation, call logs, text messages, finger taps, phone status, ambient/preferred light, data from accelerometers, gyroscopes, magnetometers, or pedometers, sleep patterns, heart rate and variability, screen behaviors like scrolling, clicking, or tapping, speech and voice modulation, battery charging frequency, navigation history, app usage, and update frequency [32]. Incorporating these data streams into AI models could allow for more personalized and adaptive interventions, particularly when used in combination with traditional psychiatric practices [53].

Voice, notably, has several important acoustic features that may be leveraged as digital biomarkers for mental health assessment, such as fluency, prosody, pitch variability, and vocal quality. The abundance of voice data collected through smartphones, virtual assistants, and telehealth visits make voice a particularly promising modality for digital phenotyping [14, 55].

Overall, digital phenotyping has the potential to revolutionize mental healthcare by providing clinicians with more comprehensive, objective data to inform diagnosis and guide treatment. However, more research and implementation studies are needed before it can have a widespread impact on clinical practice.

17.5 Applications of AI in Telepsychiatry

Although the integration of AI into mental healthcare is still an experimental field requiring further development, emerging evidence highlights its potential usefulness. AI can enhance telepsychiatry by improving diagnostic accuracy, optimizing treatment planning, and enhancing patient monitoring. AI-powered systems can analyze verbal and nonverbal cues, such as tone of voice, facial expressions, and language patterns, to assist clinicians in assessing a patient's mental state and identifying potential risk factors.

Moreover, AI algorithms can be trained to detect early warning signs of mental health crises, enabling clinicians to intervene proactively and prevent adverse outcomes. For example, AI's potential to predict and manage suicide risk has shown preliminary yet promising results, with algorithms like neural networks and gradient-boosted trees demonstrating high predictive accuracy. These models can flag at-risk individuals even when traditional assessments fall short, offering the potential to transform crisis intervention strategies [25].

In addition, AI is increasingly being incorporated into psychoeducation and psychotherapy, offering innovative approaches to mental healthcare. AI-driven platforms enhance psychoeducation by providing personalized information and resources. For example, AI chatbots can deliver tailored educational content to help individuals understand mental health conditions and develop coping strategies. These tools are accessible, scalable, and make mental health information more widely available [19].

AI-powered chatbots also offer real-time support and guidance, assisting users in managing symptoms of anxiety and depression. While they cannot replace human therapists, they provide immediate assistance and serve as supplementary resources [6]. Moreover, AI systems are being developed to deliver cognitive behavioral therapy (CBT) techniques, such as cognitive reframing, which help users identify and modify negative thought patterns. These tools are particularly beneficial for individuals who are awaiting traditional therapy sessions [19].

In summary, AI-powered chatbots and virtual assistants might serve as a first line of support in the near future, providing patients with immediate access to mental health resources, self-care strategies, and referrals to appropriate care providers. By automating certain tasks, AI can help alleviate the burden on clinicians, allowing them to focus on the more complex and nuanced aspects of patient care [2, 47]. More research and implementation studies are needed before AI can routinely be used in clinical practice, considering clinical safety and privacy.

17.6 Safety Netting and Management Plan

17.6.1 Network with Local Institution: Primary Care, Emergency, and Collaboration with Other Medical Specialists

Establishing a robust professional network with local healthcare institutions, including primary care providers, emergency services, and social service agencies, is essential for comprehensive patient care. Collaboration and mutual respect among different healthcare professionals facilitate seamless referrals, coordinated care plans, and optimal patient outcomes.

Telepsychiatry bridges gaps in mental healthcare by integrating psychiatric expertise directly into primary care settings, addressing barriers such as specialist shortages and stigma. Effective telepsychiatry requires strong interprofessional collaboration, emphasizing nonhierarchical teamwork, shared goals, and ongoing communication to support both patients and providers. Telepsychiatry consultants assist primary care providers with diagnostic clarification, medication management, and treatment planning, ensuring evidence-based care tailored to individual patient needs. While telepsychiatry enhances access, it introduces complexities, such as limited nonverbal communication and asynchronous interactions. However, where communication between referring clinician and consultant occurs at different times, access to comprehensive medical records and previous consultations is paramount for continuity of care. Clinicians should have access to electronic health record systems to review patient history, treatment plans, and relevant documentation prior to each encounter. This ensures informed decision-making, avoids duplication of efforts, promotes efficiency in remote care delivery, and contributes to reducing waiting time. Establishing clear expectations, communication protocols, and formal workflows can also address these challenges. The implementation of telepsychiatry has shown promising results in diverse primary care environments, improving care for conditions like depression and anxiety and offering tailored support for medication adherence [5].

Telepsychiatry has proven instrumental in emergency care settings, particularly during public health crises like COVID-19. Its implementation has reduced patient wait times, streamlined patient disposition, and improved access to care in underserved areas. Telepsychiatry enhances the efficiency of emergency departments (EDs) by lowering rates of inpatient admissions, decreasing the use of observation services, and mitigating ED overcrowding. It has also increased provider safety by minimizing exposure to infectious diseases and allowed for flexible staffing arrangements during crises. Despite challenges such as technology disruptions and the need for building rapport in virtual environments, telepsychiatry demonstrates significant potential to address gaps in psychiatric emergency care while improving patient and provider experiences [28].

17.6.2 Clinical Interviews, Measurement-Based Care, and Psychiatric Application

Traditional clinical interviews are crucial for gathering subjective information and building rapport with patients. However, supplementing these with measurement-based tools enhances diagnostic accuracy, treatment monitoring, and outcome assessment. Standardized assessments like the Patient Health Questionnaire-9 (PHQ-9) and the Generalized Anxiety Disorder-7 (GAD-7) provide reproducible metrics, improving consistency across practitioners and ensuring adherence to evidence-based guidelines. In addition, diagnostic interviews such as the Structured Clinical Interview for DSM Disorders (SCID) further enhance diagnostic reliability by reducing bias and ensuring comprehensive evaluation.

Measurement-based tools also play a vital role in tracking treatment progress and outcomes. Regular use of rating scales offers objective insights into symptom changes, helping clinicians make timely adjustments to therapy. For example, administering the PHQ-9 weekly can provide clear data on a patient's trajectory, allowing for more precise treatment strategies.

In telepsychiatry, these tools address challenges like limited nonverbal cues, offering structured insights that support clinical decision-making. Their digital compatibility enables easy integration into telehealth platforms, where patients can complete assessments remotely, ensuring continuous data flow. This fosters patient engagement by empowering them to track progress and participate actively in their care.

By leveraging measurement-based tools in both traditional and telepsychiatry settings, clinicians can adopt a more robust, data-driven approach to mental health care. Combining these tools with clinical interviews ensures accurate diagnoses, personalized treatments, and improved outcomes, advancing psychiatry toward more efficient and patient-centered care.

Even delicate topics in psychiatric management can be effectively addressed through telepsychiatry, with suicidality risk management serving as a prime example. The assessment and management of suicidality require a systematic and comprehensive approach, especially in remote consultations where physical observation may be limited. Clinicians should employ standardized suicide risk assessment tools, conduct thorough risk stratification, and develop safety plans tailored to individual needs. Regular follow-up and ongoing risk assessments are essential components of suicide prevention efforts. Systematic reviews and meta-analyses have shown that telehealth interventions effectively reduce suicide rates and reattempts, with high levels of patient acceptance and retention [40]. These findings align with earlier data on suicide risk management, emphasizing the importance of strategies such as emergency contact planning, access to local support resources, and the implementation of real-time safety plans customized to the patient's circumstances [26].

Of note, incorporating family members and caregivers into the treatment process can provide invaluable support and insight into the patient's condition. Clinicians should actively involve families in treatment planning, psychoeducation, and crisis intervention, fostering collaboration and resilience within the support network.

17.7 Comprehensive Investigations in Telepsychiatry: Questionnaires, Biological Monitoring, and Neuroimaging

While for physical conditions, bloodwork and other investigations are regularly used to monitor treatment and disease course, in mental health, these have less of a central role. However, they do not only play a role in excluding other causes of mental or behavioral changes, and to monitor treatment side effects, but can also inform on the clinical course of the mental disorder. For instance, weight should also be monitored in those with mental disorders. Weight loss can occur with depressive disorder, poisoning delusions, stimulants and other substance abuse, or eating disorders, and few medications (stimulants, topiramate). Weight gain can occur with eating disorders, depression with atypical features, and numerous medications, including antipsychotics, antidepressants, and mood stabilizers [45]. Also, eating disorders are unique conditions among mental disorders given their association with severe alterations in one's eating patterns. In persons suffering from eating disorders, glucose levels, complete blood count, kidney and liver function, and electrolytes should be monitored (purging, restriction, and even refeeding can alter them) [42]. Bone mineral density should be monitored in anorexia nervosa.

Besides monitoring biological markers, structured questionnaires serve as the essential tools for assessing symptom severity, functional impairment, and treatment response in psychiatric practice. Telepsychiatry platforms can facilitate the administration of standardized questionnaires, enabling efficient data collection and tracking of patient progress over time. While questionnaires or interviews do not replace the holistic assessment of a person's mental health, which should always include collection of collateral information beyond self-reported symptoms, incorporating validated measures into routine practice enhances diagnostic accuracy, treatment planning, and outcome monitoring in remote care settings.

Baseline bloodwork, including complete blood count (CBC), thyroid function tests (TSH), electrolytes, liver function tests, kidney function tests, and electrocardiography (ECG), provides valuable baseline data for psychiatric evaluation and medication management. Regular monitoring of specific medications, such as lithium, valproic acid, antipsychotics, and antidepressants, helps identify potential side effects, optimize dosing, and ensure patient safety. Also, the dose of some medications must be adjusted based on liver or kidney function, as well as comorbid conditions, and concomitant pharmacological treatments. Close collaboration between psychiatrists and primary care providers ensures comprehensive medication management and minimizes potential risks associated with long-term pharmacotherapy.

Certain clinical scenarios warrant neuroimaging studies to rule out organic pathology or structural abnormalities. Similarly, some metabolic conditions can present as and mimic symptoms of mental disorders. For instance, red flags indicating the need for brain imaging include focal neurological deficits, persistent cognitive impairment with sudden onset, new-onset seizures, or atypical psychiatric presentations. Similarly, hypoglycemia or hypothyroidism can present with confusion, or psychomotor retardation mimicking depressive symptoms or dementia. In general, confusive states, with sudden onset, disorientation, tactile, or visual hallucinations, should always pose the suspect of delirium. Persons with delirium should be assessed in hospital setting.

Overall, appropriate care also in the context of telepsychiatry cannot neglect a comprehensive assessment of a person's health, and high-quality care, including psychological treatment, should always be delivered in the context of a multidisciplinary network of mental health professionals, psychotherapists, and medical doctors.

17.8 Conclusions

Telepsychiatry has transformed the delivery of mental health services, enabling greater accessibility, continuity of care, and personalized treatment approaches. By integrating telepsychiatry into primary care, general practitioners can leverage the expertise of mental health professionals to enhance the management of psychiatric disorders in the community setting.

Primary care providers, such as general practitioners, often serve as the first point of contact for patients experiencing mental health issues, and research has shown that telepsychiatry can be an effective and reliable method for assessing a wide range of psychiatric disorders, including depression, anxiety, and post-traumatic stress disorder [52].

Further developments in telepsychiatry, such as the use of artificial intelligence and machine learning algorithms, hold promise for improving diagnostic accuracy, treatment planning, and outcome monitoring in remote care settings.

References

1. Abbs AD. Remote consultations handbook: strategies to ensure a safe and effective consultation via video or telephone. 2022.
2. Alowais SA, Alghamdi S, Alsuhebany N, Alqahtani T, Alshaya A, Almohareb SN, Aldairem A, Alrashed M, Saleh KB, Badreldin HA, Yami MSA, Harbi SA, Albekairy A. Revolutionizing healthcare: the role of artificial intelligence in clinical practice. BMC Med Educ. 2023;23(1):689. https://doi.org/10.1186/s12909-023-04698-z.
3. Boldrini T, Schiano Lomoriello A, Del Corno F, Lingiardi V, Salcuni S. Psychotherapy during COVID-19: how the clinical practice of Italian psychotherapists changed during the pandemic. Front Psychol. 2020;11:591170. https://doi.org/10.3389/fpsyg.2020.591170.
4. Brindley PG, Smith KE, Cardinal P, LeBlanc F. Improving medical communication: skills for a complex (and multilingual) clinical world. Can Respir J. 2014;21(2):89–91. https://doi.org/10.1155/2014/780270.
5. Calderone J, Lopez A, Schwenk S, Yager J, Shore J. Telepsychiatry and integrated primary care: setting expectations and creating an effective process for success. mHealth. 2020;6:29. https://doi.org/10.21037/mhealth.2020.02.01.
6. Casu M, Casu M. AI chatbots for mental health: a scoping review of effectiveness and feasibility. Appl Sci. 2024;14(13):5889. https://doi.org/10.3390/app14135889.
7. Cantor J, Schuler MS, Matthews S, Kofner A, Breslau J, McBain R. Availability of mental telehealth services in the US. JAMA Health Forum. 2024;5(2):e235142. https://doi.org/10.1001/jamahealthforum.2023.5142.
8. Conn D, Gajaria A, Madan R. Telepsychiatry: effectiveness and feasibility. Smart Homecare Technol TeleHealth. 2015;3:59. https://doi.org/10.2147/shtt.s45702.
9. Correll CU, Solmi M, Croatto G, Schneider LK, Rohani-Montez SC, Fairley L, Smith N, Bitter I, Gorwood P, Taipale H, Tiihonen J. Mortality in people with schizophrenia: a systematic review and meta-analysis of relative risk and aggravating or attenuating factors. World Psychiatry. 2022;21(2):248–71.
10. Cowan KE, McKean AJ, Gentry MT, Hilty DM. Barriers to use of telepsychiatry: clinicians as gatekeepers. Mayo Clin Proc. 2019;94(12):2510–23. https://doi.org/10.1016/j.mayocp.2019.04.018.
11. Dart EH, Whipple H, Pasqua JL, Furlow CM. Legal, regulatory, and ethical issues in telehealth technology. In: Computer-assisted and web-based innovations in psychology, special education, and health. Academic Press; 2016. p. 339–63. https://doi.org/10.1016/b978-0-12-802075-3.00013-9.
12. De Hert M, Cohen D, Bobes J, Cetkovich-Bakmas M, Leucht S, Ndetei DM, et al. Physical illness in patients with severe mental disorders. II. Barriers to care, monitoring and treatment guidelines, plus recommendations at the system and individual level. World Psychiatry. 2011;10:138–51. https://doi.org/10.1002/j.2051-5545.2011.tb00036.x.
13. Elbogen EB, Lanier M, Griffin SC, Blakey SM, Gluff JA, Wagner HR, Tsai J. A national study of zoom fatigue and mental health during the COVID-19 pandemic: Implications for future remote work. Cyberpsychology, Behavior, and Social Networking. 2022;25(7):409–415.
14. Fagherazzi G, Fischer A, Ismael M, Despotovic V. Voice for health: the use of vocal biomarkers from research to clinical practice. Digit Biomark. 2021;5(1):78–88. https://doi.org/10.1159/000515346.
15. Fassaert T, Dulmen SV, Schellevis F, Bensing J. Active listening in medical consultations: development of the Active Listening Observation Scale (ALOS-global). Patient Educ Couns. 2007;68(3):258–64. https://doi.org/10.1016/j.pec.2007.06.011.
16. Foley GN, Gentile JP. Nonverbal communication in psychotherapy. Psychiatry (Edgmont). 2010;7(6):38. https://pubmed.ncbi.nlm.nih.gov/20622944.
17. Greenhalgh T, Wherton J. Telepsychiatry: learning from the pandemic. Br J Psychiatry. 2022;220(5):257–61. https://doi.org/10.1192/bjp.2021.224.
18. Grisold W. The expanding burden of neurological disorders. Lancet Neurol. 2024;23(4):326–7. https://doi.org/10.1016/s1474-4422(24)00086-3.

19. Gutierrez G, Stephenson C, Eadie J, Asadpour K, Alavi N. Examining the role of AI technology in online mental healthcare: opportunities, challenges, and implications, a mixed-methods review. Front Psych. 2024;15:1356773. https://doi.org/10.3389/fpsyt.2024.1356773.
20. Hagi K, Kurokawa S, Takamiya A, Fujikawa M, Kinoshita S, Iizuka M, Furukawa S, Eguchi Y, Kishimoto T. Telepsychiatry versus face-to-face treatment: systematic review and meta-analysis of randomised controlled trials. Br J Psychiatry. 2023;223(3):407–14. https://doi.org/10.1192/bjp.2023.86.
21. Keuroghlian AS, Marcus PH, Neufeld J, Phillips E, Grasso C, Wozniak J. Telehealth for psychiatry and mental healthcare can improve access and patient outcomes. Nat Med. 2023;29(11):2698–700. https://doi.org/10.1038/s41591-023-02579-y.
22. Kuziemsky C, Maeder A, John O, Gogia SB, Basu A, Meher SK, Ito M. Role of artificial intelligence within the telehealth domain. Yearb Med Inform. 2019;28(01):035–40. https://doi.org/10.1055/s-0039-1677897.
23. Lauckner C, Whitten P, Holtz B. When technology alone is not enough: a discussion of a struggling telepsychiatry project and lessons from model programs; 2014. https://doi.org/10.1109/cts.2014.6867602.
24. Lawrence D, Kisely S, Pais J. The epidemiology of excess mortality in people with mental illness. Can J Psychiatry. 2010;55(12):752–60. https://doi.org/10.1177/070674371005501202.
25. Lejeune A, Le Glaz A, Perron PA, Sebti J, Baca-Garcia E, Walter M, Lemey C, Berrouiguet S. Artificial intelligence and suicide prevention: a systematic review. Eur Psychiatry. 2022;65(1):1–22. https://doi.org/10.1192/j.eurpsy.2022.8.
26. Luxton D, O'Brien K, Pruitt L, Johnson K, Kramer G. Suicide risk management during clinical telepractice. Int J Psychiatry Med. 2014;48:19–31. https://doi.org/10.2190/PM.48.1.c.
27. Moitra M, Owens S, Hailemariam M, Wilson KS, Mensa-Kwao A, Gonese G, Kamamia CK, White BJ, Young D, Collins PY. Global mental health: where we are and where we are going. Curr Psychiatry Rep. 2023;25(7):301–11. https://doi.org/10.1007/s11920-023-01426-8.
28. Natafgi N, Childers C, Pollak A, Blackwell S, Hardeman S, Cooner S, Bank R, Ratliff B, Gooch V, Rogers K, Narasimhan M. Beam me out: review of emergency department telepsychiatry and lessons learned during COVID-19. Curr Psychiatry Rep. 2021;23(11):72. https://doi.org/10.1007/s11920-021-01282-4.
29. Plana-Ripoll O, Pedersen CB, Agerbo E, Holtz Y, Erlangsen A, Canudas-Romo V, Andersen PK, Charlson FJ, Christensen MK, Erskine HE, Ferrari AJ, Iburg KM, Momen NC, Mortensen PB, Nordentoft M, Santomauro D, Scott JG, Whiteford H, Weye N, et al. A comprehensive analysis of mortality-related health metrics associated with mental disorders: a nationwide, register-based cohort study. Lancet. 2019;394(10211):1827–35. https://doi.org/10.1016/s0140-6736(19)32316-5.
30. Pogorzelska K, Chlabicz S. Patient satisfaction with telemedicine during the COVID-19 pandemic—a systematic review. Int J Environ Res Public Health. 2022;19(10):6113. https://doi.org/10.3390/ijerph19106113.
31. Prakash AV, Das S. Intelligent conversational agents in mental healthcare services: a thematic analysis of user perceptions. Pac Asia J Assoc Inf Syst. 2020;12:1–34. https://doi.org/10.17705/1thci.12201.
32. Prakash J, Chaudhury S, Chatterjee K. Digital phenotyping in psychiatry: when mental health goes binary. Ind Psychiatry J. 2021;30(2):191. https://doi.org/10.4103/ipj.ipj_223_21.
33. Priebe S, Dimić S, Wildgrube C, Janković J, Cushing A, McCabe R. Good communication in psychiatry – a conceptual review. Eur Psychiatry. 2011;26(7):403–7. https://doi.org/10.1016/j.eurpsy.2010.07.010.
34. Pygall S. Telephone triage and consultation: are we really listening? London: Royal College of General Practitioners; 2017.
35. Ramphul K. "Zoom Dysmorphia": the rise of a new issue amidst the pandemic. Acta Biomed. 2022;92(6):e2021348. https://doi.org/10.23750/abm.v92i6.12523.
36. Riedl R, Kostoglou K, Wriessnegger SC, Müller-Putz GR. Videoconference fatigue from a neurophysiological perspective: Experimental evidence based on electroencephalography (EEG) and electrocardiography (ECG). Scientific reports. 2023;13(1):18371.

37. Saxena S, Thornicroft G, Knapp M, Whiteford H. Resources for mental health: scarcity, inequity, and inefficiency. Lancet. 2007;370(9590):878–89. https://doi.org/10.1016/s0140-6736(07)61239-2.
38. Sharma G, Devan K. The effectiveness of telepsychiatry: thematic review. BJPsych Bull. 2023;47(2):82–9. https://doi.org/10.1192/bjb.2021.115.
39. Shih YH, Wang JY, Chou PH, Lin KH. The effects of treatment via telemedicine interventions for patients with depression on depressive symptoms and quality of life: a systematic review and meta-analysis. Ann Med. 2023;55(1):1092–101. https://doi.org/10.1080/07853890.2023.2187078.
40. Shoib S, Shaheen N, Anwar A, Saad A, Akr L, Saud A, Kundu M, Nahidi M, Chandradasa M, Swed S, Saeed F. The effectiveness of telehealth interventions in suicide prevention: a systematic review and meta-analysis. Int J Soc Psychiatry. 2024;70(3):415–23. https://doi.org/10.1177/00207640231206059.
41. Smits M, Dalen DV, Popping D, Bleeker R, Stommel MW, Goor HV. Designing a video consultation area for hybrid care delivery: the Garden Room with a view. Front Media. 2023;5:1198565. https://doi.org/10.3389/fdgth.2023.1198565.
42. Solmi M, Fabiano N, Clarke AE, Fung SG, Tanuseputro P, Knoll G, Myran DT, Bugeja A, Sood MM, Hundemer GL. Adverse outcomes and mortality in individuals with eating disorder-related electrolyte abnormalities in Ontario, Canada: a population-based cohort study. Lancet Psychiatry. 2024a;11(10):818–27. https://doi.org/10.1016/S2215-0366(24)00244-X.
43. Solmi M, Fiedorowicz J, Poddighe L, Delogu M, Miola A, Høye A, Heiberg IH, Stubbs B, Smith L, Larsson H, Attar R, Nielsen RE, Cortese S, Shin JI, Fusar-Poli P, Firth J, Yatham LN, Carvalho AF, Castle DJ, Seeman MV, Correll CU. Disparities in screening and treatment of cardiovascular diseases in patients with mental disorders across the world: systematic review and meta-analysis of 47 observational studies. Am J Psychiatry. 2021;178:793–803. https://doi.org/10.1176/appi.ajp.2021.21010031.
44. Solmi M, Firth J, Miola A, Fornaro M, Frison E, Fusar-Poli P, Dragioti E, Shin JI, Carvalho AF, Stubbs B, Koyanagi A, Kisely S, Correll CU. Disparities in cancer screening in people with mental illness across the world versus the general population: prevalence and comparative meta-analysis including 4 717 839 people. Lancet Psychiatry. 2020;7(1):52–63. https://doi.org/10.1016/S2215-0366(19)30414-6.
45. Solmi M, Miola A, Capone F, Pallottino S, Højlund M, Firth J, Siskind D, Holt RIG, Corbeil O, Cortese S, Dragioti E, Du Rietz E, Nielsen RE, Nordentoft M, Fusar-Poli P, Hartman CA, Høye A, Koyanagi A, Larsson H, Lehto K, Lindgren P, Manchia M, Skonieczna-Żydecka K, Stubbs B, Vancampfort D, Vieta E, Taipale H, Correll CU, ECNP Physical And meNtal Health Thematic Working Group (PAN-Health). Risk factors, prevention and treatment of weight gain associated with the use of antidepressants and antipsychotics: a state-of-the-art clinical review. Expert Opin Drug Saf. 2024b;23(10):1249–69. https://doi.org/10.1080/14740338.2024.2396396.
46. Solmi M, Seitidis G, Mavridis D, Correll CU, Dragioti E, Guimond S, Tuominen L, Dargél A, Carvalho AF, Fornaro M, Maes M, Monaco F, Song M, Shin JI, Cortese S. Incidence, prevalence, and global burden of schizophrenia – data, with critical appraisal, from the Global Burden of Disease (GBD) 2019. Mol Psychiatry. 2023;28(12):5319–27. https://doi.org/10.1038/s41380-023-02138-4.
47. Stein N. The future of population health management: artificial intelligence as a cost-effective behavior change and chronic disease prevention and management solution. MOJ Public Health. 2017;6(5):00188. https://doi.org/10.15406/mojph.2017.06.00188.
48. Tahir MJ, Waheed S, Ullah I, Ramalho R. Telepsychiatry and mental healthcare referrals: recommendations for low- and middle-income countries. Perspect Psychiatr Care. 2021;57(4):2035–6. https://doi.org/10.1111/ppc.12732.
49. Türk CB, Jafferany M. Zoom dysmorphia and increasing use of video technology: body dysmorphic disorder screening by telehealth. Prim Care Companion CNS Disord. 2022;24(4):22br03294. https://doi.org/10.4088/PCC.22br03294.

50. Viron M, Stern TA. The impact of serious mental illness on health and healthcare. Psychosomatics. 2010;51(6):458–65. https://doi.org/10.1016/s0033-3182(10)70737-4.
51. Walker ER, McGee RE, Druss BG. Mortality in mental disorders and global disease burden implications. Am Med Assoc. 2015;72(4):334. https://doi.org/10.1001/jamapsychiatry.2014.2502.
52. Wangelin BC, Szafranski D, Grös DF. Telehealth technologies in evidence-based psychotherapy. Elsevier BV; 2016. p. 119–40. https://doi.org/10.1016/b978-0-12-802075-3.00005-x.
53. Welch V, Wy TJ, Ligezka A, Hassett LC, Croarkin PE, Athreya AP, Romanowicz M. Use of mobile and wearable artificial intelligence in child and adolescent psychiatry: scoping review. J Med Internet Res. 2022;24(3):e33560. https://doi.org/10.2196/33560.
54. Yung HY, Yeung WT, Law CW. The reliability of symptom assessment by telepsychiatry compared with face to face psychiatric interviews. Psychiatry Res. 2022;316:114728. https://doi.org/10.1016/j.psychres.2022.114728.
55. Zhao Q, Fan HZ, Li YL, Liu L, Wu YX, Zhao YL, Tian ZX, Wang ZR, Tan YL, Tan SP. Vocal acoustic features as potential biomarkers for identifying/diagnosing depression: a cross-sectional study. Front Psych. 2022;13:815678. https://doi.org/10.3389/fpsyt.2022.815678.

18 Ear, Nose, and Throat Complaints in Primary Care: Assessing from a Remote Perspective

Almas Fatma, Vera Leotta, and Jacopo Demurtas

18.1 Introduction

Ear, nose, and throat (ENT) complaints are among the most common presentations in primary care, ranging from ear infections and nasal congestion to sore throats. Traditionally managed through in-person visits, the assessment and management of ENT conditions have rapidly evolved with the advent of telemedicine, especially during the COVID-19 pandemic [1]. The need to minimize physical interactions while ensuring continuity of care has underscored the importance of remote consultations in ENT, paving the way for new strategies to diagnose and manage ENT conditions effectively from a distance.

ENT is particularly well suited for remote consultations due to the nature of many upper respiratory infections and other complaints, which can often be managed initially without the need for a physical examination. In fact, early remote management approaches for ENT conditions helped establish important clinical tools, such as scoring systems for deciding whether antibiotic prescriptions are necessary [2]. Additionally, conditions such as ear infections or vertigo can often be evaluated remotely with appropriate guidance, delaying or even eliminating the need for immediate in-person care.

A. Fatma (✉)
Family Physician & Certified Digital Health Professional at Alcura Family Clinic, Navi Mumbai, India

V. Leotta
Ear, Nose, and Throat Specialist, Grosseto, Italy

J. Demurtas
Clinical and Experimental Medicine PhD Program, University of Modena and Reggio Emilia, Modena, Italy

Family Medicine Department, USL Toscana Sud-Est, Capalbio, Italy

J. Demurtas (ed.), *Remote Consultation in Primary Care*, TELe-Health,
https://doi.org/10.1007/978-3-031-89661-3_18

18.2 Common Scenarios in Remote ENT

When managing common ENT conditions such as ear infections, sore throats, or sinusitis, we may initially assume that remote assessments are inadequate. However, with proper patient collaboration and guidance, reliable findings can be obtained to support clinical decisions.

A remote consultation can be just as effective as an in-person one, provided we utilize the right techniques and involve the patient actively in the process.

While the absence of direct visualization of the ear or throat may feel limiting, modern telemedicine practices offer effective alternatives [3]. The COVID-19 pandemic has also prompted a reassessment of the necessity of routine throat examinations, highlighting the value of selective, targeted evaluations.

After completing pretriage screening to rule out emergencies, we can move forward with the remote evaluation.

Remote ENT consultations, when performed with structured guidance and patient collaboration, can provide effective assessments for conditions traditionally managed in person. In this process, the **patient becomes a key partner**, contributing through self-examinations and guided manoeuvres, such as palpating lymph nodes, inspecting the throat, or performing basic ear tests. This collaborative approach ensures that we gather essential clinical data to provide accurate advice and management remotely.

This section discusses practical approaches for evaluating ear, nose, and throat complaints, along with red flags indicating the need for urgent referral. Flowcharts and tables are included to outline decision-making pathways, aiding in remote assessments while ensuring patient safety.

18.2.1 Ear Complaints

Ear-related issues such as pain, discharge, tinnitus, and hearing loss can often be evaluated remotely with guided patient input. A structured history-taking and simple self-examination techniques allow for effective triage and management.

A structured approach is essential when addressing ear complaints remotely. The first step is to determine the **nature of the complaint**—whether it involves pain, discharge, ringing (tinnitus), or hearing loss. Based on the patient's history and reported symptoms, we can decide whether an **urgent face-to-face referral** is needed or if remote assessment will suffice.

(a) **When to Refer for Urgent In-Person Evaluation**
   - **Severe pain, discharge, or sudden hearing loss**: These may indicate serious conditions such as a **perforated eardrum**, **mastoiditis**, or **acute otitis media** with complications [4].
   - **Red flags**: Symptoms such as vertigo, high fever, swelling behind the ear (suggestive of mastoiditis), or neurological symptoms warrant immediate attention.

(b) **Remote Assessment of Milder Symptoms**

For **milder symptoms** (e.g., mild pain, fullness, or chronic tinnitus), remote assessment can proceed with guided patient self-examination and history-taking.

(c) **Techniques for Remote Ear Examination**

1. ***Hearing loss evaluation***
   - **Determine laterality**: Ask the patient to cup their hands over one ear at a time and report whether the hearing loss is **unilateral or bilateral**.
   - **Hum test** [3]: Instruct the patient to hum and note which ear hears the hum louder.
     - **Louder sound in the affected ear**: Suggests **conductive hearing loss** (e.g., fluid behind the eardrum, otitis media).
     - **Quieter sound in the affected ear**: Suggests **sensorineural hearing loss** (e.g., damage to the inner ear or nerve pathways).
     - **No difference**: Likely no hearing deficit.
     - *This test has 93% sensitivity and 100% specificity for detecting conductive hearing loss.*
2. ***Assessing pain and discharge***
   - **Tug test**: Ask the patient to gently pull on the outer ear (auricle).
     - **Pain on pulling**: Suggests **otitis externa** (infection of the ear canal).
     - **No change in pain**: More consistent with **otitis media** (infection behind the eardrum).
   - **Inspect for discharge**: Ask if the patient notices any fluid or pus draining from the ear, which may indicate **eardrum perforation** or severe infection requiring referral.
3. ***Tinnitus evaluation***
   - Ask the patient to describe:
     - **Quality**: Is it a buzzing, ringing, or whooshing sound?
     - **Frequency**: Constant or intermittent?
     - **Laterality**: Unilateral or bilateral?
   - **Middle ear involvement**: Instruct the patient to **hold their nose closed and hum**. If this worsens or alters their symptoms, it may indicate **middle ear dysfunction**.
4. ***Smartphone otoscopy***
   - If the patient has access to a **smartphone otoscope** or any other tool that may provide imaging of the ear, they can be guided to examine the **ear canal** and **tympanic membrane**. The patient can share real-time images or videos with the clinician for a better assessment of conditions like **cerumen impaction** or **eardrum perforation**.
5. ***Check for upper respiratory infections (URIs)***
   - **Recent URI symptoms** (e.g., congestion, sinus pain, sore throat) often contribute to hear complaints like **otitis media** or **Eustachian tube dysfunction**. It is crucial to explore any recent colds or sinus infections, as treating the underlying condition can resolve the ear symptoms.

6. ***Monitoring chronic hearing loss***
   - If the patient reports **progressive hearing loss**, ask about associated symptoms such as **imbalance, dizziness, or fullness** in the ear. Progressive hearing loss may involve more complex pathology, such as **otosclerosis** (involving the oval window) or **labyrinthitis**, which will require further evaluation.

- **Key Assessment Questions:**
  (i) Is the hearing loss unilateral or bilateral?
  (ii) Are there recent respiratory symptoms (cold/flu)?
  (iii) Is there dizziness or balance disturbance?

Flowchart 18.1 Remote Assessment of Ear Complaints

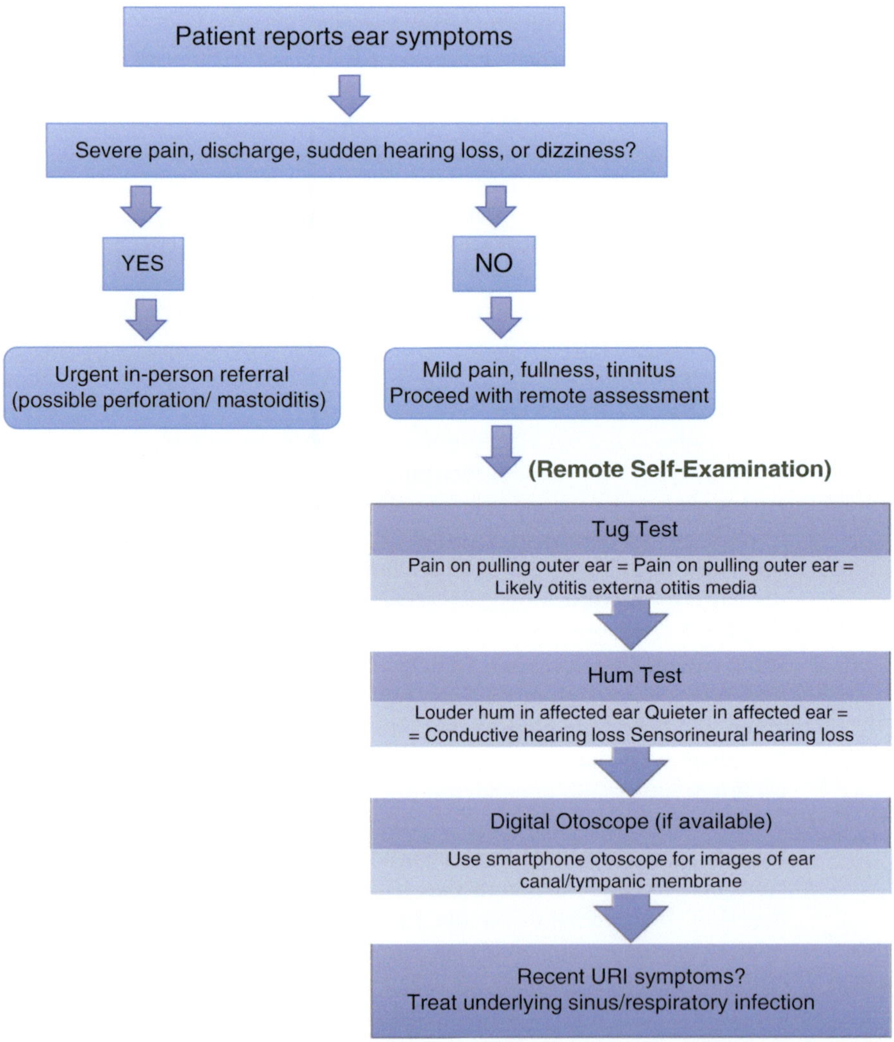

Table 18.1 Remote management of ear complaints

Symptom	Suggested action
Mild ear pain or fullness	Analgesics, monitor symptoms
Severe pain with discharge	Urgent ENT referral
Hearing loss with tinnitus	Refer for audiology if persistent
Dizziness with nausea	Monitor; consider ENT referral for vertigo symptoms

The remote assessment of ear complaints is illustrated in Flowchart 18.1, which outlines the step-by-step process for effective evaluation and triage.

Table 18.1 outlines suggested actions for managing ear complaints remotely, ranging from monitoring mild ear pain to urgent ENT referrals for severe symptoms.

By employing these simple **tests and manoeuvres** remotely, clinicians can gather useful clinical data and decide if in-person consultation is necessary. The **collaborative involvement of the patient** ensures a reliable remote assessment and improves clinical decision-making. With careful history-taking and guided self-examinations, most nonurgent ear complaints can be managed effectively through telemedicine.

18.2.2 Nose Complaints

Conditions like sinusitis, allergic rhinitis, and epistaxis (nosebleeds) are frequently encountered and, in many cases, can be managed remotely through a combination of guided self-examinations and detailed history-taking. Providing clear instructions helps the patient perform assessments independently and gather meaningful data to guide clinical decisions.

18.2.2.1 Sinusitis and Nasal Congestion

Sinus infections or nasal blockages are often associated with upper respiratory tract infections or allergies. Remote assessment can be achieved by guiding the patient through the following steps:

1. **Palpation of sinuses**
   - Ask the patient to press on the forehead (frontal sinuses) and cheeks (maxillary sinuses) to check for tenderness or pain.
   - Pain on palpation may indicate sinusitis, especially when accompanied by nasal congestion or discharge.
2. **Nasal self-examination**
   - Instruct the patient to use a flashlight or smartphone camera to inspect the nasal cavity for blockages, inflammation, or discharge.
   - Encourage them to report if the discharge is clear (allergic rhinitis) or coloured (bacterial sinusitis).
3. **Guiding questions for sinus issues**
   - Do you have a fever or facial pain?
   - Have you noticed a reduced sense of smell or taste?

– Are you experiencing headache or pressure around your eyes?
– Do your symptoms worsen when you bend forward?

For mild cases, decongestants, saline sprays, and steam inhalation may be suggested. However, if the patient reports severe symptoms or facial swelling, referral for in-person evaluation may be required.

18.2.2.2 Epistaxis (Nosebleeds)

Nosebleeds are common and can often be managed remotely, especially if the bleeding is mild or intermittent. However, severe or recurrent epistaxis may indicate an underlying issue that requires urgent care [4–6].

Remote Triage for Nosebleeds

A. **Key questions**
   - How long has the bleeding lasted?
   - How much blood has been lost?
   - Is the bleeding unilateral or bilateral?
   - How many episodes have occurred?
   - Do you feel weak or dizzy?
   - Do you have any other bleeding (e.g., gums, rectum, or bruising on the skin)?

   If the patient reports bleeding from multiple sites (e.g., hematuria, rectal bleeding, bruising), this could indicate a systemic bleeding disorder requiring urgent referral and blood tests.
B. **Possible Causes of Nosebleeds**
   - **Foreign body:** Ask if the patient suspects a foreign object lodged in the nostril.
   - **Medications:** Check for anticoagulant or antiplatelet use (e.g., warfarin, aspirin) that might impair clotting.
   - **Chronic conditions:** Assess for hypertension or clotting disorders. Although hypertension itself is not a direct cause of nosebleeds, high blood pressure may prolong bleeding episodes.

Flowchart 18.2 Remote Assessment of Epistaxis (Nosebleeds)

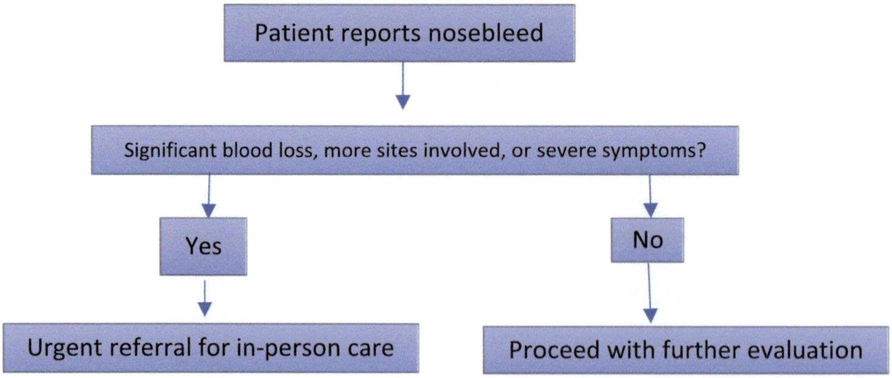

The process for remote assessment of epistaxis (nosebleeds) is detailed in Flowchart 18.2, which provides a clear framework for evaluation and management.

C. **Management of Mild Epistaxis (Nosebleeds)**

For mild cases that do not require immediate referral, advise the patient on simple self-care techniques:

(i) Pinch the nostrils firmly just below the bony part of the nose and lean forward. This prevents blood from flowing down the throat, which could cause nausea.

(ii) Apply an ice pack over the bridge of the nose to help constrict blood vessels.

(iii) Instruct the patient to avoid nose-picking, heavy lifting, or blowing the nose for at least 24 hours to prevent recurrence. If the nosebleed persists despite these measures, referral for in-person care is recommended.

Table 18.2 provides a summary of assessment methods for various nose complaints and highlights key red flags for referral, such as facial swelling and significant blood loss.

By empowering patients to participate in self-examinations and monitor symptoms, telemedicine can effectively manage many nose complaints. Careful history-taking, combined with simple at-home manoeuvres, ensures accurate remote assessments while identifying cases that require urgent in-person care.

18.2.3 Throat Complaints

Throat complaints like sore throats, swollen lymph nodes, or potential infections can be managed remotely with guided patient self-examinations, structured history-taking, and evidence-based scoring tools. Below are detailed approaches to assist remote evaluations and identify when in-person care or urgent referrals are necessary.

Table 18.2 Summary of nose complaints remote assessment

Condition	Assessment method	Red flags for referral
Sinusitis	Palpate forehead and cheeks for tenderness; inspect with flashlight or phone for discharge	Facial swelling, high fever, severe pain
Allergic rhinitis	Check for clear discharge and nasal blockage	Persistent symptoms unresponsive to antihistamines
Epistaxis	Assess bleeding duration, volume, and associated symptoms	Significant blood loss, recurrent episodes, bleeding from other sites

18.2.3.1 Palpation of Cervical Lymph Nodes

- **Instructions for the patient:**
- Ask the patient to palpate along their neck, under the jawline, and behind the ears to check for any swollen or tender lymph nodes.
- **Video demonstration:**
- Demonstrate on yourself during the consultation to improve patient compliance. If needed, request the patient to prop their phone against a stable surface for better visibility during the palpation.
- **Additional areas to assess:**
  - Tenderness over the mastoid bone
  - Discomfort around the temporal arteries
  - Pain near the roots of the upper teeth (to rule out dental involvement)

Note In case of difficulty, a family member can assist with the palpation under your guidance.

18.2.3.2 Oropharyngeal Examination

- **Video examination tips:**
- Guide the patient to use their smartphone flashlight while opening their mouth wide. Instruct them to say "ahh" to elevate the soft palate, improving visibility. If a clear view is challenging, encourage them to take a well-lit photo of the back of their throat and send it.
- **Management options:**
  - If visualization is insufficient, use scoring systems such as the **Centor Score** or **Fever PAIN** (outlined in Table 18.3) to guide treatment.
  - Consider referral to remote ENT services or in-person care if the patient has alarming symptoms.

This scoring system provides some confidence in assessing the need for antibiotics in a patient with possible bacterial (streptococcal) tonsillitis. The Royal College of Paediatrics and Child Health has recommended a pragmatic approach when it is not possible to examine the oropharynx, by starting with a baseline score of 2 [7]. Table 18.3 presents the Fever PAIN score criteria for assessing tonsillitis, which includes points for recent fever and the rapid onset of symptoms. Give one point for each of the points.

Table 18.3 Fever PAIN score for assessing tonsillitis

Criteria	Points
Fever within the last 24 hours	1
Rapid onset of symptoms (<3 days)	1
No cough or nasal congestion	1
Inflamed tonsils	1
Purulent tonsils	1

Interpretation of Scores

- **0–1:** No antibiotics needed
- **2–3:** Delayed or no antibiotics may be appropriate
- **4–5:** Immediate antibiotics should be considered

18.2.3.3 Peritonsillar Abscess (Quinsy)

A **quinsy** or peritonsillar abscess can arise as a complication of tonsillitis and may become life-threatening if left untreated. It can posteriorly obstruct the airway, necessitating immediate intervention. However, most patients can be managed conservatively, with antibiotic therapy and pain relief, provided the airway is not threatened [8].

To help differentiate between tonsillitis and quinsy, a scoring system was developed. This has been adapted following the COVID-19 pandemic to remove the need for examination of the oropharynx [3].

- ***Key questions to differentiate quinsy from tonsillitis*:**
  - Are you experiencing severe pain when swallowing?
  - Do you have difficulty opening your mouth (trismus)?
  - Is your voice altered, producing a "hot potato" sound?
  - Is there drooling or difficulty breathing?
  - Is the uvula deviated to one side?
  - Do you have ear pain (otalgia) without ear infection?
- ***Liverpool peritonsillar abscess score*:**
  - **Unilateral sore throat:** 3 points
  - **Trismus (inability to open mouth >3 cm):** 2 points
  - **Male gender:** 1 point
  - **Voice changes (hot potato voice):** 1 point
  - **Uvular deviation:** 1 point

Referral Thresholds

- **Score of 4+ *(without visual confirmation)*:** Urgent ENT referral is warranted.
- **Score of 6+ *(if oropharynx is visible):*** Referral is mandatory, given an 80% positive predictive value for quinsy.

18.2.3.4 Mumps

Mumps, a viral infection, has seen a resurgence due to declining MMR vaccination rates. It is essential to consider **mumps** as a differential diagnosis in patients presenting with unilateral or bilateral facial swelling.

- **Clinical signs of mumps:**
  - Initial swelling of a single parotid gland for 2–3 days
  - Bilateral parotid gland swelling developing later
  - Extension of swelling to the angle of the mandible and ear lobe
  - Tenderness of the affected gland
  - Earache, difficulty chewing, or trouble speaking

- **Management:**
  - Treatment is supportive, focusing on pain relief and hydration.
  - Notify public health authorities to track outbreaks.
  - Educate patients about possible complications ***(e.g., encephalitis, orchitis, meningitis)*** and advise monitoring for these symptoms.

Flowchart 18.3 Remote Assessment Flowchart for Sore Throat

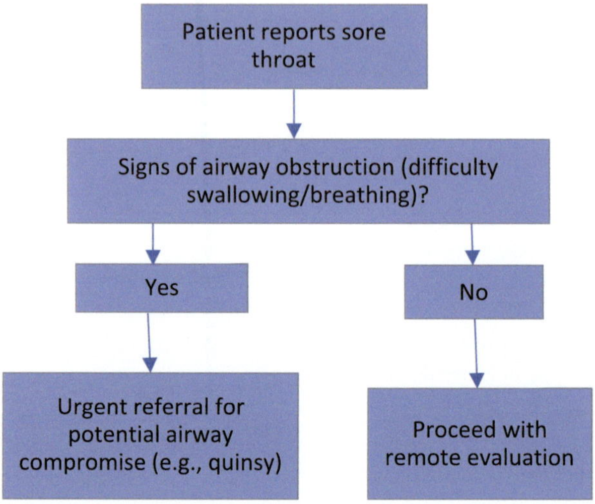

The remote assessment Flowchart 18.3 for sore throat provides a structured approach to evaluating patients with throat symptoms.

- ***Steps for Remote Oropharyngeal Examination*:**
  1. Guide the patient to inspect their throat using a smartphone flashlight.
  2. Ask them to take a deep breath and say "ahh" to elevate the soft palate.
  3. Check for redness, swelling, exudates, or uvular deviation.
  4. Use **Fever PAIN** or **Centor** score to decide on antibiotics if bacterial infection is suspected.
- ***Red Flags Requiring Immediate ENT Referral:***
  - Trismus (difficulty opening the mouth)
  - "Hot potato" voice
  - Uvular deviation
  - Drooling or inability to swallow saliva
  - Severe otalgia (referred ear pain)

By using these structured approaches, remote consultations for throat complaints can be effective, improving patient outcomes while minimizing unnecessary in-person visits.

18.3 Safety-Netting in Remote ENT Care

Safety-netting is essential in managing ENT conditions remotely to help identify serious complications early. It provides patients with clear instructions on when to seek further care if their symptoms worsen, ensuring timely intervention.

18.3.1 Conditions Requiring Urgent Referral

Table 18.4 outlines various conditions that necessitate urgent referral, detailing specific signs to watch for and the appropriate actions to take.

- ***Special considerations for children with ENT symptoms***

Young children are particularly vulnerable to complications and may have difficulty expressing their discomfort. Table 18.5 highlights safety-netting guidelines specifically for young children with ENT symptoms, emphasizing the need for early intervention and appropriate referrals. Use the safety-netting guidelines presented in the table.

Table 18.4 Conditions requiring urgent referral

Condition	Signs to watch for	Action
Mastoiditis	Swelling, redness, or tenderness behind the ear	Immediate ENT referral
Peritonsillar abscess (Quinsy)	Severe sore throat, drooling, "hot potato" voice, uvular deviation	Urgent referral to ENT specialist
Meningitis (following mumps)	Severe headache, neck stiffness, photophobia, altered consciousness	Emergency hospital referral
Epididymo-orchitis (from mumps)	Scrotal swelling, pain, fever	Urological referral
Dehydration	Inability to swallow fluids, dry mouth, dizziness, low urine output	In-person evaluation

Table 18.5 Special considerations for children with ENT symptoms

Symptom	Reason for concern	Recommended action
Bilateral ear symptoms (children <2 years)	Higher risk of middle ear infections affecting both ears	Early referral to pediatrician
Severe ear pain waking the child	Possible acute infection	Prompt evaluation
Mastoid swelling, redness, or tenderness	Indicative of mastoiditis	Immediate ENT referral
Refusal to drink fluids or swallow saliva	Risk of dehydration	Urgent face-to-face consultation
Loss of balance or dizziness	Possible inner ear involvement	ENT referral

Flowchart 18.4 Remote ENT Safety-Netting and Escalation

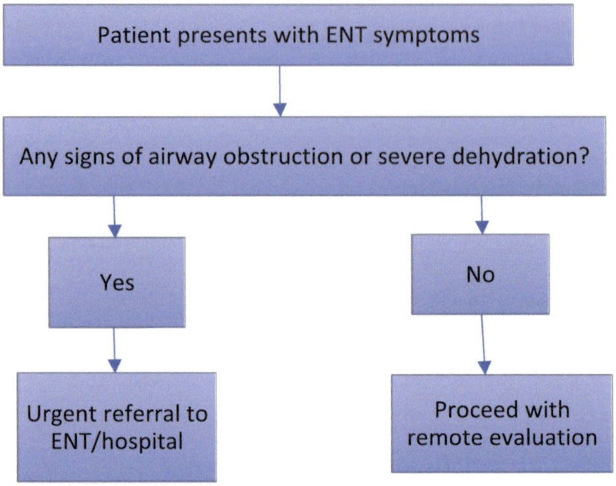

The remote ENT safety-netting and escalation Flowchart 18.4 outlines the steps for ensuring patient safety during teleconsultations.

18.3.2 Examine for Red Flag Symptoms

Table 18.6 outlines the actions to take based on the presence of red flag symptoms in various conditions, emphasizing the importance of urgent referrals for specific symptoms.

18.3.3 Remote Examination Tools for Improved Diagnosis

Many video consultation platforms now offer advanced tools, improving the quality of remote ENT consultations. Table 18.7 highlights various remote examination tools that enhance the diagnosis of ENT conditions during video consultations, showcasing their functionalities and applicable use cases. Patients can be guided to use devices listed in the table.

Table 18.6 Examination for red flag symptoms

Symptom/condition	Yes—action	No—action
Mastoiditis symptoms (swelling, pain behind the ear)	Urgent ENT referral	Continue monitoring
Oropharyngeal complaints (severe pain, drooling, uvular deviation)	Urgent ENT referral (possible quinsy)	Manage conservatively
Child <2years old with bilateral ear symptoms	Pediatric referral	Monitor and provide safety-netting instructions

- **Key benefits:**
  - Enhanced diagnostic accuracy
  - Better documentation with photos for follow-ups
  - Ability to manage more consultations remotely, reducing the need for in-person visits.

18.3.4 Differential Diagnosis of Common ENT Symptoms

Table 18.8 presents the differential diagnosis for common ENT symptoms, outlining key differentiators and investigations needed for each condition. This table helps in distinguishing between possible conditions based on overlapping symptoms in ENT, **facilitating both remote triage and referral decisions**.

Table 18.7 Remote examination tools for improved diagnosis

Tool	Functionality	Use case
Digital otoscope	Visualizes the ear canal and eardrum	Detects infections, wax buildup, or eardrum perforation
Medicam system	Provides high-quality views of throat and nasal passages	Assesses sore throat, nasal blockages, or tonsillitis
Smartphone photography	Captures images of visible pathology (e.g., tonsils, ear discharge)	Records symptoms for remote consultation and follow-up

Table 18.8 Differential diagnosis of common ENT symptoms

Symptom	Possible conditions	Key differentiators	Investigations
Ear pain (otalgia)	Acute otitis media (AOM) Otitis externa Temporomandibular joint disorder (TMJ)	AOM: Fever, bulging eardrum Otitis externa: Pain on ear manipulation TMJ: Pain on jaw movement	Otoscopy Tympanometry Jaw X-ray
Sore throat	Pharyngitis Tonsillitis Peritonsillar abscess (quinsy)	Quinsy: Uvular deviation, muffled voice Tonsillitis: Bilateral swollen tonsils Pharyngitis: Diffuse redness, no exudate	Throat swab Ultrasound (if abscess suspected)
Hearing loss	Sensorineural hearing loss Conductive hearing loss	Conductive: Improvement with tuning fork Sensorineural: No improvement Meniere's: Vertigo, tinnitus	Audiometry MRI (if central cause suspected)

(continued)

Table 18.8 (continued)

Symptom	Possible conditions	Key differentiators	Investigations
Nasal obstruction	Allergic rhinitis Nasal polyps Deviated nasal septum	Polyps: Persistent obstruction, anosmia Allergic rhinitis: Sneezing, itchy eyes Deviated septum: Unilateral blockage	Nasal endoscopy Allergy testing CT scan
Hoarseness	Laryngitis Vocal cord paralysis GERD-related laryngitis	Laryngitis: History of recent infection Vocal cord paralysis: Breathy voice GERD: Worse after meals	Laryngoscopy pH monitoring
Vertigo	Benign paroxysmal positional vertigo (BPPV) Vestibular neuritis Central vertigo	BPPV: Triggered by head movement Vestibular neuritis: Severe vertigo, no hearing loss Central: Neurological signs	Dix-Hallpike MRI Audiometry
Nasal discharge	Viral rhinitis Sinusitis CSF leak	Sinusitis: Purulent discharge, facial pain Viral rhinitis: Clear discharge, self-limiting CSF leak: Clear, watery fluid	Beta-2 transferrin test CT scan
Facial swelling	Parotitis Facial cellulitis Dental abscess	Parotitis: Pain and swelling in the parotid gland Cellulitis: Red, warm skin Dental abscess: Localized to teeth or gums	Ultrasound CT scan Dental X-ray

18.3.5 Patient Advice and Safety-Netting Instructions

Provide patients with specific guidance on when to escalate care:

- **Worsening throat pain** or development of drooling → **Call ENT specialist or visit urgent care**
- **Ear discharge lasting >48 hours** or severe pain → **Seek in-person evaluation**
- **Signs of dehydration** (dizziness, inability to drink/swallow) → **Immediate medical attention**
- **New symptoms** like high fever, stiff neck, or confusion → **Emergency referral for meningitis**

By setting clear expectations and utilizing remote tools effectively, safety-netting ensures that patients know when to seek further help, minimizing complications and improving outcomes.

18.4 Management Considerations for Remote ENT Care

Effective remote management of ear, nose, and throat (ENT) conditions requires a thorough history, patient satisfaction assessment, and careful identification of follow-up needs. Several studies have evaluated the use of telemedicine tools (phone calls, video conferencing, email, and apps) for remote follow-up in ENT care, including rhinology and general ENT cases.

18.4.1 Remote Follow-Up in Head and Neck (H&N) Patients

Studies highlight the advantages of remote follow-up, though it comes with some limitations. Table 18.9 compares remote follow-up data with face-to-face (F2F) data, highlighting significant differences in consultation duration, patient satisfaction, and the need for further evaluations. The findings indicate that remote follow-up is generally more time-efficient and cost-effective.

- **Challenges in Remote H&N Care:**
  - Some patients reported dissatisfaction due to technological issues or Internet access difficulties.
  - Staff expressed concerns about misinterpretation of email advice and potential misuse of clinician access.
  - Remote email follow-up was found beneficial for patients with speech difficulties.

Table 18.9 Comparison of remote follow-up data and face-to-face (F2F) data

Parameter	Remote follow-up data	Face-to-face (F2F) data
Delivery of biopsy results	Successfully used remote tools in 1 study	Not applicable
Need for further F2F consultation	41% (30/73) required onward referral	11.3% (9/80) required further evaluation
Touch time (consultation duration)	5.8–23.36 minutes	11.2–42.89 minutes
Patient satisfaction	Variable: High satisfaction in two studies, but lower satisfaction is reported for phone follow-ups	Higher satisfaction with in-clinic follow-ups
Cost and time savings	Remote follow-up is reported as more time-efficient and cost-effective across all studies	Less efficient than remote follow-ups

Table 18.10 Comparison of remote follow-up data and face-to-face (F2F) data

Parameter	Remote follow-up data	Face-to-face (F2F) data
Need for further F2F consultation	7.5% (19/253) and 1.5% (5/339) required referral for further testing (e.g., biopsy)	Not applicable
Referral to follow-up time	8–12 weeks with remote follow-ups	12 weeks for F2F follow-ups
Patient satisfaction	>80% reported satisfaction in two studies	Higher satisfaction with F2F consultations
Cost and time savings	Remote care preferred due to convenience and efficiency	Less convenient than remote follow-ups
Impact of COVID-19	47% of patients reported a shift in preference toward remote care due to the pandemic	Prepandemic: Higher preference for F2F care

18.4.2 Remote Rhinology Follow-Up

Rhinology patients can benefit from phone and video consultations, though certain conditions still require in-person evaluation. Table 18.10 illustrates the comparison between remote follow-up data and face-to-face (F2F) data for rhinology patients, highlighting that while remote consultations show high patient satisfaction and efficiency, certain conditions still necessitate in-person evaluations. The impact of COVID-19 is significant, with 47% of patients shifting their preference toward remote care.

- **Challenges:**
  - Lack of physical examination remains a major limitation.
  - Some consultations faced technical difficulties, affecting satisfaction.

18.4.3 Remote Follow-Up in General ENT (Adult and Pediatric Patients)

Studies show mixed results regarding the effectiveness and satisfaction with remote ENT follow-ups, especially in pediatric cases. Table 18.11 summarizes the remote follow-up data in general ENT for both adult and pediatric patients, indicating that while patient satisfaction ranges significantly, challenges such as technical issues and the need for further face-to-face consultations persist. The data highlights a notable request from caregivers for in-person reviews, particularly in pediatric case.

- **Challenges in Pediatric Remote Care:**
  - Child safeguarding is harder to evaluate remotely.
  - Technical difficulties were more common in pediatric cases, impacting both satisfaction and safety assessments.

Table 18.11 Remote follow-up in general ENT (adult and pediatric patients)

Parameter	Remote follow-up data	Challenges
Need for further F2F consultation	10% (20/200) and 45% (45/100) required F2F referral for physical exam or audiometry	Requests from caregivers for F2F reviews
Touch time (telemedicine platform)	2–21 minutes (mean: 9 minutes) using SARA platform	Not applicable
Patient satisfaction	64.6–99% satisfaction reported	Technical issues affected 42% of pediatric consultations
Staff satisfaction	Variable: Satisfied or ambivalent	Concerns about reimbursement, decision-making without physical exam, and misdiagnosis risks

- **Key Insights from Remote ENT Studies**
  - **Advantages:**

    Remote follow-ups are more time-efficient, cost-effective, and convenient compared with in-person visits.

    Many patients now prefer remote care, especially post-COVID-19.

    Remote consultations can be effective for follow-ups where physical examinations are not required.
  - **Limitations:**

    Some cases still require in-person evaluation, especially for biopsies, audiometry, or complex conditions.

    Technological literacy and access remain barriers for some patients, leading to dissatisfaction.

    Remote care may not be suitable for initial consultations in some cases, particularly pediatric evaluations.

18.5 ENT Conditions Requiring In-Person Consultation

Table 18.12 provides an overview of scenarios where remote consultation alone may be insufficient, and in-person evaluation becomes necessary for accurate diagnosis and safe management. It outlines specific ENT conditions that necessitate in-person consultations due to the limitations of remote evaluation. Conditions such as otitis media with effusion and recurrent tonsillitis require thorough physical examinations and specific investigations like tympanometry and throat swabs for accurate diagnosis and management. Additionally the table highlights the importance of face-to-face assessments, particularly in cases presenting with stridor or potential foreign body obstructions, where immediate intervention is critical.

Table 18.12 ENT conditions requiring in-person consultation

Condition	Reason for in-person visit	Examples	Investigations/ procedures needed
Otitis media with effusion (OME)	Requires otoscopic examination to assess fluid levels and evaluate eardrum mobility	Persistent ear discomfort, hearing loss	Tympanometry
Recurrent tonsillitis	Physical inspection needed to determine severity, rule out quinsy (peritonsillar abscess).	Fever, swollen tonsils, uvular deviation.	Throat swab, physical palpation of the neck
Vertigo or dizziness	Accurate differentiation between peripheral and central causes requires in-person tests (e.g., Dix-Hallpike)	Vertigo, nausea, unsteadiness	Dix-Hallpike manoeuvre, audiometry Brain MRI Neurological examination in clinic
Hearing loss	Audiometric evaluation is necessary to identify sensorineural vs. conductive hearing loss Primary cause: ear wax	Gradual or sudden loss of hearing	Pure tone audiometry, tympanometry Refer to a specialist
Epistaxis (nosebleeds)	Direct examination helps identify the bleeding site and manage recurrent or severe cases	Uncontrolled or frequent nosebleeds	Nasal endoscopy, cauterization if needed
Sinusitis with orbital complications	Immediate evaluation is required to prevent complications such as orbital cellulitis	Swelling around the eyes, blurred vision	CT scan, referral to ENT or ophthalmology
Laryngitis with stridor	Stridor suggests airway obstruction, requiring urgent in-person assessment to prevent complications	Hoarseness, difficulty breathing	Laryngoscopy, oxygen saturation check
Foreign body in ear or nose	Physical removal is essential to prevent infections or airway blockage	Ear discomfort, nasal obstruction	Foreign body removal, nasal endoscopy

18.6 Barriers and Facilitators to Remote ENT Care

Implementing remote consultations in ENT presents both challenges and opportunities. Identifying these barriers and facilitators helps promote sustainable telemedicine practices and improve patient outcomes.

18.6.1 Barriers to Remote ENT Consultations

Several barriers impact the widespread adoption of remote ENT care, including technical challenges, financial issues, and workflow adaptation. Table 18.13 outlines various barriers to the adoption of remote ENT consultations, including

Table 18.13 Barriers to remote ENT consultations

Category	Description	Details and sources
Technical infrastructure	Limited access to reliable Internet and IT support hinders teleconsultations, especially in rural areas	Poor network connectivity can lead to interruptions during remote consultations [9]
Digital literacy and training	Healthcare providers and patients often require training to use telemedicine platforms effectively	Providers must adapt clinical skills for remote care, while patients need guidance on technology use [10]
Medicolegal and ethical concerns	Lack of clear legal guidelines may create concerns around patient confidentiality, data privacy, and medical liability	Establishing policies on documentation, privacy, and liability is essential [9]
Financial sustainability	Developing sustainable reimbursement models is crucial for adoption	Initial technology investments are costly, and reimbursement models need to incentivize remote care [10]
Workflow adaptation	Integrating teleconsultations into existing healthcare workflows requires planning and adjustment	Challenges include adapting patient intake, clinical documentation, and scheduling [11]

technical infrastructure limitations and the need for enhanced digital literacy among both healthcare providers and patients. Issues such as inadequate Internet access and the necessity for training on telemedicine platforms can hinder effective remote care. Additionally, the table highlights financial sustainability challenges and workflow adaptation needs that must be addressed to promote the widespread use of teleconsultations in ENT practice.

- ***Challenges to Remote ENT in Pediatrics***
  - Remote consultations make **child safeguarding assessments more difficult**.
  - **Technical difficulties** affect pediatric care more often, with interruptions reported in 42% of remote consultations care [10].
  - Requests from caregivers often lead to in-person follow-ups for further evaluation.

18.6.2 Facilitators for Successful Implementation

Overcoming barriers requires leveraging facilitators that can enhance the delivery of remote ENT care, such as government support, advanced technology, and strategic collaborations. Table 18.14 identifies several facilitators that can enhance the implementation of remote ENT care, including government support and technological advancements. Supportive policies that promote telehealth adoption, along with user-friendly telemedicine platforms, are critical for encouraging wider acceptance and improving consultation quality. Furthermore, comprehensive education and training programs are essential for ensuring that both healthcare providers and patients are equipped with the necessary skills for effective remote consultations.

Table 18.14 Facilitators for successful implementation of remote ENT care

Category	Description	Details and sources
Government support and policy initiatives	Supportive policies that promote telehealth adoption are critical	Policies on reimbursement frameworks and liability can encourage wider adoption [12]
Technological advancements	User-friendly telemedicine platforms and digital diagnostic tools enhance consultation quality	Platforms with tools like **digital otoscopes and medicam systems** improve remote diagnosis
Education and training programs	Comprehensive training ensures that providers are skilled in telemedicine best practices	Training programs on remote consultation etiquette help both healthcare providers and patients care [10]
Collaboration and partnerships	Partnerships between healthcare institutions, tech providers, and policymakers foster innovation	Collaboration helps share knowledge, allocate resources, and develop scalable solutions [13]
Demonstrating cost-effectiveness	Evidence of time and cost savings promotes telemedicine adoption	Studies show remote follow-ups save time and reduce costs compared to face-to-face visits [14]

Table 18.15 Facilitators in action: technological solutions for remote ENT care

Technology	Use in remote ENT care	Impact
Digital otoscopes	Visualize the ear canal remotely to detect infections	Enhanced diagnosis accuracy
Medicam systems	Provide high-quality views of the throat and nasal passages	Better clinical evaluation
Smartphone photography	Patients can share photos of visible pathologies for clinician review	Improved documentation and follow-ups

- ***Facilitators in Action: Technological Solutions for ENT***

Table 18.15 outlines various technological solutions that facilitate remote ENT care, highlighting the role of digital otoscopes, medicam systems, and smartphone photography in improving diagnostic accuracy and clinical evaluation. These technologies enable enhanced documentation and follow-ups, ultimately benefiting patient care and outcomes.

18.6.3 Comparison: Barriers Versus Facilitators

Table 18.16 compares the barriers and facilitators in remote ENT care, indicating that while challenges such as poor Internet infrastructure and lack of digital literacy persist, factors like increased availability of high-speed Internet and training programs for patients and providers can promote successful implementation. Additionally, clear government policies and evidence of cost-effectiveness play crucial roles in overcoming medicolegal concerns and reimbursement challenges.

Table 18.16 Comparison of barriers and facilitators in remote ENT care

Barriers	Facilitators
Poor Internet infrastructure in rural areas	Increasing availability of high-speed internet
Lack of digital literacy in patients	Training programs for patients and providers
Medicolegal concerns over data privacy	Clear government policies addressing liability and privacy
High setup costs and reimbursement challenges	Evidence of cost-effectiveness promotes adoption
Workflow adaptation challenges	Collaboration fosters innovation and integration

18.6.4 Actionable Recommendations

- Governments and healthcare institutions should develop **supportive policies** and invest in **training programs**.
- Healthcare providers must **collaborate with technology partners** to integrate remote care effectively.
- Demonstrating the **cost-effectiveness** of remote care will encourage widespread adoption and acceptance.

By addressing these barriers and leveraging the facilitators, remote consultations can become a sustainable model for ENT care, enhancing patient outcomes and healthcare delivery.

18.7 Conclusion: Optimizing Remote ENT Management

Remote consultations in ENT have become a practical and integral part of primary care and out-of-hours general practice. While challenges remain, the evidence suggests that with appropriate tools, physician training, and patient cooperation, remote ENT management is both **feasible and effective**.

18.7.1 The Value of Remote ENT Consultations

- **Enhanced access and convenience:** Remote care expands access to healthcare, especially for patients in rural or underserved areas.
- **Time and cost savings:** Virtual follow-ups reduce travel time and expenses for both patients and providers, improving efficiency.
- **Out-of-hours triage:** Remote ENT consultations are particularly valuable in urgent care settings, where early triage can prevent complications.

18.7.2 Key Competencies and Tools for Effective Remote ENT Care

To ensure accurate diagnoses and safe management, certain **key tools** and **skills** are essential. Table 18.17 outlines the key competencies and tools necessary for effective remote ENT care, highlighting the importance of video otoscopy and video laryngoscopy in diagnosis. However, challenges such as the limited availability of these tools in primary care settings and the need for patient cooperation in guided self-examination may impact their implementation.

Finding a balance between advanced technology and basic tools will allow primary care physicians to manage ENT complaints effectively even in resource-limited environments.

18.7.3 The Importance of Safety-Netting and Referral Practices

Remote ENT care is most effective when **safety-netting protocols** are in place. These ensure that patients understand when and how to seek further medical assistance if symptoms worsen.

- **Referral criteria:** Clear guidelines for when to escalate to in-person care (e.g., persistent ear pain or worsening sore throat).
- **Self-monitoring:** Empowering patients with tools and instructions for tracking their symptoms.
- **Caregiver involvement in pediatric care:** Involving caregivers to support remote assessments for children ensures thorough monitoring.

18.7.4 Challenges to Remote ENT Care

While remote care provides many benefits, it is essential to address the challenges to achieve seamless integration. Table 18.18 presents various challenges to remote ENT care, including technical infrastructure and digital literacy issues, along with suggested solutions to address these challenges for better integration of remote services.

Table 18.17 Key competencies and tools for effective remote ENT care

Competency	Tool/technique	Availability and challenges
Video otoscopy	Visualizes the ear canal and eardrum remotely	Often unavailable in standard primary care settings [12]
Home monitoring devices—pulse oximeter	Tracks vital signs and symptoms remotely	Limited adoption due to cost and technical limitations
Guided self-examination	Patients perform self-assessment under clinician guidance	Requires patient cooperation and digital literacy

Table 18.18 Challenges to remote ENT care

Challenge	Description	Solution
Technical infrastructure	Limited Internet connectivity, especially in rural areas	Investments in reliable IT infrastructure and government support
Digital literacy	Patients and providers may struggle with telemedicine platforms.	Training programs to build confidence in technology use
Medicolegal and ethical issues	Privacy concerns and liability issues in remote care settings	Clear policies and documentation guidelines to protect both patients and providers
Clinical limitations	In some cases, a physical examination remains necessary	Judicious referral to in-person care when remote options are insufficient

18.7.5 A Balanced Approach to Remote and In-Person ENT Care

Remote consultations should complement, not replace, in-person care. **Hybrid models** combining telemedicine with face-to-face assessments are likely to offer the best outcomes, especially in the following cases:

- **Pediatric patients:** In-person care may be required for detailed evaluations or when safeguarding concerns arise.
- **Complex cases:** Patients with unclear diagnoses or persistent symptoms should be referred to ENT specialists for physical examinations.
- **Audiometry needs:** Hearing assessments and other physical tests may still necessitate in-person visits.

18.7.6 Conclusion: Unlocking the Potential of Remote ENT Care

Telemedicine has unlocked new possibilities for diagnosing and managing ENT conditions. However, success depends on **refining clinical strategies** and ensuring **patient trust** in virtual care.

- **Well-structured medical histories**, **guided virtual assessments**, and appropriate use of digital tools empower physicians to provide effective care remotely.
- **Knowing when to escalate** to in-person care is essential to avoid complications and ensure patient safety.
- Ongoing efforts to address **barriers like technical limitations, digital literacy, and medicolegal concerns** will further enhance remote ENT care delivery.

As technology evolves, remote consultations will play an increasingly prominent role in **streamlining healthcare delivery** and **improving patient outcomes**. With **supportive policies**, **collaboration across sectors**, and **continuous training**, remote ENT consultations can become a **sustainable, high-quality model of care** for both patients and providers.

References

1. Monaghesh E, Hajizadeh A. The role of telehealth during the COVID-19 outbreak: a systematic review based on current evidence. BMC Public Health. 2020;20(1):1–9. https://doi.org/10.1186/s12889-020-09301-4.
2. D'Ettorre G, Ceccarelli G, Marazzato M, Campagna G, Pinacchio C, Alessandri F, Ruberto F, Rossi G, Celani L, Scagnolari C, Mastropietro C, Trinchieri V, Recchia G, Mauro V, Antonelli G, Pugliese F, Mastroianni CM. Challenges in the management of SARS-CoV2 infection: the role of oral bacteriotherapy as a complementary therapeutic strategy to avoid the progression of COVID-19. Front Med. 2020;7:389. https://doi.org/10.3389/fmed.2020.00389.
3. Abbs AD. Remote consultations handbook: strategies to ensure a safe and effective consultation via video or telephone. 2022.
4. Akhtar M, Heukelom PV, Ahmed A, Tranter R, White E, Shekem N, Walz DF, Fairfield C, Vakkalanka JP, Mohr NM. Telemedicine physical examination utilizing a consumer device demonstrates poor concordance with in-person physical examination in emergency department patients with sore throat: a prospective blinded study. Telemed e-Health. 2018;24(10):790–6. https://doi.org/10.1089/tmj.2017.0240.
5. Carmona C, Bewick T, Macduff N, Thomas A. Suspected acute respiratory infection in over 16s: assessment at first presentation and initial management—summary of NICE guidance. BMJ. 2024;382:q339. https://doi.org/10.1136/bmj.q339.
6. Keshvardoost S, Bahaadinbeigy K, Shadman H, Tafreshi A, Baneshi MR. Design, development, and evaluation of a teleophthalmology system using a low-cost fundus camera. Acta Inf Med. 2020;28(1):12–7. https://doi.org/10.5455/aim.2019.28.12-17.
7. Kanagasabai A, Evans C, Jones HE, Hay AD, Dawson S, Savović J, Elwenspoek MMC. Systematic review and meta-analysis of the accuracy of McIsaac and Centor score in patients presenting to secondary care with pharyngitis.
8. Herzon FS. Peritonsillar abscess: incidence, current management practices, and a proposal for treatment guidelines. Laryngoscope. 1995;105(S3):1–17. https://doi.org/10.1288/00005537-199508002-00001.
9. AlKhanbashi RO, Zedan HS. Telemedicine policy availability and awareness: directions for improvement. Smart Homecare Technol TeleHealth. 2022;9:1–9. https://doi.org/10.2147/shtt.s368486.
10. Opoku D, Scott P, Quentin W. Healthcare professionals' perceptions of the benefits and challenges of a teleconsultation service in the Amansie-West District of Ghana. Telemed e-Health. 2015;21(9):748–55. https://doi.org/10.1089/tmj.2014.0210.
11. Greenhalgh T, Rosen R, Shaw SE, Byng R, Faulkner S, Finlay T, Grundy E, Husain L, Hughes G, Leone C, Moore L, Papoutsi C, Pope C, Rybczynska-Bunt S, Rushforth A, Wherton J, Wieringa S, Wood GW. Planning and evaluating remote consultation services: a new conceptual framework incorporating complexity and practical ethics. Front Digit Health. 2021;3:726095. https://doi.org/10.3389/fdgth.2021.726095.
12. Rosen R, Wieringa S, Greenhalgh T, Leone C, Rybczynska-Bunt S, Hughes G, Moore L, Shaw SE, Wherton J, Byng R. Clinical risk in remote consultations in general practice: findings from in-COVID-19 pandemic qualitative research. BJGP Open. 2022;6(3):BJGPO.2021.0204. https://doi.org/10.3399/bjgpo.2021.0204.
13. Bhutta MF, Swanepoel DW, Fagan J. ENT from afar: opportunities for remote patient assessment, clinical management, teaching and learning. Clin Otolaryngol. 2021;46(4):689–91. https://pubmed.ncbi.nlm.nih.gov/33872469/.
14. Gupta T, Gkiousias V, Bhutta MF. A systematic review of outcomes of remote consultation in ENT. Clin Otolaryngol. 2021;46:699. https://doi.org/10.1111/coa.13768.

Remote Consultation and Telemedicine for Musculoskeletal Diseases in Primary Care

19

Lee Smith and Jacopo Demurtas

19.1 Introduction

Musculoskeletal health refers to the performance of the locomotor system, comprising intact muscles, bones, joints, and adjacent connective tissues. There are greater than 150 different diseases/conditions that affect the musculoskeletal system, and these can be categorized into the following domains, impairments in the muscles, bones, joints, and adjacent connective tissues leading to temporary or lifelong limitations in functioning and participation. Musculoskeletal conditions often result in pain (acute and chronic) and limitations in mobility and dexterity, resulting in work absenteeism, sick leave, and unemployment as well as a reduction in social activities. Pain experienced in musculoskeletal structures is the most common form of noncancer pain [1].

In the treatment and management of musculoskeletal disorders multidisciplinary and multifacility treatment throughout different settings and providers (physiotherapy, rehabilitation, prehabilitation, and orthopedics; inpatient, outpatient, and home) is often required. Telemedicine is a potentially useful tool to aid in the achievement of such complex treatment and management. Indeed, for those with musculoskeletal disorders, it has been found that the adoption of telemedicine can improve clinical and patient-reported outcomes along with organizational arrangements and cost savings [2].

L. Smith (✉)
Centre for Health Performance and Wellbeing, Anglia Ruskin University, Cambridge, UK
e-mail: lee.smith@aru.ac.uk

J. Demurtas
Clinical and Experimental Medicine PhD Program, University of Modena and Reggio Emilia, Modena, Italy

Family Medicine Department, USL Toscana Sud-Est, Capalbio, Italy

J. Demurtas (ed.), *Remote Consultation in Primary Care*, TELe-Health,
https://doi.org/10.1007/978-3-031-89661-3_19

Musculoskeletal conditions are broad and to discuss each individual condition and the use of telemedicine in each case would be vast, thus, the remainder of this chapter will discuss the use of telemedicine for the following common musculoskeletal disorders, including osteoarthritis, osteoporosis, and low back pain, predominantly drawing on the most recent findings from systematic reviews and meta-analyses.

19.2 Telemedicine and Osteoarthritis

Osteoarthritis is the most common form of arthritis, affecting millions of people across the globe. It occurs when the protective cartilage that cushions the ends of the bones wears down over time and is commonly observed in the joints of the hands, knees, hips, and spine. Osteoarthritis symptoms are generally manageable; however, the damage to joints cannot be reversed. Regular participation in physical activity, maintaining a healthy weight and receiving targeted treatments can slow progression of the disease and improve pain and joint function [3].

Numerous studies have been carried out on telemedicine and osteoarthritis. One systematic review and meta-analysis aimed to identify telerehabilitation strategies attributing to the improvement of pain and physical function outcomes in patients with knee osteoarthritis. A total of six randomized controlled trials (RCTs; $n = 734$) incorporating eight different telerehabilitation strategies were included. The duration of the interventions ranged from 1 to 48 weeks, and sample sizes ranged from 20 to 350 patients. The results showed that RCTs that provided telerehabilitation were found to be more effective than conventional treatments for improving pain ($P = 0.003$; standardized mean difference [SMD] −0.21, 95% CI −0.35 to −0.07), but not physical function ($P = 0.24$; SMD −0.09, 95% CI −0.25 to 0.06). Furthermore, this systematic review and meta-analysis indicated that there is no significant correlation between different telerehabilitation strategies and the pain and physical function of patients with knee osteoarthritis [4].

Another systematic review and meta-analysis aimed to evaluate the effectiveness of Internet-based telehealth programs in the management of patients with hip or knee osteoarthritis. A total of 21 studies were included in the meta-analysis. The pooled results showed that Internet-based telehealth had a superior effect on increasing function (SMD 0.30, 95% CI 0.23–0.37, $P < 0.001$), relieving pain (SMD −0.27, 95% CI −0.34 to −0.19, $P < 0.001$), and improving self-efficacy for pain (SMD 0.21, 95% CI 0.08–0.34, $P < 0.001$) compared to the conventional intervention group. It was also observed that Internet-based telehealth with exercise (one domain of physical activity) can significantly alleviate pain and improve function and self-efficacy. However, interestingly, Internet-based telehealth with cognitive-behavioral therapy only had the effect of reducing pain [5].

Another review aimed to identify and discuss the modes of service delivery and technologies in telerehabilitation programs for patients with knee osteoarthritis. A total of 38 studies were included. Four modes of telerehabilitation service delivery were identified: phone-based, video-based, sensor-based, and expert system–based telerehabilitation. The intervention services provided in the studies included information, training, communication, monitoring, and tracking. Video-based telerehabilitation programs were frequently used. Among the identified services, information and educational material were introduced in 25% of the studies. The study concluded that video-based telerehabilitation programs can be considered the best alternative solution to conventional treatment [6].

19.3 Telemedicine and Osteoporosis

Osteoporosis is a bone disease that develops when bone mineral density and bone mass decreases, or when the structure and strength of bone changes. This can lead to a decrease in bone strength that can increase the risk of fractures [7]. Osteoporosis is a leading cause of fractures in postmenopausal women and in older men. Osteoporotic fractures happen most often in bones of the hip, vertebrae in the spine, and wrist [7].

One review aimed to discuss the evidence for remote healthcare delivery in the context of osteoporosis during the COVID-19 pandemic. It was found that within the context of osteoporosis management, there is some limited evidence to suggest telemedicine approaches are acceptable to patients and unclear evidence on whether telemedicine approaches support informed drug adherence. Multiple gaps in the evidence were identified pertaining to the acceptability and benefits of using telemedicine in populations with hearing, cognitive, or visual impairments and in those with low levels of health literacy. The study concluded that there is an urgent need for further health service evaluation and research to address the impact of remote healthcare delivery during COVID-19 outbreak on patient care, and in the longer term, to identify acceptability and cost- and clinical-effectiveness of remote care delivery on outcomes of relevance to people living with osteoporosis [8].

While there is an absence of systematic reviews and meta-analysis on telemedicine and osteoporosis, many individual studies do exist covering a range of outcomes. One study aimed to understand the experiences, benefits, and challenges associated with receiving osteoporosis care by telemedicine from the patient perspective. A mixed methods study design whereby both a quantitative component (mailed survey) and qualitative component (30-min telephone interviews) were conducted simultaneously. In addition to reporting survey data, thematic analysis was applied to interview data. The study found that participants were comfortable with virtual technology and perceived that their quality of care by telemedicine was comparable to in-person visits. Expressed benefits included the convenience of timely care close to home, reduced burden of travel and costs, and enhanced sense of confidence with being assessed by an osteoporosis specialist. Perceived barriers included poor follow-up with allied health professionals in the telemedicine program (e.g., physiotherapist) and coordination of tests and investigations. Many participants indicated interest in an osteoporosis self-management program, with content focusing on diet and lifestyle factors [9]. Another study aimed to assess the acceptability of teleconsultations across five dimensions for osteoporosis care among patients who started or continued with teleconsultations after the COVID-19 pandemic. They then explored the patient characteristics associated with these perceptions. The degree of acceptability of teleconsultations was overall good across the 80 respondents and the five domains. Some heterogeneity in perceptions emerged with respect to teleconsultations substituting for in-person visits, negatively impacting continuity of care and reducing the length of consultations. Overall, acceptability was not affected by patient characteristics with a few exceptions related to treatment time and familiarity with the teleconsultation service modality (i.e., length of osteoporosis treatment and number of telecommunications experienced by the patient) [9].

19.4 Telemedicine and Low Back Pain

Low back pain (LBP) describes pain between the lower edge of the ribs and the buttocks. It can be acute or chronic and impact anyone regardless of demographics. Regardless of the type and stage of LBP, rehabilitation is essential in pain management and to support patients returning to activities of daily life. However, specialized care pathways may be needed for specific LBP.

One systematic review [10] sought to identify all clinical trials and cohort studies that utilized some type of synchronous telehealth intervention for the virtual management of LBP. Interestingly, the search revealed a single unblinded, noninferiority trial comparing a synchronous telehealth interaction with standard, in-person care. This significant literature gap and lack of clinical trials studying synchronous telehealth interventions for LBP is somewhat surprising. The field of LBP is in desperate need of a solution to increase access points for care and faster referral of patients to a nonsurgical provider. There are conditions for which management via telehealth has begun to thrive, and the authors of this systematic review hypothesized that LBP was no different. Ultimately, this focused area of research is still in its infancy. We call on the scientific arena to implement more projects in the domain of telehealth and LBP.

When assessing LBP, several red flags must be considered, to exclude a cauda equina syndrome: loss of bowel or bladder control, severe or progressive leg weakness, saddle anesthesia (altered sensation when wiping following toileting or weird sensation in the inner part of thighs), and loss of power or sensation in one or both legs. If any of these red flags are present, urgent/emergency referral to hospital is warranted [11].

19.5 Guidance for Clinicians

19.5.1 Preparing the Setting

When assessing musculoskeletal conditions remotely, either by phone or video, the setup conditions must be considered after a thorough history taking. Patients should have enough space to demonstrate their movements (i.e., to walk so gait can be evaluated). The patient needs to be equipped with a smartphone camera to allow thorough evaluation from a distance.

If there are signs or symptoms suggesting severe conditions, like sepsis or trauma, the patient should still be referred to an in-person consultation [12].

19.5.2 Performing the Consultation

The key elements of the musculoskeletal examination—*look, feel, and move*—remain applicable during remote consultations. However, if there are any concerns about a possible bony injury or nonaccidental injury, a face-to-face referral is essential [11].

19.5.2.1 Look

The consulting clinician should ask the patient to use their phone or camera to provide a close-up view of the affected body parts. The clinician should observe for signs of swelling, redness, muscle waste, or any evidence of trauma. The assessment of other joints should also be carried out, particularly those above and below the affected area, as well as the contralateral joint. Additionally, the clinician should request a side view from the patient to help evaluate any swelling in the joint [11].

19.5.2.2 Feel

To feel the affected body parts, the clinician should instruct the patient to position the phone to the side, freeing both their hands. This will allow them to palpate their own joints and report any warmth, crepitus on movement, or tenderness. Time should be taken to guide the patient in precisely locating any areas of tenderness, which will achieve a more accurate diagnosis. Additionally, the patient should be asked to feel the joints in different positions to assess whether this affects reported tenderness [11].

19.5.2.3 Move

To move the affected body parts, the patient should be instructed to step back from the camera so that one can observe both left and right sides to identify any asymmetry. The patient should then be asked to move the affected limbs, which will allow for the assessment of pain, range of motion, and function. Evaluating the patient's ability to stand on one leg is a useful screening test for lower limb fractures, as it eliminates compensation from the healthy limb. The clinician should request the patient to walk to the back of the room and back again to assess their gait. The clinician should demonstrate the desired movements to guide the patient and ensure they perform the actions correctly [11].

Considering the general indications given, remote consultation may be a viable approach for managing certain musculoskeletal conditions in primary care, particularly for conditions involving minor sprains, acute LBP, and follow-up care [13].

Some districts where remote consultations may provide useful information are the shoulder and the knee, often affected by several disorders, such as calcific tendinitis, instability, and osteoarthritis [14, 15]. Face-to-face consultation remains essential for more severe or complex conditions, significant trauma or other 'red flag' symptoms [11].

19.6 Shoulder Examination

In a remote setting, the shoulder examination can be challenging, but key elements can still be assessed. Movement patterns can be observed by watching the patient. The range of motion and any significant asymmetry in shoulder height or scapular positioning can be noted. The patient can be instructed to grip their arm and pull upward to assess for impingement, and they may also be asked to demonstrate specific movements like overhead reach and cross-body adduction [16, 17]. Additionally, a variant of the Neer or Hawkins Kennedy test, without using the examiner's hands but relying on the patient, can be performed to assess impingement conditions [18].

The examiner may ask the patient to put their contralateral hand on the affected shoulder or elbow and identify the area of greatest tenderness or pain with movement. Other maneuvers are possible, depending on the expertise of both the clinician and the patient.

While palpation of the shoulder is limited in the remote setting, the patient can be guided to locate and palpate structures like the acromioclavicular joint, the biceps tendon, and the greater tuberosity, reporting any tenderness.

19.7 Knee Examination

The knee examination can still be viable in remote consultations, relying on patient feedback and indications [14]. The patient can demonstrate movements like knee flexion and extension, allowing the examiner to observe the range of motion, quality of movements, and any gross instability or crepitus. Additionally, the patient may be instructed to perform a single-leg stance test to assess quadriceps/patellar tendon strength and stability. Other maneuvers, such as assessing joint-line tenderness or checking for ligamentous laxity, could be suggested, with the patient providing immediate feedback regarding any pain or instability.

While a remote evaluation may not be as comprehensive as an in-person examination, it can still provide valuable information to guide initial management and determine the need for further in-person evaluation [11, 15].

Other districts and joints may be assessed as well, depending on patients' collaboration and examiner's skills.

19.8 Conclusions

There is a growing and emerging body of scientific literature in relation to musculoskeletal disorders and telemedicine. However, the distribution of the research across the most predominant musculoskeletal conditions is uneven. While there are multiple nuances in the findings in the scientific literature in relation to telemedicine and musculoskeletal disorders, overall, the literature suggests a role and that patients generally accept such an approach. However, there is a true sparsity of research in some important areas in relation to telemedicine and musculoskeletal disorders. Thus, the authors of this chapter call on the academic and clinical audience to divert time and research into understanding the true potential of telemedicine across all musculoskeletal conditions.

Remote examinations of musculoskeletal disorders are often possible and viable, giving information to the examiner and permitting a grand triage of many conditions. While possible, remote consultation and telemedicine application of musculoskeletal complaints is not adequately supported by literature findings.

References

1. Liu S, Wang B, Fan S, Wang Y, Zhan Y, Ye D. Global burden of musculoskeletal disorders and attributable factors in 204 countries and territories: a secondary analysis of the global burden of disease 2019 study. BMJ Open. 2022;12(6):e062183.
2. Foni NO, Costa LAV, Velloso LMR, Pedrotti CHS. Telemedicine: is it a tool for orthopedics? Curr Rev Musculoskelet Med. 2020;13:797–801.
3. Peterson LS. Mayo clinic guide to arthritis: managing joint pain for an active life. Rosetta Books; 2020.
4. Xiang W, Wang JY, Ji BJ, Li LJ, Xiang H. Effectiveness of different telerehabilitation strategies on pain and physical function in patients with knee osteoarthritis: systematic review and meta-analysis. J Med Internet Res. 2023;25:e40735.
5. Wang HN, Luo P, Liu S, Liu Y, Zhang X, Li J. Effectiveness of internet-based telehealth programs in patients with hip or knee osteoarthritis: systematic review and meta-analysis. J Med Internet Res. 2024;26:e55576.
6. Naeemabadi M, Fazlali H, Najafi S, Dinesen B, Hansen J. Telerehabilitation for patients with knee osteoarthritis: a focused review of technologies and teleservices. JMIR Biomed Eng. 2020;5(1):e16991.
7. https://www.niams.nih.gov/health-topics/osteoporosis.
8. Paskins Z, Crawford-Manning F, Bullock L, Jinks C. Identifying and managing osteoporosis before and after COVID-19: rise of the remote consultation? Osteoporos Int. 2020;31:1629–32.
9. Palcu P, Munce S, Jaglal SB, Allin S, Chishtie JA, Silverstein A, Kim S. Understanding patient experiences and challenges to osteoporosis care delivered virtually by telemedicine: a mixed methods study. Osteoporos Int. 2020;31:351–61.
10. Bise CG, Cupler Z, Mathers S, Turner R, Sundaram M, Catelani MB, et al. Face-to-face telehealth interventions in the treatment of low back pain: a systematic review. Complement Ther Clin Pract. 2022;50:101671.
11. Abbs AD. Remote consultations handbook: strategies to ensure a safe and effective consultation via video or telephone; 2022.

12. Shaver J. The state of telehealth before and after the COVID-19 pandemic [review of the state of telehealth before and after the COVID-19 pandemic]. Prim Care. 2022;49(4):517. Elsevier BV. https://doi.org/10.1016/j.pop.2022.04.002.
13. Cliffe S, Stevenson K. Patient experiences of virtual consultation during COVID 19: a musculoskeletal service evaluation. Musculoskelet Care. 2020;19(3):380. Wiley. https://doi.org/10.1002/msc.1534.
14. Murray T, Murray G, Murray JRD. Remote musculoskeletal assessment framework: a guide for primary care. Cureus. Cureus, Inc. 2021;13(1):e12778. https://doi.org/10.7759/cureus.12778.
15. Portnoy JM, Waller M, Elliott T. Telemedicine in the era of COVID-19. J Allergy Clin Immunol Pract. 2020;8(5):1489. Elsevier BV. https://doi.org/10.1016/j.jaip.2020.03.008.
16. Marreez YMAH, Forman MD, Brown SR. Physical examination of the shoulder joint—part I: supraspinatus rotator cuff muscle clinical testing. OFP. 2013;5(3):128. Elsevier BV. https://doi.org/10.1016/j.osfp.2013.01.005.
17. Tennent TD, Beach WR, Meyers JF. A review of the special tests associated with shoulder examination [review of a review of the special tests associated with shoulder examination]. Am J Sports Med. 2003;31(1):154. SAGE Publishing. https://doi.org/10.1177/03635465030310011101.
18. McFarland EG, Garzon-Muvdi J, Jia X, Desai P, Petersen SA. Clinical and diagnostic tests for shoulder disorders: a critical review [review of clinical and diagnostic tests for shoulder disorders: a critical review]. Br J Sports Med. 2009;44(5):328. BMJ. https://doi.org/10.1136/bjsm.2009.067314.

Abdominal Examination and Complaints: Triage and Remote Consultation

20

Francesco Di Gennaro, Luisa Frallonardo, Giacomo Guido, and Jacopo Demurtas

20.1 Introduction

In medical practice, abdominal examinations have traditionally required in-person evaluations due to the complexity of accurately diagnosing abdominal complaints. Many believe that without a direct examination, physicians risk overlooking serious conditions. But is an in-person evaluation always essential? In some healthcare settings and countries, logistical limitations hinder prompt access to in-person abdominal assessments, especially for complaints involving the gastrointestinal tract, urinary tract, or nearby anatomical structures. In these situations, telemedicine and remote consultation tools serve as valuable alternatives, allowing initial evaluations and decision-making regarding the need for further care [1–4]. While physical exams remain essential in primary care, healthcare providers must adapt to remote consultations by relying on a combination of patient-reported symptoms, vital signs, and observable signs via video or phone [5–9]. Notably, patients with certain abdominal complaints do not always need face-to-face assessment; with an adequate remote examination and appropriate guidance, these cases can often be managed safely without in-person visits. The COVID-19 pandemic demonstrated that in-person visits could be minimized effectively, with many abdominal complaints addressed through virtual means, as shown in studies highlighting reduced patient referrals and hospitalization rates for specific conditions during the pandemic.

F. Di Gennaro (✉) · L. Frallonardo · G. Guido
Clinic of Infectious Diseases, Department of Precision and Regenerative Medicine and Ionian Area (DiMePRe-J), University of Bari Aldo Moro, Bari, Italy
e-mail: francesco.digennaro1@uniba.it

J. Demurtas
Clinical and Experimental Medicine PhD Program, University of Modena and Reggio Emilia, Modena, Italy

Family Medicine Department, USL Toscana Sud-Est, Capalbio, Italy

J. Demurtas (ed.), *Remote Consultation in Primary Care*, TELe-Health,
https://doi.org/10.1007/978-3-031-89661-3_20

20.2 Abdominal Examination in Remote Consultation

The abdominal examination is a critical component of the physical evaluation, providing valuable insights into the underlying condition. While conducting a comprehensive in-person examination is ideal, healthcare providers can still obtain useful information through a remote assessment. During a remote consultation, the healthcare provider should guide the patient through a series of self-examination maneuvers, while also observing the patient's responses and any visual cues that may be available [10–17].

Below you can find the key steps for a remote abdominal examination:

20.2.1 Palpation

Instructing the patient to identify the precise location of their abdominal pain is a fundamental step in remote abdominal examination. Ask the patient to use a single finger to point directly to the center of their pain, as this helps in localizing the discomfort more accurately. This method is generally more effective if the patient is standing, as gravity can affect abdominal positioning, potentially revealing or relieving certain types of discomfort. The patient can then perform a self-palpation while lying down, ideally on a firm surface, dividing their abdomen into six zones: top, middle, bottom, left, right, and center. This division allows the patient to focus on one area at a time, making it easier to detect specific points of tenderness or discomfort.

When the patient encounters a tender area and reflexively avoids it, this can be indicative of guarding, a clinical sign often associated with conditions that cause peritoneal irritation, such as appendicitis or diverticulitis. It is important to emphasize to the patient that they should avoid applying excessive pressure and instead focus on light palpation. In some cases, healthcare providers can guide the patient to palpate the renal angle (costovertebral angle) by lying down and gently pressing with their fingertips near the lower ribs on each side of the back. The patient should report back on any pain, discomfort, or tenderness felt during this process, as well as confirm the specific area they palpated, to ensure clarity and precision in the self-examination.

During remote consultations, ensuring that both the examiner and the patient accurately agree on the region of pain is crucial, especially when visual cues are limited, such as in a telephone consultation without video. In these cases, guiding the patient step-by-step is essential. Provide clear, simple instructions, ensuring that the approach is tailored to the patient's reported symptoms, age, sex, and any known comorbidities. Encourage the patient to describe their pain in detail, noting if it is sharp, dull, radiating, or cramping, and whether it fluctuates with movement, eating, or lying down.

Differences in understanding and defining abdominal regions can complicate remote diagnosis. Research has shown that telephone triage providers may misinterpret or misjudge the patient-reported location of pain or tenderness, as patients and healthcare providers may have differing conceptualizations of abdominal anatomy [14]. To minimize this risk, it may be useful to describe landmarks in plain language or ask the patient to think in terms of common references, such as "above or below the belly button" or "near the hip bones."

After establishing the location of pain, assessing its severity using a numerical rating scale can be informative. Ask the patient to rate their pain on a scale from 0 to 10, with 0 representing no pain and 10 the worst pain imaginable. This quantification can help monitor changes over time and provide a baseline for follow-up discussions. Additionally, asking the patient to compare their pain level to other familiar experiences may enhance clarity. If the pain is severe or unrelenting, or if other red-flag symptoms (such as fever or nausea) are present, an in-person evaluation may be necessary, as these signs could indicate more serious underlying pathology.

Finally, instructing patients on techniques for self-assessment fosters their active involvement in their healthcare, empowering them to participate in the examination and communicate more effectively about their symptoms. This approach not only aids the provider in making a more accurate assessment but also helps patients feel more engaged and informed throughout the process, which is particularly valuable in remote settings.

20.2.2 Abdominal Bloating

Abdominal bloating is a frequent complaint in primary care, often described by patients as a sensation of fullness, tightness, or distension in the abdomen. During a remote consultation, patients can be instructed to palpate their abdomen gently and identify any areas of tenderness or enlargement. This self-assessment can help healthcare providers gain insight into the nature and location of the bloating [10]. Patients should be encouraged to describe their symptoms, noting whether the bloating feels like a generalized sensation across the entire abdomen or is localized to specific quadrants. It can also be helpful to ask the patient to rate the severity of their bloating on a numerical scale from 1 to 10, with 10 representing the most intense sensation of fullness or discomfort [1].

In some cases, patients may observe a sudden increase in abdominal girth or even changes in how their clothes fit, such as a tighter belt or waistband. This is an important distinction, as a sudden change in belt size often suggests bloating rather than gradual weight gain. Bloating can be caused by a variety of factors, from dietary triggers and functional gastrointestinal disorders to more serious underlying conditions. Persistent or recurring bloating should be approached with caution and considered a red flag, as it may indicate underlying pathology, such as gastrointestinal obstruction, ascites due to liver disease, or even malignancy [1].

Differentiating between benign and concerning forms of bloating requires careful consideration of associated symptoms and the timing of the bloating. For instance, bloating that improves after passing gas, having a bowel movement, or belching is generally associated with functional gastrointestinal disorders, such as irritable bowel syndrome (IBS) or simple indigestion, and is less likely to be linked to severe conditions. In contrast, bloating that persists despite these measures, or that is accompanied by other concerning symptoms (such as weight loss, nausea, vomiting, or changes in bowel habits), warrants further investigation. Providers should inquire about the patient's eating patterns, specific foods or beverages that may exacerbate bloating, and any recent lifestyle changes that could impact gastrointestinal function.

A crucial aspect of managing bloating remotely is understanding its onset, duration, and progression over time. For instance, sudden or acute bloating, especially when accompanied by sharp or persistent pain, may suggest a more urgent condition like bowel obstruction or appendicitis, necessitating in-person assessment. In cases where bloating has been a recurring issue for weeks or months without other concerning symptoms, a conservative approach that includes dietary modifications and lifestyle counseling may be appropriate.

The concept of a "test of time" can also be valuable in remote management. Advising patients to monitor their symptoms over a set period, with instructions to seek follow-up if there is no improvement, can help differentiate self-limiting cases from those requiring further investigation [3]. Additionally, providing clear instructions for follow-up, such as a callback or telemedicine check-in, allows for continuous monitoring, especially if symptoms escalate [17]. This safety-netting strategy is particularly beneficial in telemedicine, where direct reassessment is not always immediately available.

Finally, lifestyle recommendations can play a key role in managing bloating remotely. Patients experiencing functional bloating may benefit from dietary adjustments, such as reducing intake of gas-producing foods (e.g., beans, lentils, carbonated drinks), and adopting smaller, more frequent meals to reduce abdominal distension. Educating patients on the potential effects of dietary triggers, stress management, and regular physical activity can empower them to take an active role in managing their symptoms. However, it is important for providers to clarify that if bloating persists or worsens despite these measures, or if additional red-flag symptoms appear, a face-to-face consultation or further diagnostic testing should be promptly considered.

20.3 Urinary Tract Infections and Bladder Pain

Urinary tract infections (UTIs) are among the most frequently encountered infections in primary care settings, affecting millions of people each year. Women are disproportionately affected due to anatomical factors that make bacterial ascent into the urinary tract more likely. In particular, sexually active women, postmenopausal women, and individuals with diabetes or immunosuppression are at higher risk. The condition can range from uncomplicated cystitis to more severe infections such as pyelonephritis, which can have significant morbidity if left untreated [11]. NICE guidelines permit the remote diagnosis and management of uncomplicated UTIs in nonpregnant women under the age of 65, especially if they present with classic symptoms such as dysuria (painful urination), frequency, and urgency, typically without the need for urine microscopy [18]. However, healthcare providers should exercise caution with older patients, men, pregnant women, and those with atypical presentations, as these groups are more susceptible to complications and may require closer monitoring or in-person evaluation.

In remote consultations, healthcare providers need to conduct a thorough history-taking to establish a probable diagnosis. They should inquire about risk factors, including recent sexual activity, use of spermicides, and previous history of UTIs, which may increase the likelihood of recurrent infections. UTIs in men, although less common, often indicate underlying structural abnormalities or chronic prostatitis and therefore require further investigation rather than remote management alone. Providers should also consider the possibility of asymptomatic bacteriuria in older people or pregnant patients, which, while generally not treated in most populations, does warrant treatment in pregnancy due to the risk of progression to pyelonephritis and associated pregnancy complications.

20.3.1 Recognizing Symptoms and Severity Remotely

A comprehensive assessment of urinary symptoms is crucial in a remote setting to determine the severity and potential complications of the infection. The provider should ask the patient detailed questions about classic UTI symptoms, including:

- *Frequency*: Increased frequency of urination, particularly if accompanied by a burning sensation.
- *Dysuria*: Pain or discomfort during urination, which is a hallmark symptom of cystitis.
- *Urgency*: A strong, sudden need to urinate that may be difficult to control.
- *Hematuria*: Blood in the urine, which can indicate a more severe infection or inflammation in the urinary tract.
- *Changes in urine odor or color*: Cloudy or foul-smelling urine may be suggestive of a bacterial infection.

Additionally, asking about systemic symptoms, such as fever, chills, or flank pain, is important for identifying patients at risk of more serious infections like pyelonephritis. Flank pain, particularly when unilateral and accompanied by fever or chills, may suggest an ascending infection reaching the kidneys. In these cases, the patient should be advised to seek immediate in-person care, as pyelonephritis often requires hospitalization and intravenous antibiotics.

Patients should also be asked about any underlying conditions that could complicate the course of a UTI, such as diabetes, immunosuppressive therapy, or recent catheterization, as these factors increase the risk of complicated infections. In older patients, atypical presentations are common; symptoms like confusion, weakness, or generalized discomfort, rather than localized urinary symptoms, may be the primary indicators of a UTI in this population. If such atypical signs are present, in-person assessment may be needed to prevent complications, including sepsis.

20.3.2 Antibiotic Stewardship and Remote Prescribing

With the rise of antimicrobial resistance, judicious antibiotic prescribing has become increasingly critical. In cases of uncomplicated cystitis in nonpregnant women with no complicating factors, narrow-spectrum antibiotics, such as nitrofurantoin, are typically the preferred choice due to their high efficacy against common uropathogens and their relatively low risk of promoting resistant strains [11]. When prescribing antibiotics remotely, healthcare providers should ensure the patient understands the importance of adhering to the prescribed course to prevent resistance and recurrence. Additionally, for patients with frequent recurrent UTIs, nonantibiotic prophylactic measures, such as increased hydration, cranberry products, and postcoital voiding, can be discussed as preventive strategies.

In situations where symptoms are mild and the patient prefers to avoid immediate antibiotics, a "delayed prescription" approach may be considered. This involves providing the patient with a prescription but advising them to delay filling it for 48 h to see if symptoms improve spontaneously. This strategy has been shown to reduce antibiotic use in some cases without compromising clinical outcomes. Providers should educate patients on monitoring symptoms and instruct them to fill the prescription if symptoms persist or worsen.

For complicated or recurrent infections, a urine culture is generally recommended to guide appropriate antibiotic selection. In patients who present with recurrent UTIs, healthcare providers should consider factors that may predispose to reinfection, such as sexual activity or certain forms of contraception, and provide tailored advice on preventive strategies. When managing recurrent infections remotely, providers can also discuss the option of low-dose prophylactic antibiotics for patients with frequent episodes, though this should be approached cautiously to avoid resistance.

20.3.3 Safety-Netting and Follow-Up for UTIs

Safety-netting plays an essential role in remote management of UTIs. Patients should be provided with clear information on when to seek further care, especially if symptoms do not improve within 48–72 h of starting antibiotics or if they worsen. Key warning signs that should prompt immediate medical attention include [14, 16]:

- *High fever*: Persistent fever, especially above 38.5 °C, may indicate progression to pyelonephritis.
- *Severe back or flank pain*: This could suggest kidney involvement, necessitating urgent intervention.

- *Persistent hematuria*: Continued presence of blood in the urine may warrant further investigation for conditions beyond simple cystitis, including renal stones or malignancies.
- *General malaise or confusion*: Particularly in older patients, generalized symptoms or mental status changes could signal sepsis, requiring prompt evaluation.

Providing structured follow-up through scheduled telemedicine check-ins can be beneficial, particularly for older or high-risk patients. This allows healthcare providers to reassess symptom resolution and reinforce medication adherence, thus minimizing the risk of recurrence and complications. For recurrent UTI patients, remote consultations offer an opportunity to discuss long-term management strategies, including lifestyle modifications, hydration, and avoidance of bladder irritants (e.g., caffeine, alcohol) to support urinary health.

For men and older patients with atypical symptoms or recurrent UTIs, providers should maintain a low threshold for in-person assessment or referral to a urologist, as these cases may indicate underlying structural or functional abnormalities that require specialist care. Education on the importance of completing the full course of antibiotics and following up if symptoms return is crucial in preventing recurrent infections and mitigating the risk of developing antibiotic resistance.

In summary, the remote management of UTIs requires a structured approach that incorporates detailed history-taking, judicious antibiotic prescribing, and effective safety-netting. By educating patients on symptom recognition and ensuring appropriate follow-up, healthcare providers can manage uncomplicated UTIs effectively while minimizing unnecessary in-person visits and supporting antibiotic stewardship.

20.4 Common Infectious Abdominal Pathologies

Infections affecting the abdominal area can lead to significant morbidity if not managed promptly. Remote consultations provide an initial avenue for assessing symptoms, but healthcare providers must recognize the limitations of remote diagnosis in conditions that may rapidly worsen [19]. Below are some common infectious abdominal pathologies that require careful evaluation and may necessitate in-person assessment.

20.4.1 Appendicitis

Appendicitis is one of the most common and time-sensitive abdominal emergencies, often requiring prompt surgical intervention. The classic presentation of appendicitis includes periumbilical pain that migrates to the right lower quadrant, typically accompanied by symptoms such as nausea, loss of appetite, and low-grade fever. During a remote consultation, providers should ask patients about these hallmark symptoms, specifically the characteristic "migration" of pain and any increase in severity over time.

In some cases, rebound tenderness or pain on movement may be elicited by asking the patient to apply gentle pressure to the right lower abdomen and then release it quickly, though this can be challenging without direct guidance. Appendicitis can rapidly progress to perforation if untreated, leading to peritonitis and sepsis, which carry significant risks. Therefore, patients suspected of having appendicitis should be advised to seek immediate in-person assessment, ideally in an emergency setting [7]. In children and older patients, appendicitis may present with atypical symptoms, making remote assessment particularly challenging in these populations. Providers should maintain a low threshold for referral in these cases to prevent delay in diagnosis and treatment.

20.4.2 Diverticulitis

Diverticulitis, an inflammatory condition affecting the diverticula (small pouches) within the colon, commonly presents with left lower quadrant pain, fever, and altered bowel habits, such as constipation or diarrhea. Patients with known diverticulosis (the presence of diverticula) are at risk of developing diverticulitis, especially with advancing age and dietary factors. Remote consultations can help in assessing mild cases, especially in patients with a history of similar episodes who can recognize early symptoms [15, 23].

For mild diverticulitis, remote management may involve dietary modifications, such as a temporary switch to a low-residue or liquid diet to allow the colon to rest, along with advice on increased hydration. In certain cases, antibiotics may be prescribed remotely, but providers should carefully assess for any red flags, such as severe pain, inability to tolerate oral intake, or fever exceeding 38.5 °C, which would indicate a need for in-person evaluation. Complications of diverticulitis, such as abscess formation or perforation, require hospitalization and potentially surgical intervention. Providers should educate patients on recognizing worsening symptoms and emphasize the importance of follow-up [23].

20.4.3 Hepatitis Infections

Hepatitis infections, caused primarily by hepatitis A, B, and C viruses, often manifest with a range of abdominal symptoms, including right upper quadrant discomfort, nausea, and jaundice. Hepatitis A is typically transmitted via the fecal-oral route and is more common in areas with inadequate sanitation, while hepatitis B and C are primarily bloodborne and can lead to chronic liver disease. The remote assessment of hepatitis can be challenging, as many patients initially present with nonspecific symptoms like fatigue, malaise, and nausea, which overlap with other conditions.

For patients reporting dark urine, pale stools, and jaundice, a physical examination may be warranted to assess for hepatomegaly or right upper quadrant tenderness, indicative of liver inflammation. Providers should inquire about recent travel history, sexual activity, or intravenous drug use, as these are risk factors for hepatitis transmission. If hepatitis is suspected, laboratory testing is essential to confirm the diagnosis and assess liver function. In cases where jaundice or other severe symptoms are present, patients should be referred for immediate evaluation due to the risk of acute liver failure in certain types of hepatitis [27]. Remote follow-up may be useful for monitoring stable chronic hepatitis cases and educating patients on lifestyle changes to support liver health.

20.4.4 Gastroenteritis

Gastroenteritis, an inflammation of the gastrointestinal tract often caused by viral or bacterial infections, presents with symptoms such as diarrhea, abdominal cramping, vomiting, and sometimes fever. While viral gastroenteritis typically resolves on its own, bacterial forms (e.g., those caused by *Salmonella*, *Shigella*, or *E. coli*) can be more severe and may require antibiotic treatment. Remote assessment should focus on evaluating dehydration risk, especially if the patient reports frequent vomiting or diarrhea. Instructing the patient to monitor for signs of dehydration, such as dry mouth, reduced urine output, and lightheadedness, can help guide decisions about whether further care is needed. Persistent symptoms or the presence of blood in stools warrant an in-person assessment [15].

20.5 Abdominal Pain Red Flags and Safety-Netting in Remote Consultations

20.5.1 Identifying Red Flags

Any unexpected weight loss, persistent vomiting, inability to tolerate fluids or food, severe abdominal pain, hematemesis (vomiting blood), or melena (black, tarry stools indicative of gastrointestinal bleeding) should prompt an immediate face-to-face assessment or urgent referral to secondary care. These symptoms can signal serious underlying pathologies, such as gastrointestinal bleeding, obstruction, or malignancy, that require prompt intervention [3, 4, 7]. This recommendation is particularly critical for vulnerable populations, such as pregnant women, where additional comorbidities may increase the risk of complications. For pregnant patients, abdominal pain and associated symptoms should always be approached cautiously, given the potential for unique conditions such as ectopic pregnancy, preeclampsia, or placental abruption, which require specialized care and rapid evaluation.

Red-flag symptoms that should prompt urgent assessment include:

- *Unexplained weight loss*: Sudden, unintended weight loss may signal malignancy, chronic infection, or inflammatory bowel disease.
- *Persistent vomiting*: Inability to retain food or fluids can lead to dehydration and electrolyte imbalances, particularly in young children and older adults.

- *Severe or sudden onset pain*: Acute, intense pain, especially if localized, could indicate a surgical emergency, such as appendicitis, bowel obstruction, or ischemic bowel.
- *Hematemesis and Melena*: Vomiting blood or black, tarry stools suggest gastrointestinal bleeding, which requires immediate intervention.
- *Signs of systemic infection*: Fever, chills, and fatigue, in combination with abdominal symptoms, may indicate a spreading infection, such as sepsis secondary to peritonitis or pyelonephritis.

Instructing patients to recognize these red flags and seek immediate care if they arise is crucial for safe remote management. For example, a patient experiencing unrelenting pain that disrupts sleep or impairs daily activities should not delay seeking evaluation, as this could indicate serious pathology. Similarly, unexplained fever accompanied by abdominal pain warrants further investigation to rule out infections or inflammatory conditions.

20.5.2 Safety-Netting for Remote Abdominal Pain Consultations

Safety-netting involves setting clear expectations for patients on when to seek further help. For abdominal complaints managed remotely, provide patients with specific instructions on which symptoms or changes should prompt immediate reassessment. Patients should be advised to monitor their symptoms closely, particularly if they were mild or vague during the initial consultation, as many serious conditions begin with nonspecific symptoms that can escalate over time.

For example:

- *Mild but persistent abdominal pain*: Advise patients to monitor pain that remains mild but persists beyond 24–48 h, as it may be a sign of early appendicitis or diverticulitis.
- *Onset of fever in previously afebrile patients*: Patients who develop fever after an initial consultation should be advised to seek in-person assessment, as this could indicate an infection.
- *Escalation of symptoms in older or high-risk patients*: For older adults and patients with comorbidities, worsening abdominal symptoms should prompt immediate evaluation due to higher risks of complications and atypical presentations.

Examples of conditions that could develop over time include:

- *Ovarian Cysts*: If a patient has a suspected or known ovarian cyst, they should be advised that pain may intensify, especially with movements such as jumping or sudden physical exertion. Increasing pain or signs of acute discomfort could indicate cyst rupture or torsion, both of which require urgent assessment.

- *Appendicitis*: In suspected cases of appendicitis, the patient should be instructed to monitor for pain that shifts to the right lower quadrant, specifically to the area just above the hip. This migration of pain, combined with worsening intensity, often signifies that the condition is progressing and may soon require surgical intervention. In children, asking to do a star jump, with their hands lifted, may indicate a peritoneal irritation. If they can do this, they are unlikely to be suffering from peritoneal inflammation.
- *Pyelonephritis*: Patients with symptoms suggestive of a urinary tract infection who begin to feel generally unwell, develop vomiting, or experience flank pain (especially if accompanied by fever and chills) should be evaluated for pyelonephritis. This kidney infection can cause significant morbidity if left untreated and may necessitate hospital admission for intravenous antibiotics.
- *Peritonitis*: If a patient reports increased pain with simple movements, particularly in the abdomen, peritonitis should be considered. Peritonitis, indicative of inflammation or infection of the peritoneal lining, is a late sign in many abdominal pathologies and requires immediate emergency care.

Peritonism, a sign of peritoneal inflammation, is generally a concerning indicator of advanced abdominal pathology, such as perforation or peritoneal infection [20, 21]. In remote consultations, it is crucial to evaluate for this sign, even though direct examination is limited. Providers can instruct patients to perform a simple maneuver: asking them to draw in their abdomen (suck in their umbilicus) and then expand it outward as far as possible. Observing any expressions of pain during this maneuver or any reported sharp discomfort can serve as an indirect assessment for peritoneal irritation. If peritoneal involvement is suspected based on this or other findings, the patient should be advised to seek immediate referral to emergency or secondary care rather than undergoing further primary care evaluation, as this condition requires urgent intervention [22, 23].

Providers should document safety-netting instructions carefully to ensure clarity and consistency, especially in remote settings. Additionally, scheduling a follow-up consultation, either by phone or video, within a specified timeframe can be beneficial for monitoring cases that are not immediately concerning but may develop over time. Reinforcing education on symptom recognition empowers patients to take an active role in monitoring their health and reduces the risk of delayed diagnosis in serious cases.

20.6 Conclusions and Take-Home Messages

The ability to conduct thorough abdominal examinations and manage related complaints remotely has become essential in modern primary care. The shift toward telemedicine, accelerated by the COVID-19 pandemic, has pushed healthcare providers to adapt traditional examination techniques and diagnostic frameworks for virtual settings. Telemedicine offers a valuable platform for initial assessments, especially for common, uncomplicated conditions. However, it also presents unique challenges, particularly in ensuring that serious cases are promptly recognized and directed toward in-person care when needed.

Remote assessments have proven effective for managing conditions such as uncomplicated urinary tract infections, mild gastroenteritis, and functional gastrointestinal complaints. A well-structured approach that integrates detailed history-taking with guided self-examination can yield valuable insights without necessitating an in-person visit [22]. This approach not only enhances patient accessibility but also reduces the strain on healthcare facilities by minimizing unnecessary hospital visits. Nevertheless, in complex or atypical cases—such as those involving severe or persistent pain, jaundice, unexplained weight loss, or systemic symptoms—providers should maintain a low threshold for recommending face-to-face evaluation to rule out serious pathology [1, 13, 24–27].

Key Takeaways for Remote Abdominal Assessment and Management

1. *Adaptation of Traditional Techniques*: Traditional abdominal examination methods can be effectively adapted for remote consultations. By guiding patients through self-examination techniques and carefully interpreting their descriptions, providers can gather crucial diagnostic information. Instructions for patients should be clear and specific, with providers ready to adapt their approach based on each patient's unique context, including age, comorbidities, and ability to follow instructions. This adaptability is fundamental in maximizing diagnostic accuracy and supporting patient confidence in telemedicine.
2. *Emphasis on Safety-Netting*: In remote settings, robust safety-netting is essential. Providers should offer explicit guidance on which symptoms warrant escalation and advise patients to seek further care if they experience any worsening or new symptoms. For abdominal complaints, this is particularly important given that serious conditions can initially present subtly. Safety-netting reinforces patient autonomy and empowers individuals to make informed decisions about their health while providing a safety cushion against the limitations of remote assessment.
3. *Awareness of Red Flags*: Recognizing red flags is crucial in remote abdominal evaluations. Symptoms like unexplained weight loss, persistent vomiting, severe abdominal pain, hematemesis, or signs of systemic infection (e.g., fever, chills, malaise) are indicators of potential serious underlying conditions that require prompt in-person evaluation. By training patients to recognize these red flags and act on them, healthcare providers can reduce the risk of delayed diagnosis and potential complications, ensuring timely intervention for cases that need urgent attention.
4. *Antibiotic Stewardship*: In managing remote cases of uncomplicated UTIs, it is crucial to adhere to guidelines that advocate for selective and judicious use of antibiotics. By prescribing narrow-spectrum antibiotics, such as nitrofurantoin, only when clearly indicated, providers can help reduce antimicrobial resistance and promote sustainable healthcare practices. Additionally, educating patients

on the importance of completing their prescribed antibiotic course enhances treatment efficacy and minimizes recurrence.

5. *Optimizing the Role of Telemedicine*: Remote management of abdominal complaints offers a valuable solution for reducing unnecessary in-person visits, especially when providers are equipped with effective remote assessment techniques and digital diagnostic tools. Telemedicine allows for more efficient use of healthcare resources, optimizing the capacity of healthcare systems to manage high-demand situations while maintaining patient safety and care quality. The convenience and accessibility of telemedicine also promote continuity of care, as patients are more likely to seek timely advice when barriers to access are reduced.
6. *Empowering Patient Education and Self-Care*: One of the key advantages of remote abdominal assessment is the opportunity to engage patients actively in their own care. By educating patients on self-assessment techniques, symptom monitoring, and preventive measures, providers can encourage patients to take a proactive approach to managing their health. This education is particularly important for recurrent conditions, such as UTIs, where lifestyle modifications and hygiene practices can play a significant role in preventing recurrence. Patient empowerment not only enhances adherence to treatment plans but also fosters trust and satisfaction in the healthcare process.
7. *Integration of Telemedicine with In-Person Care*: Telemedicine should not be viewed as a standalone solution but rather as a complementary component of a comprehensive healthcare approach. For conditions that can initially be managed remotely, follow-up consultations may be scheduled to reassess progress or refer to in-person care if symptoms escalate. This integrated approach ensures continuity and enables healthcare providers to address evolving health concerns in a timely manner, optimizing outcomes for patients with abdominal complaints.

Final Thoughts

The use of telemedicine to manage abdominal and urinary complaints marks a significant advancement in primary care, offering a flexible and efficient alternative to traditional in-person assessments. However, the success of remote care relies on a structured approach that combines detailed history-taking, patient education, and a high degree of vigilance for potential red flags. By adapting traditional examination skills for remote settings, healthcare providers can offer high-quality, patient-centered care while reducing the burden on healthcare systems.

Telemedicine is now an indispensable tool in modern healthcare, promoting accessibility, efficiency, and safety. Through the thoughtful integration of telemedicine with conventional care practices, providers can create a responsive and adaptive healthcare environment that meets the needs of diverse patient populations. By blending established clinical knowledge with innovative virtual approaches, healthcare providers can deliver comprehensive, effective care and help patients navigate their symptoms with confidence and clarity.

References

1. Abbs J. Remote abdominal examination techniques in primary care. J Telemed Telecare. 2022;28(4):218–25.
2. Alter MJ, Seeff LB. Hepatitis C: management and treatment in primary care. N Engl J Med. 2000;345(3):259–64.
3. Almond S, Summerton N. Red flags in abdominal pain and their importance in remote consultations. Br J Gen Pract. 2009;59(558):489–91.
4. Benziger CP, et al. Telemedicine in abdominal pain management: emerging trends and insights. Glob Health Sci Pract. 2020;8(2):209–14.
5. Drekonja DM, et al. Diagnosis and management of UTIs in telemedicine. Ann Intern Med. 2013;158(2):135–40.
6. Escobedo AA, et al. Giardiasis and Amebiasis: management and prevention. Infect Dis Clin N Am. 2016;30(3):779–808.
7. Fitzgerald JE, et al. Approaches to suspected appendicitis in remote consultation. Br Med J. 2018;360:k759.
8. Finucane TE, et al. Symptom-based approach in telemedicine for UTI diagnosis. J Gen Intern Med. 2019;34(10):2025–30.
9. Ghany MG, et al. Chronic hepatitis B and C: comprehensive review for practitioners. Hepatology. 2020;71(1):54–64.
10. Gogălniceanu P, et al. Effective techniques in self-assisted abdominal examination. Med Teach. 2015;37(11):1015–21.
11. Gupta K, et al. Management of cystitis in outpatient settings. Clin Infect Dis. 2011;52(5):e103–20.
12. Hay AD, et al. UTI management and antibiotic stewardship in primary care. J Antimicrob Chemother. 2013;68(11):2516–23.
13. Jones CH, et al. Safety-netting advice for abdominal pain in telemedicine. Fam Pract. 2013;30(5):543–50.
14. Kamin RA, et al. Challenges in telephone triage for abdominal pain. Acad Emerg Med. 2003;10(3):344–8.
15. Kirk M, et al. Bacterial gastroenteritis: recognition and management guidelines. Clin Gastroenterol. 2015;43(4):467–77.
16. Lemon SM, et al. Understanding hepatitis infections in primary care. J Viral Hepat. 2018;25(2):170–82.
17. Mitchell RK. Implementing follow-up protocols for abdominal bloating in remote care. J Fam Med. 2014;31(4):345–51.
18. National Institute for Health and Care Excellence. Guidelines for urinary tract infection management. London: NICE; 2021.
19. Neal RD, et al. Understanding red flags in abdominal pain: a review for remote consultations. J Clin Med. 2015;4(7):89–102.
20. Strate LL, et al. Diverticulitis management in primary care. J Clin Gastroenterol. 2012;46(9):735–43.
21. Petri WA, et al. Amebiasis and parasitic infections: a primary care approach. Am J Med. 2000;108(5):554–9.
22. Rogers BA, et al. Cholangitis and biliary infections: recognition and management in primary care. J Hepatobiliary Pancreat Surg. 2018;25(2):156–64.
23. Smith MA, et al. Telemedicine and reduced hospital visits during COVID-19. Health Aff. 2022;41(2):221–9.
24. Summerton N. Understanding test of time in remote abdominal pain assessments. Br J Gen Pract. 2009;59(559):506–7.
25. Thielman NM, Guerrant RL. Clinical aspects of gastroenteritis. Clin Infect Dis. 2004;39(9):1278–83.
26. Wong CL, et al. Spontaneous bacterial peritonitis: a guide for telemedicine providers. J Hepatol. 2013;58(5):1019–27.
27. World Health Organization. Guidelines on hepatitis and chronic liver disease management. Geneva: WHO; 2021.

Remote Consultation and Telemedicine in Pediatrics 21

Jacopo Ceradini, Renato Cutrera, Alessandro Onofri, Sergio Bella, Fabrizio Drago, Riccardo Schiaffini, Anna Maria Caterina Musolino, Paolo Alfieri, Rachele Adorisio, and Massimiliano Raponi

21.1 Background

Telemedicine is a widely recognized tool in the management and treatment of pediatric patients with chronic diseases [1–3]. The recent pandemic has shed light on the vulnerabilities of healthcare systems, including disparities in access due to geographic and socioeconomic status, waiting list for diagnostic tests and outpatient care, and a lack of synergy between hospital care and community-based health services [4].

The increased prevalence of pediatric patients suffering from chronic diseases and the vulnerabilities of the healthcare systems needs some adjustment in how healthcare services are structured and organized [5]. Technological advancements play a role in reshaping healthcare delivery by shifting the emphasis from hospitals to communities through innovative care models that prioritize individual needs and global access to healthcare services. In this setting, telemedicine plays a pivotal role in ensuring access to care in remote areas, providing access to specialized services and promoting collaboration among different specialized physicians and healthcare professionals for a better continuity of care in managing chronic conditions [2].

Furthermore, telemedicine has the potential to involve the patient himself/herself in self-management solutions and remote monitoring, thus enhancing his/her quality of life, supporting early referral to hospital and also early discharge [1–2].

J. Ceradini (✉) · R. Cutrera · A. Onofri · S. Bella · F. Drago · R. Schiaffini
A. M. C. Musolino · P. Alfieri · R. Adorisio · M. Raponi
Bambino Gesù Children's Hospital, IRCCS, Rome, Italy
e-mail: jacopo.ceradini@opbg.net; renato.cutrera@opbg.net; alessandro.onofri@opbg.net; sergio.bella@opbg.net; fabrizio.drago@opbg.net; riccardo.schiaffini@opbg.net; amcaterina.musolino@opbg.net; paolo.alfieri@opbg.net; rachele.adorisio@opbg.net; massimiliano.raponi@opbg.net

J. Demurtas (ed.), *Remote Consultation in Primary Care*, TELe-Health,
https://doi.org/10.1007/978-3-031-89661-3_21

The advances in the management of chronic diseases in the pediatric population have not only increased life expectancy but also the need of personalized and timely care in those patients; therefore, telemedicine and remote care have emerged not only as solutions to reduce hospital stays and related stress but also associated costs [6–7]. At present, telemedicine initiatives in children too often remain at experimental or prototype stage with limited case studies [7–9]. The recently published guidelines and operational models for telemedicine are a step forward to further facilitate the transition from experimental to systematic use of telemedicine services in the pediatric setting [1–3]. Even if the implementation of the current guidelines in clinical practice is fragmented, it is crucial to identify the best indicators capable of describing the performance of the different telemedicine and telehealth initiatives to foster their future use in children [1, 10]. Table 21.1 summarizes the health, social, and economic benefits associated with the adoption of telemedicine in the pediatric context and the potential obstacles [2].

The recent COVID-19 pandemic highlighted the necessity to maintain continuous and accessible care for pediatric patients who present acute symptoms. This has led to the exploration and development of different approaches to replace the traditional face-to-face assessment of pediatric patients. The alternative strategies that have emerged can be summarized in three key interventions: (1) teleconsultation between pediatricians/caregivers; (2) virtual visits and remote monitoring; and (3) consultation between pediatricians and specialist consultants, via telecommunication. The pediatrician/caregiver teleconsultation has been initially used by primary care pediatricians, and it is supported by the pediatrician's comprehensive understanding of the child's health coupled with the sociocultural context of the caregiver [11–12]. To expand this practice to healthcare providers, such as hospital pediatricians, continuity of care physicians, and specialists, it is crucial to establish how to share details on the child's health and sociocultural status and that of their caregiver [13]. Teleconsultation and telemonitoring through video calls or quick sharing of multimedia files like images and audio recordings can further enhance the

Table 21.1 The health, social, and economic benefits associated with the adoption of telemedicine in the pediatric context and the potential obstacles

Advantages	Obstacles
Reduction in economic costs for families	Difficulty performing the physical examination
Reduction in patient absences from school	Inability to urgently perform laboratory tests or imaging studies
Reduction in parental absences from work	Lack of direct doctor–patient interaction
Facilitation of regular frequency of clinical checkups	Inability to provide nursing or physiotherapy support
Automatic collection of clinical and research data	Digital divide between families
Cost reduction for the National Health System	

communication between physicians, healthcare professionals, and caregivers and can facilitate the sharing of information alongside traditional telephone consultations [14]. Additionally, promoting the adoption of existing telemonitoring devices providing data such as oxygen saturation levels, heart and respiratory rate, etc., can further improve the remote assessment of pediatric patients. When logistical, environmental factors or the patients' clinical condition hampers the possibility of teleconsultation, a possible solution is the use of an integrated system, where the patients' medical history, test results, and the actual physical and clinical evaluation conducted by a primary care pediatrician are recorded. Integration of these data to teleconsultation will make more effective and efficient the medical response to the patients' health needs, even in acute/subacute conditions.

21.2 Teleconsultation for Pediatric Patients

Teleconsultation is generally conducted using a commercial teleconferencing tool accessible via PC or smartphone, with the link sent after obtaining consent and providing information regarding privacy [15], digital literacy, and the limitations of the tool. Follow-up teleconsultation is authorized in health service of Lazio, Italy, only for patients with an identified clinical condition during the initial visit to evaluate their progress. Usually, consultation is supported by patients' caregivers, notably parents or other members of the family. Nevertheless, it is important that the consultations are not only based on third parties but also consider the child/pediatric patient perspective and evaluate their speech and characteristics by directly involving them in the consultation. It is also important to assess the setting in which the consultation is held. Literature reports experience of telephone triage [16] in which the setting of the consultation and direct speaking with the patient changed the potential advice given by the physician [17]. Telemedical tools allow for consideration of the context in which observations are made. For example, dyspnea observed in an open environment during recreational activity will be evaluated differently than the same symptom observed at home. Similarly, a call made in a restaurant during a meal will be assessed differently compared to a televisit in a patient's bedroom where they are unable to swallow food or water.

21.3 Execution Method

After patient identification and verification of device functionality, a medical history is reviewed from the day of discharge. The interview focuses on the evolution of respiratory symptoms and the appearance of new symptoms. Nutritional status, sleep–wake rhythm, adherence to discharge instructions, and proper management of home therapy are assessed, such as correct use of aerosol therapy and effective nasal hygiene, particularly in infants [17].

21.4 Physical Examination

The physical examination involves assessing the general condition, the psychological state, and the child's interaction with the environment. Respiratory dynamics are examined by directing the camera toward the child, preferably using natural light. HD cameras generally allows for a good view of intercostal and jugular retractions, nasal flaring, and nodding (use of the sternocleidomastoid muscles for breathing). Skin and mucous membrane color are evaluated by adjusting the camera for optimal lighting. Hydration status and capillary refill can be assessed with the HD camera [16].

During the teleconsultation, weight and vital signs (temperature, heart rate, respiratory rate, oxygen saturation) are also assessed.

Numerous low-cost commercial devices can aid caregivers in recording these parameters. Another central aspect of teleconsultation is educating the caregiver to detect early signs of clinical deterioration. Teleconsultation also allows for the sharing of multimedia content, enabling caregivers to send synchronous video or audio recordings of significant events, such as a productive cough or bronchospasm. The teleconsultation should conclude with the establishment of a follow-up diagnostic-therapeutic plan, such as a follow-up with the primary care pediatrician or a day hospital appointment.

In the second section of the chapter, we will discuss the application of telemedicine in specific pediatric subsets. Table 21.2 highlights the opportunities and

Table 21.2 Opportunities and challenges associated with telemedicine in different settings

Chronic disease	Application	Limits
Pneumology and allergology	Pneumology and allergology screening, and monitoring of asthma and other chronic lung diseases	Difficulty of carrying out a complete physical examination remotely, beyond a simple inspection through monitors and video cameras
Cystic fibrosis	Monitoring of oxygen saturation, weight, respiratory function, and compliance to therapy	Inability to perform sputum cultures; difficulty in early diagnosis of respiratory exacerbations
Cardiology	Teleassistance, teleconsultation, telemonitoring, and teleecography in patients with known heart diseases or heart failure	Absence of structured and standardized organizational models
Diabetology	Telemonitoring of health data and empowerment of the patient and family to achieve good glycemic control	Absence of structured and standardized organizational models
Neurology and child neuropsychology	Monitoring of clinical symptoms and efficacy of antiepileptic treatment, teleconsultation (doctor–physician or doctor–technician) for neuroradiological diagnostic aspects, psychiatric and physiological consultation in emergency	Difficulty in initial assessment in patients with neuromuscular disorders, autoimmune disorders, and autism and in children under 1 year of age

challenges associated with telemedicine as reported by leading Italian pediatric hospitals, particularly in the management of respiratory diseases, cardiac arrhythmias, and neuropsychiatric conditions [2, 5, 20–23].

21.5 Telemedicine in Specific Pediatric Settings: Pneumology

Technological progresses in the management of pediatric patients with chronic respiratory failure resulted in improved survival rates, but children may be dependent on mechanical ventilation or require other complex devices and often require complex home management. During the COVID-19 pandemic, children with complex medical conditions faced multiple disruptions to their care, including interruptions in specialist care, in therapeutic and rehabilitative services, and in home care. Several studies have highlighted the benefits of telemedicine for monitoring children on home mechanical ventilation with growing interest in using remote monitoring in this setting [5].

To minimize the interruption of crucial clinical services, a telemedicine strategy involving teleconsultations and telemonitoring to assist pediatric patients on long-term home mechanical ventilation would be helpful. Teleconsultations allow healthcare providers to interact with patients and their families/caregivers via video calls. It also facilitates communication and actively involves caregivers. Telemonitoring allows physicians to monitor patients' health remotely by accessing ventilation data through web platforms connected to their equipment. This teleconsultation and telemonitoring program acts in addition to the standard of care for medically complex children on long-term mechanical ventilation. These patients often require other devices such as gastrostomy and enteral pumps, as they have multisystemic diseases involving multiple organs. The home ventilation devices used allows to remotely track ventilation patterns and detect any issues. It is evident that telemedicine has transformed healthcare management for children dependent on long-term home mechanical ventilation [5]. This approach has been shown to improve access to care, patient quality of life, and facilitation of family involvement in decision-making processes [5].

Telemedicine allows constant remote monitoring of the child's condition through connected medical devices that transmit data to healthcare personnel. This practice can reduce the need for frequent hospital visits, alleviating logistical and psychological burdens on families. Particularly, medically complex children typically have high technological dependency and often require extensive care. Families at home often experience difficulties managing various daily clinical and care-related issues. In this context, telemedicine has shown high potential, as it allows for closeness to families and supports healthcare personnel caring for the patient at home. In our case, the use of telemedicine with remote monitoring of ventilator data has also allowed for better management of the ventilatory equipment, with periodic retraining for caregivers on usage methods and specific needs (humidity level, interface problems, etc.). A key aspect of activity is parental and caregiver education. Through teleconsultations, it has been possible to improve learning to safely and appropriately manage respiratory support at home. In this way, family autonomy is promoted, reducing dependence on external assistance, particularly hospital-based assistance.

The use of telemedicine in long-term mechanically ventilated patients offers several significant advantages, improving the efficiency of patient management and contributing to overall care quality. Telemedicine allows for constant remote monitoring of the vital conditions of mechanically ventilated patients, enabling accurate and timely surveillance of vital parameter changes such as respiratory rate, oxygen saturation, and heart rate.

Remote ventilator monitoring adds the possibility of assessing ventilation trends, particularly regarding adherence to device use, the presence of air leaks, and residual ventilation events. Data can be transmitted to healthcare providers in real time without requiring the patient's physical presence, alleviating the discomfort and costs associated with travel. The logistical aspect is often crucial for medically complex children. Their movements are burdensome and complex, and the possibility of reducing scheduled hospital visits represents added value and an important achievement for many families. Patients continued with scheduled follow-up visits and admissions for their underlying condition. The use of teleconsultations and remote ventilator monitoring has led to a reduced need for emergency department visits and unplanned admissions. The use of telemedicine tools with medically complex patients has supported caregivers and home care personnel throughout the care process. The telemedicine team, composed of a physician, respiratory therapist, and nurse, has interacted with home-based professionals, allowing for better connection between the hospital and the community.

Telemedicine also allows for the involvement of experts from other disciplines, ensuring a multidisciplinary approach to treating children with complex conditions.

Families enrolled [5] have shown high satisfaction with the telemedicine care offered; this tool has allowed for the enhancement of care offered with the standard of care, improving healthcare for patients with complex chronic conditions. In addition to teleconsultations, the project includes telemonitoring and, in some more stable cases, even remote adjustment of ventilator parameters. Remote ventilator monitoring has already proven useful in various contexts in adult patients. In the pediatric population, it has been shown to improve adherence to home ventilator use after initiation and to enhance family empowerment in device use.

It should be emphasized that, despite the numerous advantages, telemedicine does not completely replace physical care in certain circumstances. Only patients already known to the unit, in current follow-up, were included in the project. No initial visits were ever conducted via teleconsultation. Telemedicine tools also require technological adequacy of infrastructures and connectivity, which is sometimes lacking and affects the quality of remote care. This limitation results in reduced inclusivity of such tools and hinders access to care for population segments that would sometimes be the most in need.

The use of telemedicine in the context of medically complex children on long-term home mechanical ventilation represents a step forward in optimizing care. Through this mode, more accessible, personalized, and efficient medicine is achieved, significantly improving the quality of life for patients and their families.

21.6 Telemedicine in Specific Pediatric Settings: Cystic Fibrosis

The telemedicine initiative for cystic fibrosis provides remote assistance to some of the patients followed in children's hospitals. It includes the monitoring of parameters related to the respiratory function (such as spirometry results, heart rate, and oxygen saturation) using instruments capable of conducting a spirometry test within 5 min [18–20].

The process initiated when a patient is deemed suitable for inclusion in the project involves drafting a request to be submitted to the local Health Authority, which must accept to purchase or lease the requested kit. Once the request is accepted, the patient will have all the necessary equipment available to proceed with parameter monitoring [20–21].

The key points that the project aims to always maintain and adhere to are:

- Use of innovative and user-friendly instruments
- Monitoring of symptoms and other psychophysical conditions of the patient, not exclusively respiratory parameters
- Availability for telephone conversations between healthcare personnel and the patient
- Sharing of results among the doctor, nurse, and patient

21.7 Pediatric Teleconsultation Following Emergency Department Discharge

In Italy's largest children's hospital, follow-up teleconsultation has been implemented to provide timely and secure discharge for patients admitted to the emergency department and hospitalized for a relatively short duration, typically around 2–3 days. These patients generally came with respiratory tract infections, such as pneumonia and bronchiolitis during the winter season, and dehydration/gastroenteritis during the summer season.

The use of telemedicine can help streamline patient care pathways and offer parents a valuable opportunity to receive specific training from home. This training is crucial for managing the patient, particularly in ensuring adherence to therapy and preventing unnecessary readmissions to the hospital.

After the teleconsultation, a satisfaction survey link is sent to the patient/parent, where it is recommended to separate technological aspects from educational and medical care aspects. At the end of the entire process, a process/outcome evaluation should be conducted using direct or proxy indicators, such as rehospitalization rates, repeated admissions, and teleconsultations resulting in emergency department visits.

21.8 Telemedicine in Specific Pediatric Settings: Cardiology

Pediatric patients with pacemakers or implantable cardioverter-defibrillators (ICDs) are monitored and regularly sent data via telemedicine regarding their device functionality or any occurrence of arrhythmias and signs of retention linked to heart failure exacerbation [22]. Additionally, patients with implantable loop recorders (ILRs) experiencing unexplained palpitations, near-syncope, syncopal events, or severe arrhythmogenic conditions are monitored at home due to being at high risk.

If there are recordings indicating an issue with the device or malfunction in urgent transmissions signaling system or if severe arrhythmia is detected, the patient's family should be promptly contacted. Advise them to seek immediate medical attention at the nearest emergency department.

21.9 Telemedicine in Specific Pediatric Settings: Diabetology

Pediatric patients with diabetes may be followed up with interesting results remotely [23]. To enhance care, telemedicine service for diabetes consultations, focused on monitoring and offering treatment recommendations to children and teenagers with Type 1 Diabetes and other forms of childhood diabetes, were implemented [24]. This includes tracking of blood sugar levels and insulin therapy using technological devices such as glucose sensors with external transmitters, insulin pumps, and hybrid insulin delivery systems. These devices allow for data transfer to computer platforms. During telemedicine diabetes visits, standard procedures are followed, including reviewing history, assessing home blood glucose, monitoring data via computer platforms, providing suggestions for better glycemic control, and offering comprehensive guidance on managing specific situations like low blood sugar levels, physical activity, and other health issues.

Additionally, diabetology specialists offer support to children and adolescents showing symptoms that may indicate the onset of Type 1 diabetes or other types of childhood diabetes. Families can seek advice from hospital specialists if symptoms like urination, thirstiness, and sudden weight loss are observed in children throughout the day.

21.10 Telemedicine in Specific Pediatric Settings: Neurology and Neuropsychiatry

Follow-up tele-visits for patients with behavioral disturbances but without any anticonservative ideas, typically within the context of syndromic and nonsyndromic intellectual disabilitiesm, were provided in pediatric hospitals. These follow-ups have primarily aimed at verifying previous prescriptions made during day hospital/clinic sessions and monitoring the patient's clinical progress. These patients are often very fragile and struggle to wait their turn in the waiting room, especially when faced with extended wait times due to the physician managing concurrent emergencies. Evaluating patients remotely and within their familial context often provides clearer insights into the patient's clinical trajectory. Initially, families were somewhat hesitant to adapt to this new remote modality, fearing that it might compromise the quality of follow-up care. Remote activities also allow for better appointment scheduling for physicians, as not being physically present permits greater flexibility in coordination with families.

21.11 Conclusion

Telemedicine in pediatric care offers significant benefits, particularly in improving access to healthcare for children, especially in rural areas. It facilitates continuous monitoring for chronic conditions, reducing the need for frequent travel to healthcare facilities. Additionally, telemedicine alleviates the burden on hospitals by decreasing in-person visits for minor ailments and follow-up, allowing healthcare providers to concentrate on more severe cases.

This approach is particularly effective for managing chronic conditions, enhancing treatment adherence, and enabling timely interventions. Moreover, it plays a crucial role in delivering mental health services, providing children with support in a comfortable environment, which improves accessibility and increases the frequency of treatments. In summary, while telemedicine is a valuable complement to traditional pediatric care, enhancing accessibility and quality, it is essential to address technological, ethical, and training challenges to optimize its implementation, ensuring a patient-centered approach that meets the specific needs of pediatric patients.

References

1. Esposito S, Rosafio C, Antodaro F, Argentiero A, Bassi M, Becherucci P, Bonsanto F, Cagliero A, Cannata G, Capello F, Cardinale F, Chiriaco T, Consolaro A, Dessì A, Di Mauro G, Fainardi V, Fanos V, Guarino A, Li Calzi G, Lodi E, Maghnie M, Manfredini L, Malorgio E, Minuto N, Modena MG, Montori R, Moscatelli A, Patrone E, Pescio E, Poeta M, Ravelli A, Spelta M, Suppiej A, Vai S, Villa L, Zanini R, Botti R, Gaddi AV. Information and training on the use of telemedicine in pediatric population: consensus document of the Italian Society of Telemedicine (SIT), of the Italian Society of Preventive and Social Pediatrics (SIPPS), of the Italian Society of Pediatric Primary Care (SICuPP), of the Italian Federation of Pediatric Doctors (FIMP), and of the Syndicate of Family Pediatrician Doctors (SIMPeF). J Pers Med. 2023;13(2):314. https://doi.org/10.3390/jpm13020314. PMID: 36836548.
2. Esposito S, Rosafio C, Antodaro F, Argentiero A, Bassi M, Becherucci P, Bonsanto F, Cagliero A, Cannata G, Capello F, et al. Use of telemedicine healthcare systems in children and adolescents with chronic disease or in transition stages of life: consensus document of the Italian Society of Telemedicine (SIT), of the Italian Society of Preventive and Social Pediatrics (SIPPS), of the Italian Society of Pediatric Primary Care (SICuPP), of the Italian Federation of Pediatric Doctors (FIMP) and of the Syndicate of Family Pediatrician Doctors (SIMPeF). J Pers Med. 2023;13:235. https://doi.org/10.3390/jpm13020235.
3. Esposito S, Rosafio C, Antodaro F, Argentiero A, Bassi M, Becherucci P, Bonsanto F, Cagliero A, Cannata G, Capello F, Cardinale F, Chiriaco T, Consolaro A, Dessì A, Di Mauro G, Fainardi

V, Fanos V, Guarino A, Li Calzi G, Lodi E, Maghnie M, Manfredini L, Malorgio E, Minuto N, Modena MG, Montori R, Moscatelli A, Patrone E, Pescio E, Poeta M, Ravelli A, Spelta M, Suppiej A, Vai S, Villa L, Zanini R, Botti R, Gaddi AV. Use of telemedicine healthcare systems in pediatric assistance at territorial level: consensus document of the Italian Society of Telemedicine (SIT), of the Italian Society of Preventive and Social Pediatrics (SIPPS), of the Italian Society of Pediatric Primary Care (SICuPP), of the Italian Federation of Pediatric Doctors (FIMP) and of the Syndicate of Family Pediatrician Doctors (SIMPeF). J Pers Med. 2023;13(2):198. https://doi.org/10.3390/jpm13020198. PMID: 36836432; F Ferro et al Impact of telemedicine on health outcomes in children with medical complexity: an integrative review European Journal of Pediatrics (2021) 180:2389–2400.

4. Castillo-Rodenas M, Vicente Gómez JÁ, Fuster-Casanovas A, Miró Catalina Q, Vidal-Alaball J, López SF. Impact of COVID-19 on the pediatric primary care model in Catalonia: analysis of changes in the number and type of face-to-face and remote visits. JMIR Pediatr Parent. 2024;7:e49943. https://doi.org/10.2196/49943. PMID: 38532544.
5. Onofri A, Pavone M, De Santis S, Verrillo E, Caggiano S, Ullmann N, Cutrera R. Telemedicine in children with medical complexity on home ventilation during the COVID-19 pandemic. Pediatr Pulmonol. 2021;56(6):1395–400. https://doi.org/10.1002/ppul.25289.
6. Dev V, Mittal A, Joshi V, Meena JK, Dhanesh Goel A, Didel S, Pareek P, Misra S, Singh K. Cost analysis of telemedicine use in paediatric nephrology-the LMIC perspective. Pediatr Nephrol. 2024;39(1):193–201. https://doi.org/10.1007/s00467-023-06062-1. Epub 2023 Jul 24. PMID: 37488241.
7. McWilliams T, Hendricks J, Twigg D, Wood F, Giles M. Telehealth for paediatric burn patients in rural areas: a retrospective audit of activity and cost savings. Burns. 2016;42(7):1487–93. https://doi.org/10.1016/j.burns.2016.03.001. Epub 2016 Aug 26. PMID: 27575678.
8. Mosquera RA, Avritscher EBC, Pedroza C, Lee KH, Ramanathan S, Harris TS, Eapen JC, Yadav A, Caldas-Vasquez M, Poe M, Martinez Castillo DJ, Harting MT, Ottosen MJ, Gonzalez T, Tyson JE. Telemedicine for children with medical complexity: a randomized clinical trial. Pediatrics. 2021;148(3):e2021050400.
9. Lee KH, Pedroza C, Avritscher EBC, Mosquera RA, Tyson JE. Evaluation of negative binomial and zero-inflated negative binomial models for the analysis of zero-inflated count data: application to the telemedicine for children with medical complexity trial. Trials. 2023;24(1):613. https://doi.org/10.1186/s13063-023-07648-8. PMID: 37752579.
10. Folk JB, Valencia-Ayala C, Holloway ED, Anvar S, Czopp A, Tolou-Shams M. Feasibility and acceptability of a family-based telehealth intervention for families impacted by the child welfare system: formative mixed methods evaluation. JMIR Form Res. 2024;8:e57939. https://doi.org/10.2196/57939.
11. Neves AL, Burgers J. Digital technologies in primary care: implications for patient care and future research. Eur J Gen Pract. 2022;28:203–8.
12. Krupinski EA, Bernard J. Standards and guidelines in telemedicine and telehealth. Healthcare. 2014;2:74–93.
13. Sheikhtaheri A, Kermani F. Telemedicine in diagnosis, treatment and management of diseases in children. Stud Health Technol Inform. 2018;248:148–55.
14. Smaradottir BF, Berntsen GKR, Fensli RW. How to enhance digital support for cross-organisational health care teams? A user-based explorative study. J Health Eng. 2020;2020:8824882.
15. Ricci G, Gibelli F, Bailo P, Caraffa AM, Nittari G, Sirignano A. Informed consent in paediatric telemedicine: challenge or opportunity? A scoping review. Healthcare (Basel). 2023;11(10):1430. https://doi.org/10.3390/healthcare11101430. PMID: 37239716; PMCID: PMC10218595.
16. Wagner R, Lima TC, Silva MRTD, Rabha ACP, Ricieri MC, Fachi MM, Afonso RC, Motta FA. Assessment of pediatric telemedicine using remote physical examinations with a mobile medical device: a nonrandomized controlled trial. JAMA Netw Open. 2023;6(2):e2252570. https://doi.org/10.1001/jamanetworkopen.2022.52570. PMID: 36729459; PMCID: PMC9896296.

17. McConnochie KM. Potential of telemedicine in pediatric primary care. Pediatr Rev. 2006;27(9):e58–65. https://doi.org/10.1542/pir.27-9-e58. PMID: 16950936.
18. Calthorpe RJ, Smith S, Gathercole K, Smyth AR. Using digital technology for home monitoring, adherence and selfmanagement in cystic fibrosis: a state-of-the-art review. Thorax. 2020;75:72–7.
19. Tagliente I, Trieste L, Solvoll T, Murgia F, Bella S. Telemonitoring in cystic fibrosis: a 4-year assessment and simulation for the next 6 years. Interact J Med Res. 2016;5(2):e11. https://doi.org/10.2196/ijmr.5196. PMID: 27142963; PMCID: PMC4870389.
20. Federici A, De Marchis M, Alghisi F, Fiocchi AG, Bella S. Telemonitoring for cystic fibrosis patients of Bambino Gesù Children's Hospital during COVID-19. Clin Ter. 2022;173(5):440–2. https://doi.org/10.7417/CT.2022.2460. PMID: 36155730.
21. De Biase RV, Cristiani L, Paglia C, Alghisi F, Giordani B, Lucidi V, Bella S. Clinical and microbiological monitoring of cystic fibrosis patients, three years of follow-up via tele-medicine: an empirical research. Clin Ter. 2020;171(5):e381–4. https://doi.org/10.7417/CT.2020.2244. PMID: 32901778.
22. Silvetti MS, Saputo FA, Palmieri R, Placidi S, Santucci L, Di Mambro C, Righi D, Drago F. Results of remote follow-up and monitoring in young patients with cardiac implantable electronic devices. Cardiol Young. 2016;26(1):53–60. https://doi.org/10.1017/S1047951114002613. PMID: 25585614
23. Tornese G, Schiaffini R, Mozzillo E, Franceschi R, Frongia AP, Scaramuzza A, On Behalf of Hcl Expert Pathway Pediatric Group, The Diabetes Study Group of The Italian Society for Pediatric Endocrinology. Telemedicine in the time of the COVID-19 pandemic: results from the first survey among Italian Pediatric Diabetes Centers. Healthcare (Basel). 2021;9(7):815. https://doi.org/10.3390/healthcare9070815. PMID: 34203306; PMCID: PMC8304480.
24. Tornese G, Schiaffini R, Mozzillo E, Franceschi R, Frongia AP, Scaramuzza A, Diabetes Study Group of the Italian Society for Pediatric Endocrinology and Diabetes. The effect of the COVID-19 pandemic on telemedicine in pediatric diabetes centers in Italy: results from a longitudinal survey. Diabetes Res Clin Pract. 2021;179:109030. https://doi.org/10.1016/j.diabres.2021.109030. Epub 2021 Aug 28. PMID: 34461140; PMCID: PMC8438313.

Remote Consultation and Triage in Older People

22

Nicola Veronese, Jacopo Demurtas, Carlo Custodero, Virginia Boccardi, Pinar Soysal, and Stefania Maggi

22.1 Introduction

The so-called silver tsunami is upcoming, demographic is changing, and a huge number of older people with different stages of functioning and disabilities are rising and can cause several trouble to healthcare systems and services. As we age, the complexity of managing health conditions increases significantly. Older adults often face a range of interrelated challenges, including multiple chronic conditions such as cardiovascular disease, diabetes, and osteoporosis. For instance, Isik et al. found in their experience that in an older people population the frequency of polypharmacy was 54.5%, urinary incontinence 47.6%, malnutrition 9.6%, depression

N. Veronese (✉)
Saint Camillus International University of Health Sciences, Rome, Italy
e-mail: nicola.veronese@unicamillus.org

J. Demurtas
Clinical and Experimental Medicine PhD Program, University of Modena and Reggio Emilia, Modena, Italy

Family Medicine Department, USL Toscana Sud-Est, Capalbio, Italy

C. Custodero
Department of Interdisciplinary Medicine, "Aldo Moro" University of Bari, Bari, Italy

V. Boccardi
Division of Gerontology and Geriatrics, Department of Medicine and Surgery, University of Perugia, Perugia, Italy

P. Soysal
Department of Geriatric Medicine, Faculty of Medicine, Bezmialem Vakif University, Istanbul, Turkey

S. Maggi
National Research Council (CNR), Aging Section, Padova, Italy

J. Demurtas (ed.), *Remote Consultation in Primary Care*, TELe-Health,
https://doi.org/10.1007/978-3-031-89661-3_22

35.1%, dementia 21.6%, falls 33.6%, sarcopenia 31.7%, and frailty 28.3%. While 20% of cases in the 60–69 year age group did not have any syndromes, 48% of cases in ≥80 years had more than four syndromes simultaneously.

These chronic illnesses frequently coexist, requiring careful coordination of treatments, medications, and lifestyle adjustments. In addition to these physical conditions, cognitive impairment—ranging from mild cognitive decline to more severe forms like dementia—can complicate health management further. Mental health issues are also prevalent in this population, with depression and anxiety being common, often underdiagnosed, and linked to the broader challenges of aging. The intersection of mental health and chronic illness adds another layer of complexity to care, as psychological well-being significantly impacts physical health outcomes. Finally, many older adults experience functional limitations, such as reduced mobility, diminished sensory capabilities, and difficulties with activities of daily living (ADLs). These limitations require adaptive strategies to ensure that individuals can maintain as much independence as possible while adhering to their treatment plans. In the context of remote consultation, these challenges become even more pronounced. Managing complex health needs through telemedicine can be difficult due to technological barriers, limited access to proper digital tools, and the need for clear communication in assessing both cognitive and functional abilities. Remote consultations, while a valuable resource, demand tailored approaches to accommodate the unique needs of older adults, ensuring that comprehensive care remains effective despite the distance [1].

Healthy ageing is promoted nevertheless, and more and more older persons are living with disabilities and often alone because of the fall of the family model. Sometimes they can rely on formal or informal caregivers, and sometimes just on themselves. Digital medicine strategies can provide effective and economic solutions for these patients, and telemedicine, including remote consultation with a physician, a nurse, or a paramedic, can be one of the services that could improve these patients' conditions.

Literature on this topic showed that older adults with cognitive impairment or dementia can benefit from telemedicine interventions [2]; these digital health solutions offer a unique opportunity to improve the care and management of these vulnerable populations, providing both clinical and practical support in a range of settings.

Telemedicine platforms enable remote monitoring of chronic conditions and cognitive decline, allowing healthcare providers to track patients' health status more frequently and intervene earlier when issues arise. This continuous monitoring can be particularly beneficial for those with dementia or mild cognitive impairment (MCI), who may struggle to recognize or communicate their own symptoms. Early detection of changes in health, behavior, or cognitive function can lead to more timely adjustments in care plans and medication, ultimately enhancing the quality of care. Additionally, these interventions provide a way to offer guidance and education directly to the patient and their caregivers. With telemedicine, caregivers can be actively involved in consultations, even when they are not physically present. This is particularly valuable as caregiving is often a shared responsibility, with family members balancing multiple roles.

While the benefits are clear, it is essential that telemedicine solutions are designed with user-friendly interfaces and are accessible for older adults, considering potential limitations such as reduced digital literacy, sensory impairments, and technological access. Efforts must be made to ensure these platforms are as inclusive and adaptable as possible, so that older adults and their caregivers can fully engage with the tools available.

For instance, in chronic disease management, one of the most common conditions in older populations, teleconsultation can be a useful tool to connect patients, providers, and caregivers, aiming to improve self-care and reduce the need for in-person visits [3, 4].

However, disparities in access to telemedicine for older adults exist. According to a study, the odds of using telemedicine services via videoconference are lower for people aged 65 or older compared to those aged 64 or younger [5]. This is due to several reasons: older adults may have lower digital literacy, vision, or hearing impairments, and be less comfortable with technology [6]. Moreover, those with low socioeconomic status and limited Internet access may have even more difficulties in accessing remote consultations.

This chapter will offer a comprehensive overview of the current evidence on remote consultation and triage for older adults in primary care, emphasizing both the potential benefits and the challenges associated with these approaches [5–7].

22.2 Challenges of Remote Consultation in Older People

Conducting remote consultations with older patients presents unique challenges that require heightened attention to detail and a tailored approach to address their specific needs. Older adults often exhibit vague or nonspecific symptoms, which may be difficult to assess accurately without an in-person examination. This, combined with potential impairments such as hearing loss, visual deficits, or cognitive decline, complicates the ability to gather a clear clinical picture during a remote interaction. Furthermore, older patients frequently present with multiple coexisting conditions that can mask or overlap with other symptoms, making accurate diagnosis and management more complex. The lack of in-person cues, such as body language or subtle physical signs, means that clinicians must rely more heavily on detailed verbal communication and careful questioning to understand the patient's condition. In many cases, remote consultations involve a third party, such as a family member or caregiver, who mediates the interaction. While this can be helpful for gathering information, it also introduces additional layers of complexity. The indirect nature of these consultations can make it harder for healthcare providers to directly engage with the patient and fully assess their individual needs and preferences. Caregivers may unintentionally filter or misinterpret information, making the diagnostic process more difficult. To address these challenges, clinicians must adopt a more holistic and adaptive approach, being mindful of the need for clearer communication, more in-depth patient histories, and greater reliance on caregiver input when necessary. Technological limitations, such as inadequate Internet access or unfamiliarity with digital tools, can also further hinder the consultation process, requiring additional flexibility and patience.

22.2.1 Blurred Symptoms

Often symptoms may be milder in frail older adults, whereas minor illnesses may be disabling and critical. Try to focus on how the person that you are examining "looks" based on their previous history and if available on the feedback of relatives or former caregivers. Some illnesses like respiratory tract infections, delirium, and urinary tract infections in older adults may have more atypical presentations.

Try to gather data on the pharmacotherapies as often older people are on polypharmacotherapy, and this may be directly linked to frailty. Also, many of the symptoms presented by older people may be directly or indirectly linked to therapy and its adverse events.

One of the main challenges of remote consultation in older people is the difficulty in comprehensively assessing their health status. Older people often present atypical symptoms, which can make it challenging for the healthcare provider to identify and address the underlying condition [4]. For example, an older patient may present with confusion or fatigue rather than the more classic symptoms of an illness.

22.2.2 Third-Party Consultations

Complicating this is the fact that communication can be challenging. Older patients may have speech, hearing, or vision difficulties that interfere with communication, and they may have cognitive impairments that limit their ability to participate fully in the telehealth encounter [4, 5]. In some cases, the healthcare provider may need to rely on information provided by a caregiver or family member rather than directly from the patient [6].

When dealing with older adults in a remote consultation, it must be ensured to get information from the actual patients, not just from the caller. Often, consultations for older people are handled, especially when they feel sick, by a relative or caregiver. Nevertheless, the importance of gathering information directly from the patient has to be stressed. As reported in the literature, in remote consultation by phone, physicians, nurses, and paramedics rely on verbal and paraverbal cues, while in video and face-to-face consultation also on nonverbal cues and clues. This is of paramount importance. When taking a call, the handler has to carefully appreciate the paraverbal cues of the patient (does he/she seem in pain? In danger? How ill does he/she seem?) and consider not just verbal information. So, even if the patient seems unable to talk, for instance, this applies to people with dementia or severe cognitive impairment, the handler must hear their voice and gather information from that source: the tone, the rhythm, the quietness, or the agitation can reveal a lot.

- How is he/she breathing
- Pain
- Weakness
- Confusion
- Shivers…

22.2.3 Communicational Issues

Limitations and communication challenges must be identified and overtaken through an efficient and empathic dialogue with the patient, as much as possible.

Older patients may often be affected by conditions of impairment that should be considered. A hearing loss, or acoustic impairment, may impact severely on the communication ability of the patient and impair their social life and finally negatively affect their quality of life. To cope with this problem, the healthcare professional must learn proper communication techniques. Vision impairment, or visual disability, represents another common issue that can influence the ability of the patient to interact during a remote consultation.

Cognitive impairment or dementia are other common conditions in the older population, which may significantly change the ability of the patient to clearly understand the questions and provide coherent answers.

These limitations highlight the need for the healthcare provider to be adaptable and to use a variety of communication techniques when conducting a remote consultation with an older patient.

On the other hand, while handling a consultation, using a loud tone of voice may impact how the handler is perceived, due to the modifications in the paraverbal cues given. It is also to remember that talking too loudly, even in conditions of hearing impairment, may be considered impolite and impair the outcome of the consultation.

22.3 Opportunities in Remote Assessment

Despite the challenges, remote assessment of older adults offers several promising opportunities that can enhance both accesses to care and the quality of healthcare delivery. These opportunities, if leveraged correctly, can greatly benefit this population by improving monitoring, reducing barriers to healthcare, and enabling more comprehensive, continuous care. Remote consultations can significantly increase access to healthcare, particularly for older adults who may have mobility issues, live in rural or underserved areas, or find travel difficult due to health constraints. Telemedicine reduces the need for in-person visits, ensuring that patients can access care from the comfort of their homes, thus minimizing logistical challenges like transportation or waiting times. Technologies such as remote monitoring devices, wearables, and telehealth platforms enable continuous tracking of vital signs and other health metrics (e.g., blood pressure, glucose levels, heart rate). These tools provide real-time data, allowing healthcare providers to identify potential health issues early and intervene before they become more severe. This is particularly useful for managing chronic conditions prevalent among older adults, such as diabetes, hypertension, or heart disease. Remote assessment allows caregivers to be more actively involved in the healthcare process, ensuring they can participate in consultations and better understand treatment plans. This collaborative model improves the management of care for older adults, especially those with cognitive impairments or mobility limitations, as caregivers play a vital role in ensuring adherence to medication, monitoring symptoms, and managing day-to-day healthcare needs. Remote assessment tools allow for personalized care plans tailored to the specific needs of each patient. These consultations can be scheduled more frequently without the constraints of travel, providing flexibility to adjust treatments or medication regimens based on the patient's ongoing condition. This personalization can be enhanced by integrating data analytics from remote monitoring devices, offering clinicians a clearer picture of the patient's overall health over time. Regular remote assessments provide the opportunity for early detection of health problems, including subtle changes in symptoms or functional decline, which might go unnoticed during infrequent in-person visits. Early identification of these issues can lead to timely interventions, potentially preventing hospitalization or worsening of chronic conditions. Remote consultations also open the door to greater mental health support for older adults, particularly those who may be experiencing social isolation or depression. Telepsychiatry and counselling services can provide regular check-ins and emotional support, addressing a critical need for older adults who may otherwise lack access to mental health services. Regular communication via telehealth can also help mitigate the psychological effects of isolation by creating more frequent human contact, even if it's virtual. Remote assessments can reduce the burden on healthcare systems by allowing for more efficient use of resources. Minor or routine check-ups that do not require physical examinations can be handled remotely, freeing up in-person appointments for more complex or urgent cases. This model can help streamline healthcare services and ensure that older adults receive the right level of care at the right time.

22.3.1 Triage

A fast yet effective evaluation of patients symptoms and signs may be done remotely, either by telephone or video consultation [5, 6, 8]. A good triage can determine the urgency of the situation and guide the patient to the most appropriate level of care, reducing in-person visits and increasing access to primary care.

Silver triage evaluations for acute but nonurgent conditions and acute exacerbations of chronic diseases could represent a first line of remote care for the older population with significant benefits. A quick remote assessment of the general conditions, breathing, mental status, and vital signs can help to determine the severity of the situation and whether an in-person visit is needed.

Remote triage can provide an opportunity to screen and evaluate patients without the need for travel, which may be challenging for older adults with limited mobility or transportation options. By triaging patients remotely, healthcare providers can better allocate resources and direct patients to the most appropriate level of care, whether that is an in-person visit, a telehealth consultation, or self-care guidance.

The literature data show that remote triage and telephone consultations have significant potential to improve health outcomes in older adults, by providing prompt access to care and facilitating more appropriate resource utilization. The experience with the so-called Silver Triage, by Jones et al., suggests that geriatrician-led telephone triage may improve the care of older people by preventing unnecessary hospitalization and has been well received by paramedics [9]. In the cited experience, researchers organized a remote second-level triage service for frail older people, in which a teleconsultation is made with paramedics on the scene to inform their decision-making on appropriate referral of older patients, suggesting the best solution for each case: emergency department referral, hospital at home, or other safe alternatives. It has been shown in other experiences that this approach can reduce the number of older people requiring emergency department attendance and subsequent admission to hospital [10].

For instance, the use of remote consultations for managing urinary tract infections in older adults has been associated with a reduction in emergency department visits and hospitalization rates [8].

22.3.2 Remote Comprehensive Geriatric Assessment (CGA)

As illustrated in the literature [11, 12], telemedicine can enable Comprehensive Geriatric Assessment (CGA) to be performed remotely, leveraging digital technologies like video consultations or remote monitoring. In this way, older people can be assessed comprehensively at home, without the need to travel, which is particularly beneficial for frail or functionally limited older adults.

A recent review by Faust et al. on geriatric telemedicine concluded that both real-time video consultations and asynchronous home monitoring can enable CGA, with the potential to improve quality of care, enhance accessibility, and reduce healthcare costs.

A CGA can be performed remotely and may be extremely important when dealing with older patients by phone or video, to determine whether they have or do not have a certain level of impaired function and disability, and, considering that these tools explore multiple dimensions, to detect the healthcare and social aspects that are more impaired.

The use of CGA remotely has been boosted particularly since the COVID-19 pandemic when a large part of vulnerable older adults risked being excluded from geriatric consultation services or lost to the follow-ups due to restriction measures and fear of contagion [13]. Technological advancements and continuous refinement of optimal modalities to apply virtual CGA enables early detection of disease, to monitor for change of functional, cognitive, nutritional, and social status, to deliver personalized care, to check the adherence to the treatment plan, and finally to optimize healthcare resources for better health outcomes [14].

Some experiences demonstrated that this approach may be feasible and well accepted by older adults [13].

For example, an adapted telephone-administered version of a CGA-based tool as the Multidimensional Prognostic Index (MPI), called TELE-MPI has been recently validated. This instrument offers useful prognostic information exploring eight domains of the CGA: (1) basal activity of daily living (ADL); (2) instrumental activities of daily living (IADLs); (3) mobility through three simple questions evaluating the abilities to transfer from bed to chair or wheelchair, walking, and going up and down the stairs; (4) cognitive status with the Short Portable Mental Status Questionnaire (SPMSQ); (5) nutritional status using the Mini Nutritional Assessment Short Form (MNA-SF); (6) burden of comorbidities investigated by the Cumulative Illness Rating Scale-comorbidity index (CIRS-CI) and assigning 1 point to each health problems/diseases that are so severe to require chronic drug therapies in 13 aspects of health; (7) polypharmacy with the number of medications; and (8) cohabitation status. The TELE-MPI showed strong agreement with the standard form, being able to predict risk of falls and psychiatric disorders in community-dwelling older adults [15]. Moreover, in another study, a self-administered geriatric assessment smartphone application, the electronic geriatric assessment bundle (e-GAB), has been developed and validated to screen for problems in cognition, mood, sensory systems, urinary continence, nutrition, functional capacity, balance and risk of falls, frailty, sleep, pain, home safety and social problems, showing good reliability compared to the standard CGA instruments [16].

In the near future telemedicine might also offer the opportunity to get a CGA from direct environmental monitoring in daily life rather than using conventional questionnaires [17].

Obviously, these approaches cannot completely substitute the clinical examination and the multidisciplinary standard CGA but may overcome some barriers for the CGA application in general practice and help to spread the CGA concept to a wider audience.

22.3.3 Medication Review and Deprescribing

When handling remote consultation for older adults, it is fundamental to pay attention to the patients' pharmacological therapy, trying to identify potential issues, reduce inappropriate polypharmacy, and check for adherence and safety.

Given the association between drug consumption, depression, and cognitive impairment highlighted in some studies [18], special attention should be devoted to the medications, their interactions and potential side effects, which may impact on the mental health and function of older patients [18].

Remote access and telehealth experiences may represent an excellent opportunity for medication review and deprescribing, empowering the clinician to promote safer and more appropriate pharmacological management, especially for vulnerable older patients hardly reached by traditional healthcare services [18].

A recent review pointed out that remote medication review can decrease harmful polypharmacy and improve patient safety, especially when combined with other telehealth interventions [19]. Telehealth can enable clinicians to assess older patients' medication regimens, adherence, side effects, and interactions, and then work with the patient and caregivers to optimize the medication management through shared decision-making and targeted deprescribing [20].

22.3.4 Continuity of Care

During the COVID-19 pandemic, remote care via telehealth has been particularly relevant to ensure continuity of care for the older population, who face higher risks from in-person visits. Telehealth solutions have enabled continuous monitoring, timely adjustment of care plans, and early detection of deterioration, thus preventing costly acute care episodes and maintaining older adults in their homes and communities [19].

Integrated home-based care models combining remote monitoring, virtual consultations, and community-based services have shown promising results in supporting older adults with chronic conditions and functional impairments. Such models allow clinicians to proactively identify problems, adjust care plans, and coordinate across the care continuum, while providing older adults and caregivers with accessible, personalized support.

Robust systems for data sharing, care coordination, and interdisciplinary collaboration are essential to harness the full potential of telehealth for continuity of care in older populations.

Safe monitoring of parameters may be done, sometimes with telemedicine monitoring tools or in presence, convening hospital admissions and consultations only when necessary and avoiding unneeded exposure of frail older patients to healthcare settings.

22.4 Conclusions

In summary, remote consultation and triage represent valuable tools for enhancing both the management and accessibility of primary care for older adults, particularly when the inherent challenges of communication and assessment are addressed with care and precision. The ability to remotely assess patients allows healthcare providers to triage more efficiently, accurately evaluate the urgency of medical conditions, and direct patients to the appropriate level of care. This not only ensures timely interventions but can also reduce the strain on healthcare resources by minimizing unnecessary hospital visits and admissions, ultimately contributing to better health outcomes. To maximize the effectiveness of remote healthcare for the older population, it is crucial to integrate these efforts with complementary approaches. Remote monitoring can offer continuous oversight of chronic conditions, providing real-time data to alert clinicians to potential issues before they escalate. A comprehensive geriatric assessment, conducted remotely, allows for a holistic understanding of a patient's physical, mental, and social health, which is key to addressing the multifaceted needs of older adults. Medication reviews, facilitated through telemedicine, ensure that polypharmacy risks are managed and that medication regimens are optimized for safety and effectiveness. Additionally, strategies to ensure continuity of care, such as regular follow-ups and caregiver involvement, are critical in maintaining consistent, patient-centered care over time. By combining these remote healthcare strategies, the care delivered to older adults can be significantly improved, fostering a more accessible, efficient, and personalized approach that addresses both immediate health concerns and long-term well-being.

References

1. Harper MS. Behavioral, social and mental health aspects of home care for older Americans. Home Health Care Serv Q. 1989, February 22;9(4):61–124. https://doi.org/10.1300/j027v09n04_05.
2. Marešová P, Tomsone S, Lameski P, Madureira J, Mendes A, Zdravevski E, Chorbev I, Trajkovik V, Ellen M, Rodil K. Technological solutions for older people with Alzheimer's disease: review. Curr Alzheimer Res. 2018, August 15;15(10):975–83. https://doi.org/10.2174/1567205015666180427124547.
3. Fadzil NHM, Shahar S, Rajikan R, Singh DKA, Ludin AFM, Subramaniam P, Ibrahim N, Vanoh D, Ali NM. A scoping review for usage of Telerehabilitation among older adults with mild cognitive impairment or cognitive frailty. MDPI. 2022, March 28;19(7):4000. https://doi.org/10.3390/ijerph19074000.
4. Goins RT, Kategile U, Dudley KC. Telemedicine, rural elderly, and policy issues. J Aging Soc Policy. 2002, September 20;13(4):53–71. https://doi.org/10.1300/j031v13n04_04.
5. Zhai Y. A call for addressing barriers to telemedicine: health disparities during the COVID-19 pandemic. Psychother Psychosom. 2020, June 4;90(1):64–6. https://doi.org/10.1159/000509000.
6. NACNS White Paper on Telehealth Competency for the Clinical Nurse Specialist: Gap Analysis and Recommendations. Clin Nurse Spec. 2022, January 1;36(1):E1–7. https://doi.org/10.1097/nur.0000000000000650.
7. Chuna YJ, Patterson P. A suggestion for future research on interface design of an internet-based telemedicine system for the elderly. Work. 2012, January 1;41:353–6. https://doi.org/10.3233/wor-2012-0181-353.
8. Roberts L, Osborn-Jenkins L. Delivering remote consultations: talking the talk. Musculoskelet Sci Pract. 2021, April 1;52:102275. https://doi.org/10.1016/j.msksp.2020.102275.
9. Jones HT, Teranaka W, Hunter P, Gross L, Conroy S. What is the impact of a pre-hospital geriatrician led telephone 'Silver Triage' for older people living with frailty? Eur Geriatr Med. 2023, May 23;14(5):977–81.
10. Newberger R, Braithwaite S. EMS prioritization of response. 2020, August 16. https://www.statpearls.com/articlelibrary/viewarticle/31804/
11. Albornoz SCD, Sia K, Harris A. The effectiveness of teleconsultations in primary care: systematic review. Fam Pract. 2021, July 19;39(1):168–82. https://doi.org/10.1093/fampra/cmab077.

12. Carmona C, Bewick T, Macduff N, Thomas A. Suspected acute respiratory infection in over 16s: assessment at first presentation and initial management—summary of NICE guidance. BMJ. 2024, March 11;384:q339. https://doi.org/10.1136/bmj.q339.
13. Loewenthal J, DuMontier C, Cooper L, Frain L, Waldman LS, Streiter S, Cardin K, Tulebaev S, Javedan H, Orkaby AR, Hshieh T. Adaptation of the comprehensive geriatric assessment to a virtual delivery format. Age Ageing. 2021;50(2):597–8. https://doi.org/10.1093/ageing/afaa257.
14. Wu X, Freeman S, Miyagi M, Park U, Nomura K, Ebihara S. Comprehensive geriatric assessment in the era of telemedicine. Geriatr. Gerontol. Int. 2024;24:67–73. https://doi.org/10.1111/ggi.14705.
15. Custodero C, Senesi B, Pinna A, Floris A, Vigo M, Fama M, Mastropierro V, Sabbà C, Prete C, Pilotto A. Validation and implementation of telephone-administered version of the Multidimensional Prognostic Index (TELE-MPI) for remote monitoring of community-dwelling older adults. Aging Clin Exp Res. 2021 Dec;33(12):3363–3369. https://doi.org/10.1007/s40520-021-01871-6. Epub 2021 May 18. PMID: 34002336; PMCID: PMC8128686.
16. Rasheedy D, Mohamed HE, Saber HG, Hassanin HI. Usability of a self-administered geriatric assessment mHealth: cross-sectional study in a geriatric clinic. Geriatr. Gerontol. Int. 2021;21:222–8. https://doi.org/10.1111/ggi.14122.
17. The Japan Geriatrics Society Geriatric Medical Practice Committee, Nomura K, Ebihara S, Ikebata Y, et al. Japan Geriatrics Society "Statement for the use of telemedicine in geriatric care: Telemedicine as a complement to in-person medical practice": Geriatric medical practice committee consensus statement. Geriatr. Gerontol. Int. 2022;22:913–6. https://doi.org/10.1111/ggi.14490.
18. Faber LM, Scheicher ME, Soares E. Depressão, Declínio Cognitivo e Polimedicação em idosos institucionalizados. Revista Kairós-Gerontologia. 2017, June 30;20(2):195. https://doi.org/10.23925/2176-901x.2017v20i2p195-210.
19. Ngaruiya N, Orwa D, Waiganjo P. Towards a deployment model for emonitoring of geriatric persons in rural developing countries: Case of Kenya. 2017, May 1. https://doi.org/10.23919/istafrica.2017.8102353.
20. Hovey L, Kaylor MB, Alwan M, Resnick HE. Community-based telemonitoring for hypertension management: practical challenges and potential solutions. Mary Ann Liebert Inc. 2011, October 1;17(8):645–51. https://doi.org/10.1089/tmj.2011.0027.

Remote Consultation in Primary Care During Emergencies

23

Domenico Penna, Maria Vittoria Dubbini, Erik Lagolio, and Ilaria Rossiello

23.1 Introduction

Integrating remote consultation is a pivotal yet understudied frontier in primary care during crises and emergencies. The recent pandemic has shown the increasing importance of remote consultation tools in every medical setting. However, there is limited scientific evidence on using these tools during emergencies in primary care. Nonetheless, the available research data can give us insights into possible applications and potential benefits. This chapter tries to clarify the role of remote consultation within emergency primary care, exploring its advantages and delineating its limitations. In the following paragraphs, the remote consultation's impact in emergencies will be analyzed through the lens of appropriateness increment, efficiency increment, cost reduction, management improvement, specific situations management, infectious emergencies management, interdisciplinary collaboration enhancement, and the identification of limitations.

D. Penna (✉) · M. V. Dubbini
Transfusion Medicine Service, Azienda Ospedaliera Marche Nord, San Salvatore Hospital, Pesaro, Italy

E. Lagolio
Italian College of General Practitioners and Primary Care, Florence, Italy

General Practitioner and referral of NOVA MEDICA FINALESE medical center in Finale Ligure, Savona Province, Italy

I. Rossiello
General Practitioner AST3 Montecosaro, Marche, Italy

J. Demurtas (ed.), *Remote Consultation in Primary Care*, TELe-Health,
https://doi.org/10.1007/978-3-031-89661-3_23

23.2 Appropriateness Increment

The primary role of remote consultation in primary care during emergencies is to optimize access to the healthcare system by acting as a filter capable of selecting appropriate cases. This function is crucial because it limits inappropriate access and overcrowding of emergency services, allowing for better management of cases that require immediate attention. It is important to note that a significant percentage of emergency facility visits are inappropriate, and remote consultation tools provide valuable additional clinical information and help general practitioners distinguish cases to be sent to emergency services from those that require outpatient management or remote monitoring. Considering the speed of remote initial assessments, these tools also encourage patients to contact their primary care physician for a preliminary evaluation before going to the emergency room. In a report from the Health Foundation on the role of telemedicine in primary care in England during the COVID-19 epidemic, Geraldine Clarke, Paris Pariza, and Arne Wolters examined how the implementation of this service significantly impacted the activation of the emergency system. In particular, the three authors demonstrated that using remote consultation by general practitioners served as a filtering function, reducing the number of emergency room visits during the period under analysis [1]. An article published in the *British Journal Of General Practice* further emphasized how the implementation of remote consultation, especially video consultation, was perceived by general practitioners as a valuable tool for improving the initial triage of patients [2].

23.3 Efficiency Increment

Several studies have also highlighted how remote consultation in primary care settings during emergencies can make the emergency response system more efficient [2, 3]. While this tool does not replace in-person care, remote consultation ensures a timelier response, reducing delays in responding to emergencies.

Thanks to this tool, general practitioners, who already have various clinical information about the patient, can perform an initial assessment and manage immediate clinical problems, coordinating with other healthcare providers if necessary. In this setting, the preliminary assessment by the general practitioner is valuable not only for providing initial clinical guidance to the patient but also because it can activate subsequent diagnostic and therapeutic hospital pathways, reducing emergency room waiting times based on the severity of the clinical condition. Furthermore, this tool plays a crucial role in continuity of care because, in addition to providing a preliminary assessment, it allows for effective follow-up of patients after the initial intervention, reducing the risk of complications and providing patients with continuous contact with the healthcare system. In this way, it is possible to ensure better care and a reduction in the occupancy time of high-intensity care beds.

23.4 Cost Reduction and Management Improvement

The increase in efficiency and appropriateness of the emergency system ultimately results in cost reduction and better management of resources for the entire healthcare system.

Cost reduction is achieved through the prevention of inappropriate access and the consequent reduction of operational costs (personnel, equipment, and facilities), while improved efficiency results from a more efficient distribution of human resources, with medical expertise being used more judiciously, focusing immediately on severe clinical cases.

Remote consultation in primary care settings during emergencies can generate complex positive effects, influencing the healthcare system at multiple levels.

23.5 Specific Situations Better Management

There are specific situations where the ability to conduct remote consultations with one's physician is critical because it proves to be a particularly suitable tool for addressing specific issues. To begin with, a key role played by remote consultation in the setting of primary care during emergencies is to ensure access to qualified and fast healthcare in remote areas (islands, mountain communities, rural areas with limited connectivity to reference cities), in particular situations (patients in prison or quarantine), or in cases where patients are unable to travel (isolated or mobility-impaired patients). Remote consultation is accessible at any time and location with Internet connectivity. A recent study showed that these features have already been crucial in specific settings, such as providing acute pediatric care in regions with low pediatric healthcare facility density [4]. With this tool, general practitioners can provide initial medical care and monitor patients' clinical conditions, preventing the interruption of care and activating the rest of the emergency response system simultaneously.

23.6 Infectious Emergencies Better Management

Remote consultation can also be particularly useful in infectious emergencies. As demonstrated in the recent COVID-19 epidemic, this tool is highly versatile and practical in global healthcare emergencies. During such crises, remote consultation services can be rapidly implemented to manage the increasing number of patients requiring medical assistance. In this setting, remote consultation helps limit the spread of pathogens by reducing physical contact between patients and between patients and healthcare providers. At the same time, this tool ensures the ability to monitor the pathogen's spread and advise patients in isolation or quarantine [5]. These actions result in increased safety for healthcare personnel who can continue to work without being exposed to the pathogen and continuous monitoring of clinical cases, allowing for a more precise and rapid distinction between urgent patients to be sent to the emergency room and patients who can be managed remotely with appropriate precautions. This tool thus guarantees adequate healthcare response in epidemic settings, not only by reducing the pathogen transmission rate among patients but also by ensuring the safety of healthcare personnel by reducing the risk of infection [6–9].

23.7 Interdisciplinary Collaboration Improvement

Remote consultation also facilitates interdisciplinary collaboration among physicians of different specialties [10]. For example, in emergencies, a general practitioner can consult with specialists in real time to evaluate complex cases. This multidisciplinary approach helps improve the quality of care and reduces the need for transfers to hospital facilities, optimizing resource utilization. In this regard, some national and international experiences have already been realized. Of particular interest is the "Online Cardiology" project, which has shown that offering the possibility of real-time consultation between general practitioners and cardiovascular disease specialists through remote consultation has improved care pathways, communication between hospital and nonhospital healthcare facilities, and reduced outpatient and emergency room visits [11].

Equally compelling projects are also carried out in settings different from primary care, which are now being closely monitored for their potential applicability in this setting. For example, a remote consultation protocol has been recently proposed to improve decision-making in cases of acute abdomen. The project involved a group of emergency physicians and surgeons tasked to conduct remote consultations in specific clinical situations based on a precise diagnostic and therapeutic protocol proposed by the World Society of Emergency Surgeons. This project significantly impacted on healthcare costs related to tests, admissions, surgeries, and unnecessary transfers [12]. Applying similar standardized protocols in combination with remote consultation could improve decision-making in primary care during emergencies. These protocols can guide general practitioners in evaluating and managing emergency patients, allowing them to make informed decisions in real time. The interdisciplinary development of such protocols could optimize remote consultation in this complex clinical setting.

23.8 Limitations of Primary Care Remote Consultation During Emergencies

So far, we have analyzed the potential of remote consultation in primary care settings during emergencies, but we must remember the limitations of this tool. The analysis of limitations is crucial for correctly identifying the setting of the application of remote consultation services, to ensure that they represent appropriate support for daily clinical activities [13].

The first and most important limitation of remote consultation in emergencies is the inability to perform a complete physical examination and monitor vital signs, which makes it challenging to manage severe cases.

Therefore, if one of the possible advantages of this tool is the ability to act as a filter to reduce inappropriate access to the emergency system, on the other hand, the implementation of such a tool in the setting of primary care must include the possibility of activating the same system quickly in cases of absolute necessity (severe traumas, heart attacks, strokes) that require immediate care that can only be provided in a hospital setting [14].

A second limitation that could compromise the benefits of improving the efficiency of the emergency system offered by remote consultation is the need for healthcare providers to develop specific skills in using this tool. It is necessary to train general practitioners in effective communication with patients, which is particularly complex in the setting of high emotional activation, as well as in effective communication with emergency healthcare providers. Such communication should be facilitated by specific training and supported by appropriate decision algorithms [15].

A third limitation concerns the initial costs of starting a remote consultation service. It should be remembered that implementing such a system requires an initial investment in creating an infrastructure that guarantees data privacy and security and provides each physician with the necessary technology to work effectively. Furthermore, managing a portion of the emergency-urgent system within primary care settings must stay manageable for the involved healthcare providers. Other investments should be, therefore, directed to hiring the additional physicians needed to satisfy the new job requirements [16].

Finally, to ensure the adequate accessibility and equity of a widespread remote consultation service, especially in emergency settings, it is necessary to not only ensure the availability of stable Internet connections in the areas where the service is implemented but also to facilitate access for people of different genders, ages, ethnicities, socioeconomic statuses, and residence in rural or urban areas [17].

23.9 Summary

As summarized in the diagram of functions of remote consultation in primary care during emergencies (Fig. 23.1), this chapter has examined the role and features of remote consultation in primary care during emergencies. Despite limited scientific evidence, the analysis of the studies conducted has allowed us to highlight the importance and complexity of this tool. As seen in the previous paragraphs, remote consultation serves various functions.

First and foremost, it contributes to quickly distinguishing cases to be sent to the emergency room from those that can be managed on an outpatient basis or remotely, thus acting as a filter that selects appropriate cases to be sent to emergency services and reduces overcrowding of these facilities [1, 2]. This action, in turn, allows for the concentration of more resources on patients requiring immediate attention due

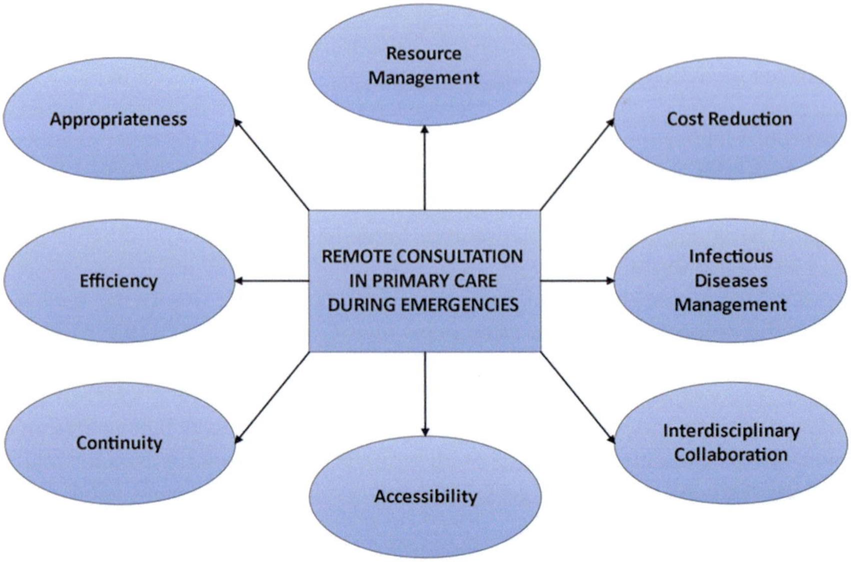

Fig. 23.1 Diagram of functions of remote consultation in primary care during emergencies

to severe clinical conditions, increasing the performance of the entire healthcare system.

Second, remote consultation makes the emergency response system more efficient [3]. This service guarantees, in fact, both rapid activation and a more targeted assessment of clinical cases, as general practitioners can conduct a more precise preliminary assessment thanks to the clinical information they already possess. This assessment helps activate subsequent diagnostic and therapeutic pathways more precisely, ensuring a faster and more appropriate response to individual clinical conditions. All of this would result in cost reduction and better healthcare resource management.

Third, remote consultation is particularly suitable for addressing specific situations. This tool is valuable in situations characterized by limited accessibility or in infectious healthcare emergencies [4–9].

Finally, remote consultation encourages interdisciplinary collaboration among physicians of different specialties and the creation of specific diagnostic-therapeutic algorithms in a complex emergency setting. In the coming years, attention should focus on these aspects to develop a remote consultation service that can effectively address future healthcare emergencies [10–12]. In conclusion, remote consultation in primary care during emergencies can significantly improve the efficiency of the emergency system; however, it is essential to address and overcome the associated limitations to maximize its potential benefits in providing high-quality healthcare.

References

1. Clarke G, Pariza P, Wolters A. https://www.health.org.uk/news-and-comment/charts-and-infographics/how-are-total-triage-and-remote-consultation-changing-the-us. 2020 Dec 3.
2. Payne RE, Clarke A. How and why are video consultations used in urgent primary care settings in the UK? A focus group study. BJGP Open. 2023;7(3):BJGPO.2023.0025. https://doi.org/10.3399/BJGPO.2023.0025.
3. Libreros-Peña L, Quintero JA, Gelves A, et al. Telemedicine consultation for emergency patients' attention: a clinical experience from a high complex university hospital from Latin America. BMC Health Serv Res. 23, 559 (2023). https://doi.org/10.1186/s12913-023-09520-6; BJGPO.2023.0025. https://doi.org/10.3399/BJGPO.2023.0025.
4. Beyer A, Moon K, Penndorf P, et al. Triage through telemedicine in paediatric emergency care-Results of a concordance study. PLoS One. 2022;17(5):e0269058. https://doi.org/10.1371/journal.pone.0269058.
5. Tarn DM, Hintz C, Mendez-Hernandez E, et al. Using virtual visits to care for primary care patients with COVID-19 symptoms. J Am Board Fam Med. Feb 2021;34(Supplement):S147–51. https://doi.org/10.3122/jabfm.2021.S1.200241.
6. Khairat S, Meng C, Xu Y, et al. Interpreting COVID-19 and virtual care trends: Cohort study. JMIR Public Health Surveill. 2020;6:e18811. https://doi.org/10.2196/18811.
7. Rockwell KL, Gilroy AS. Incorporating telemedicine as part of COVID-19 outbreak response systems. Am J Manag Care. 2020;26:147–8. https://doi.org/10.37765/ajmc.2020.42784.
8. Lurie N, Carr BG. The role of telehealth in the medical response to disasters. JAMA Intern Med. 2018;178:745–6. https://doi.org/10.1001/jamainternmed.2018.1314.
9. Greenhalgh T, Koh GCH, Car J. Covid-19: a remote assessment in primary care. BMJ. 2020;368:m1182. https://doi.org/10.1136/bmj.m1182.
10. Aghdam MRF, Vodovnik A, Hameed RA. Role of telemedicine in multidisciplinary team meetings. J Pathol Inform. 2019;10:35. https://doi.org/10.4103/jpi.jpi_20_19.
11. Cainelli L, Moretti M, Bonmassari R. Efficacy of remote consultation between hospital cardiologists and primary care in cardiovascular disease management: the "Cardiologia in linea" project in Trentino. Italy G Ital Cardiol (Rome). 2023;24(6):432–5. https://doi.org/10.1714/4041.40202.
12. De Simone B, Ansaloni L, Sartelli M, et al. The Video-Consulting Emergency protocol: a proposition from the World Society of Emergency Surgery members for the initial management of non-traumatic acute abdomen. Minerva Chir. 2019;74(3):189–94. https://doi.org/10.23736/S0026-4733.18.07963-4.
13. Vodička S, Zelko E. Remote consultations in general practice – a systematic review. Zdr Varst. 2022;61(4):224–30. https://doi.org/10.2478/sjph-2022-0030.
14. Jin MX, Kim SY, Miller LJ, Behari G, Correa R. Telemedicine: current impact on the future. Cureus. 2020;12(8):e9891. https://doi.org/10.7759/cureus.9891.
15. Witkowska-Zimny M, Nieradko-Iwanicka B. Telemedicine in emergency medicine in the COVID-19 pandemic-experiences and prospects-a narrative review. Int J Environ Res Public Health. 2022;19(13):8216. https://doi.org/10.3390/ijerph19138216.
16. Greenhalgh T, Rosen R, Shaw SE, et al. Planning and evaluating remote consultation services: a new conceptual framework incorporating complexity and practical ethics. Front Digit Health. 2021;3:726095. Published 2021 Aug 13. https://doi.org/10.3389/fdgth.2021.726095.
17. Liddy C, Joschko J, Guglani S, et al. Improving equity of access through electronic consultation: a case study of an econsult service. Front. Public Health. 7:279. https://doi.org/10.3389/fpubh.2019.00279.

Remote Consultation on Family Violence in Primary Care

24

Raquel Gomez Bravo, Carmen Fernández Alonso, Vinicius Jobim Fischer, Sajaratulnisah Othman, and Jennifer Neil

24.1 Remote Consultation on Family Violence

The purpose of this chapter is to explore the role of teleconsultation in addressing family violence, intimate partner violence (IPV), and related forms of abuse within primary care settings. It aims to provide healthcare professionals with practical guidance on conducting remote consultations that prioritize patient safety,

R. G. Bravo (✉)
Centre Hospitalier Neuro-psychiatrique (CHNP), Rehaklinik, Ettelbruck, Luxembourg

Department of Behavioural and Cognitive Sciences, University of Luxembourg, Esch-sur-Alzette, Luxembourg
raquel.gomezbravo@chnp.lu

C. F. Alonso
Spanish Scientific Society of Family and Community Medicine, Valladolid, Spain
mcfernandeza@saludcastillayleon.es

V. J. Fischer
Student Services, University of Luxembourg, Esch-sur-Alzette, Luxembourg

Centre Hospitalier Neuro-psychiatrique (CHNP), Rehaklinik, Ettelbruck, Luxembourg
Vinicius.fischer@uni.lu

S. Othman
Faculty of Medicine, Universiti Malaya, Kuala Lumpur, Malaysia
e-mail: sajar@um.edu.my

J. Neil
Department of General Practice, Monash University, Clayton, VIC, Australia

Department of General Practice and Primary Care, University of Melbourne, Parkville, VIC, Australia
e-mail: Jennifer.neil@monash.edu

J. Demurtas (ed.), *Remote Consultation in Primary Care*, TELe-Health,
https://doi.org/10.1007/978-3-031-89661-3_24

confidentiality, and cultural sensitivity. The chapter also addresses the unique challenges and specific strategies needed for effective telehealth assessments, screening, and intervention in cases of violence, ultimately expanding access to care for vulnerable populations.

Family violence, also known as domestic violence, encompasses a range of violent or threatening behaviors within families. It includes physical, sexual and psychological violence, economic, religious abuse, and reproductive abuse, among others. Research indicates that different forms of violence often coexist. Physical intimate partner violence is commonly accompanied by sexual and emotional abuse. Psychological/emotional violence and coercive control whereby the abuser obtains control through credible threats is more challenging to identify due to its less visible consequences [1, 2]. Nonetheless, these can be as detrimental as physical violence [3]. In addition, previous research indicates that psychological violence is uniquely associated with various stress-related conditions (e.g., irritable bowel syndrome and chronic pain) as well as mental health issues (e.g., posttraumatic stress disorder, major depression), often having a greater impact than physical violence [4, 5].

Family violence can affect various members of a household, including children, older people, and disabled individuals [1, 2, 6, 7]. Intimate partner violence IPV is the most prevalent form of family violence globally, with 1 in 3 women experiencing physical and/or sexual violence by a partner or nonpartner in their lifetime, approximately 736 million [7–11]. Violence against women has been declared a "global health problem of epidemic proportions" by the World Health Organization (WHO). It constitutes a severe violation of human rights, resulting in significant physical, mental, sexual, and social consequences. In extreme cases, it can lead to femicide, homicide, or suicide [11, 12].

Family violence is a global issue that also affects men and children [13–15] (Table 24.1).

Despite its prevalence, most cases of family violence go unrecognized, undisclosed, or unreported, often represented by the image of an iceberg. The visible cases are typically the most severe, with many more hidden beneath the surface. Factors preventing disclosure include shame, stigma, guilt, fear of repercussions, and cultural/religious beliefs. Societal victim-blaming attitudes further complicate disclosure and access to help [1, 16, 17].

During conflicts and disasters, violence against women, children, and vulnerable populations tends to increase. The collapse of basic services and changes in administration and data collection exacerbate the issue, leading to even lower rates of disclosure and reporting [12, 18, 19]. This happened during the COVID-19

Table 24.1 Prevalence of family violence

1 in 3 women experience physical and/or sexual violence by a partner or nonpartner in their lifetime
1 in 10 men has experienced intimate partner or sexual violence
1 in 4 adults experienced physical abuse in childhood
1 in 4 women and 1 in 13 men were sexually abused in childhood
1 in 6 elderly individuals suffer some form of abuse annually

pandemic, with the UN Women's Executive Director, Phumzile Mlambo-Ngcuka, referring to it as the "shadow pandemic." Lockdowns, reduced mobility, increased isolation, stress, and economic uncertainty turned many homes into environments where violence and abuse were more likely to occur [20].

The systematic review by Chan et al. highlights that telehealth interventions show promise in reducing psychological distress among IPV survivors and could be a valuable tool for identifying IPV victimization, especially when in-person consultations are not feasible [21]. However, it is essential to clarify that routine screening for IPV is not currently recommended due to a lack of proven improvement in outcomes, as indicated by the Cochrane systematic review and meta-analysis by O'Doherty et al. (2014). Instead, *casefinding* is the preferred approach, which involves inquiring about IPV based on clinical judgment and contextual cues rather than through systematic screening [22].

There is still no consensus on systematic screening for IPV [1, 24]. Nonetheless, when indicators of possible abuse are present, there is growing support for incorporating routine questions, as endorsed by scientific organizations and reflected in WHO guidance. The WHO emphasizes listening to patients in a nonjudgmental manner and validating their experiences when they disclose IPV [1, 24]. This approach, grounded in empathy and patient-centered care, aligns with established protocols that prioritize response capacity and support within health and social care systems. Moreover, even in the absence of clear indicators, the high prevalence of IPV—affecting approximately one-third of women—and persistently low detection rates suggest that many affected individuals either do not exhibit warning signs or are not identified by healthcare providers. In this context, routinely asking all patients about IPV does not appear excessive or irresponsible, provided that appropriate safety measures and support systems are in place [1, 24]. Further research is needed to evaluate the effectiveness of telehealth in IPV interventions and to clarify its role in supportive, patient-driven case finding [22].

24.2 Healthcare Services and Training Gap

Data show that abused women use healthcare services more frequently than nonabused women and often identify healthcare providers as the most trusted professionals for disclosing abuse. However, despite increased awareness over the last decade, about 80% of health professionals have never received training on managing and addressing domestic violence [23]. Such context highlights the significant gap between the severity of the problem and the training provided to frontline healthcare professionals. In response, the World Health Organization (WHO) and the National Institute for Health and Care Excellence have published guidelines emphasizing the need to improve education for these professionals [23].

Family violence is a complex issue requiring sustained efforts from governments, communities, and individuals. The general public also plays a vital role in addressing it, as recognizing warning signs in daily interactions with colleagues, family members, and friends is essential to prevention and intervention efforts.

24.3 Consultation

Addressing family violence requires a multidisciplinary approach, with healthcare professionals in primary health care often serving as the first—and sometimes only—point of contact [23]. In traditional in-person consultations, asking open-ended questions like "How are things going at home?" can create a safe space for potential victims or survivors to open up. However, in telehealth settings, open-ended questions may not always be safe, as it's unclear who else might be present on the other end of the line.

To ensure safety, it's essential to first assess the patient's environment by asking questions such as, "Are you alone?" or "Is it safe for you to answer questions about your family situation?" This initial step can help establish a secure setting for further discussion, allowing the healthcare provider to proceed appropriately and prioritize the patient's confidentiality and well-being.

The WHO recommends the LIVES approach for continuing conversations about domestic violence [24]:

- Listen closely with empathy and no judgment.
- Inquire about needs and concerns.
- Validate experiences by showing belief and understanding.
- Enhance safety.
- Support connection with additional services.

Conducting teleconsultations for cases involving family violence involves several specific steps to ensure effective communication, safety, and appropriate support (Fig. 24.1).

In a teleconsultation, especially when assessing sensitive topics like family violence, IPV (intimate partner violence), trafficking, or FGM (female genital mutilation), the structure of the assessment must be tailored to the limitations of the virtual setting. Table 24.2 presents a general framework for conducting a *structural assessment during teleconsultation* for such complex cases, ensuring safety, privacy, and comprehensive care.

Fig. 24.1 Structured process for conducting teleconsultations in family violence cases

Table 24.2 General framework for conducting a structural assessment during teleconsultation

Structural assessment
1. *Pre-consultation preparation*
Review patient history: If possible, review the patient's medical and social history before the consultation to better understand their context and any previous indicators of abuse or violence
Understand telehealth limitations: Recognize that physical exams are not possible in telehealth settings; rely on verbal and visual cues. Be prepared to offer follow-up care or referrals if in-person assessment is necessary
Technology setup: Use a secure, encrypted telehealth platform (e.g., Zoom with end-to-end encryption, Doxy.me, or other HIPAA-compliant services). Test the technology prior to the session to minimize technical issues. *For phone consultations*, consider using no caller ID to protect the patient's privacy
Setting up a safe time and modality: Prearrange a safe time for the consultation, such as during a morning walk or a grocery trip, where the patient feels secure to speak freely. For phone calls, confirm that the patient's surroundings allow them to talk safely, and for video calls, ensure they can clear their web browser history afterward to maintain privacy
Setting setup: Choose a private, quiet, and comfortable space for conducting the consultation. Position electronic devices for clear visibility and sound quality, using support material to stabilize the equipment if needed
Training: Ensure all staff are trained in recognizing signs of abuse and in the use of the teleconsultation platform. Familiarize yourself with local resources and legal requirements for handling such cases
Suggestion for EMR enhancement: Consider implementing an *EMR checklist and decision-support tool* to aid in cases of abuse and violence, including:
Checklist of signs and symptoms: Guide for recognizing abuse indicators
Trauma-informed question prompts: Safe, context-sensitive inquiry prompts
Quick-access training links: Resources for abuse recognition and trauma-informed care
Follow-up alert options: Reminders for continuity and in-person follow-up
Quick exit/black screen mechanism: An instant screen close for patient safety (urgent exit / screen black mechanism)
2. *Establishing privacy and safety*
Confirm a safe space: At the start of the teleconsultation, ensure the patient is in a private and safe environment where they can speak freely without fear of being overheard. Begin with yes/no questions to confirm privacy, such as, "Are you alone?" or "Is it safe to talk right now?" If the response is positive, you can continue with more open-ended questions, like, "Are you in a place where you feel comfortable talking privately?"
Ask about potential risks: For sensitive issues like family violence or FGM, check if anyone else is present or if there is a risk of someone overhearing the conversation. This can be done with a yes/no format to confirm safety
Initial contact and safety check.
Contact information:
Collect multiple forms of contact information in case the call is interrupted
Verify the identity of the person you're consulting with to ensure confidentiality
Safety verification:

(continued)

Table 24.2 (continued)

Structural assessment
Ask yes/no questions to determine if they are in a safe place to talk and if they can speak freely
Use nonverbal cues, like head nodding or hand signals, if verbal communication is not safe
Have a prearranged signal for the individual to indicate if someone enters the room or if they need to end the call suddenly
The Signal for Help (Fig. 24.2), launched by the Canadian Women's Foundation during the pandemic, is a one-handed sign that can be used to silently ask for help, especially in the presence of an abuser. Learning and sharing this sign can raise awareness and enable more victims/survivors to ask for help safely
3. *Conducting the teleconsultation: rapport building and trauma-informed approach*
Introduction and consent:
Introduce yourself in a nonjudgmental and compassionate manner and explain the purpose of the call. Acknowledge that discussing health, trauma, or abuse can be difficult
Obtain informed consent for the teleconsultation, explaining confidentiality and the limits of it, especially regarding mandatory reporting requirements which will be different in each jurisdiction
Set expectations: Explain what will happen during the consultation, reassure the patient that the conversation is confidential, and let them know they can stop or pause the conversation at any time
Cultural sensitivity: Be aware of and respectful toward cultural or religious beliefs, particularly in cases involving FGM or trafficking
Building rapport:
Use a warm, empathetic tone to build trust
Allow the individual to share their story at their own pace. Never pressurize anyone to disclose
IPV victims may be frequently seen in telemedicine visits, but additional steps should be taken to ensure their needs are met in addition to safe disclosure methods, providers should consider additional needs related to social concerns, stress, and physical health. Given the burgeoning use of telemedicine, steps should be taken to prepare for such visits so this complexity can be appropriately and safely addressed
Pay attention to nonverbal cues: Because teleconsultations limit physical examination, pay attention to nonverbal cues, including discomfort, hesitation, or signs of distress.
4. *General health inquiry*
Start with broad questions: Begin with general questions about the patient's overall health to create a sense of normalcy and ease the patient into the consultation:
"How have you been feeling lately?'
"Are there any specific health concerns you'd like to discuss today?"
There are distinct approaches and structures for assessing different types of family violence, IPV (intimate partner violence), and trafficking during a teleconsultation. Each type of violence has its own complexity, and while many core principles remain the same (e.g., ensuring privacy and safety, sensitive and trauma-informed care), the specifics of assessment can vary based on the type of violence being addressed. Here are some key differences in assessment approaches in teleconsultation settings.
5. *Focused assessment based on type of violence or abuse*
A. *Intimate partner violence (IPV)/gender-based violence*
Indirect screening for abuse: Ask questions that allow the patient to disclose abuse safely, particularly if the abuser might be nearby.

(continued)

Table 24.2 (continued)

Structural assessment
"How do you feel about your relationships at home?"
"Do you ever feel unsafe or controlled by your partner?"
"Are you afraid of your partner?"
Risk of harm: Assess the immediate risk of harm and explore safety planning
Emotional and physical assessment:
Assess for signs of emotional, psychological, and physical abuse, as well as any control over finances, social interactions, or communication
Inquire about immediate safety and any injuries
Ask about the frequency, type, and history of the abuse
Identify if children are involved and their safety
Tailored interventions:
Focus on resources specific to IPV, such as shelters, referrals to family violence organizations, legal aid, and safety planning. The assessment should explore the immediate risk to the patient and potential options for leaving an abusive situation
B. *Family violence (IPV, elder abuse, child abuse, and FGM, among others)* [24, 25]
An assessment should be holistic, covering all possible types of abuse (physical, emotional, neglect) and asking questions about living conditions, caregiver dynamics, and support networks
Vulnerability:
The patient (whether an elder or dependent adult) may be more vulnerable and less able to self-report
Explore financial exploitation and control over their resources
Evaluate their physical and cognitive abilities
Vulnerability assessment: Ask questions about caregiving, living arrangements, and general well-being
"How are things at home? Are you receiving the care you need?"
"Have you experienced any changes in your physical or mental health recently?"
Providers should carefully observe *nonverbal cues* and involve external agencies as needed
Caregiver and family dynamics: Understanding the family structure and caregiver dynamics is key in identifying abuse. The assessment may need to explore the health and capability of caregivers and any patterns of neglect or isolation
C. *Human trafficking*
Risk of exposure: Victims of trafficking may not be in control of their environment during the teleconsultation, and they may face severe repercussions if they disclose their situation
Specific indicators:
The assessment must be attuned to red flags specific to trafficking, such as restricted movement, lack of identification, or an unusual dependence on a companion (who may be the trafficker). Look for indicators of coercion, restricted movement, and lack of personal freedom
Ask about living and working conditions
Check for control over personal documents and finances
Look for red flags: Ask subtle questions about the patient's control over their own life, movement, and communication:
"Are you able to make your own decisions about work, finances, and where you live?"
"Do you feel you have control over your daily activities?"

(continued)

Table 24.2 (continued)

Structural assessment
Legal and social services: The response to trafficking requires a multidisciplinary approach involving law enforcement, social services, and trafficking-specific support systems. Questions should aim to assess the immediate risk and needs for legal intervention or extraction
D. *Female genital mutilation (FGM)*
Sensitive inquiry: Approach FGM carefully by first building trust and asking open-ended questions:
"Some women from certain backgrounds have had medical procedures like FGM. Would you feel comfortable discussing your experience?"
Physical and psychological impact: Ask about any ongoing health issues (pain, infections, reproductive health) and emotional distress.
6. *Mental health and psychological well-being*
Screen for trauma and stress: For all types of violence or abuse, ask about mental health:
"How have you been feeling emotionally?"
"Do you ever feel anxious, depressed, or overwhelmed by your situation?"
Nonverbal cues: In a virtual setting, pay close attention to body language, tone of voice, and facial expressions that may indicate distress or hesitation.
7. *Safety planning, risk assessment, support and resources*
Immediate safety:
For cases of IPV or ongoing violence, assess whether the patient is currently safe or at risk of further harm:
"Are you in immediate danger? Do you have a safe place to go if needed?"
Create a safety plan:
Work with the patient to create a basic safety plan if there is a risk of harm, tailored to the individual's situation, including emergency contacts and safe locations
Discuss discreet ways to seek help, such as using code words or hidden messages (text, email, hotlines)
Resource accessibility: Ensure that victims have access to local and national resources, such as hotlines, legal aid, and mental health services, and provide discrete follow-up options (email, text)
8. *Referrals and follow-up care*
Provide contact information for local resources such as shelters, legal aid, hotlines, and counseling services
Offer to connect them directly if they are comfortable with that
Physical health referrals: If the patient has physical symptoms or needs further care, refer them to a specialist for an in-person consultation (e.g., gynecologist for FGM, trauma specialist for IPV)
Mental health support: Offer referrals to mental health professionals, including therapists trained in trauma, PTSD, or domestic violence
Social services and legal aid: In cases of trafficking, IPV, or FGM, connect the patient with appropriate legal and social services for protection, housing, or legal intervention
9. *Education and empowerment*
Provide information: Share information about the health risks related to their condition (e.g., long-term effects of FGM, legal rights for IPV victims). Ensure this is done in a way that respects their cultural background and beliefs
Empower decision-making: Encourage the patient to make informed decisions about their health and safety. Avoid pressuring them into any specific course of action

(continued)

Table 24.2 (continued)

Structural assessment
10. *Follow-up plan*
Establish a follow-up: Offer a follow-up appointment to monitor the patient's situation and ongoing safety and ensure they are getting the support they need
Provide discreet communication options: Depending on the patient's safety situation, offer discreet ways to communicate between consultations (email, text) if returning for a virtual or in-person consultation may be unsafe
11. *Documentation and confidentiality*
Record observations and findings: Document the patient's history, symptoms, and disclosures in a confidential and trauma-informed manner
Accurate records:
Document the consultation thoroughly and securely, noting any signs of abuse and the individual's statements
Ensure that records are stored in a secure, confidential manner
Confidentiality: Respect the individual's privacy and only share information as required by law or with their explicit consent
Legal considerations:
For cases involving abuse, be aware of mandatory reporting laws in your jurisdiction and comply with it, but also consider the patient's safety when disclosing information
Inform the individual of your duty to report if necessary, ensuring they understand what this involves
Key considerations for teleconsultation:
Limited physical examination: Since teleconsultations do not allow physical exams, rely heavily on verbal inquiry and encourage patients to seek in-person care if necessary
Privacy and confidentiality: Ensure that teleconsultation platforms are secure, and emphasize confidentiality to the patient
Cultural competence: Be respectful of cultural differences and ensure that any guidance or recommendations are aligned with the patient's values and beliefs
Ethical practices:
Assure a nonjudgmental space, where victims feel comfortable disclosing sensitive information
Maintain nondiscrimination and respect for the individual's autonomy
Provide support in a nonjudgmental manner
Conclusion:
The assessment structure in teleconsultations for any type of violence and abuse should prioritize the patient's safety, privacy, and well-being. By following this structured approach, healthcare providers can offer comprehensive, trauma-informed care while navigating the limitations of virtual settings

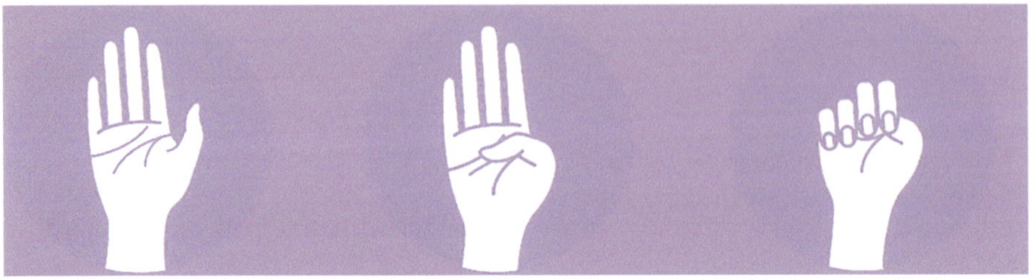

Fig. 24.2 Signal for help (Canadian Women's Foundation). (Reproduced with permission. Source: https://canadianwomen.org/signal-for-help-work/)

24.4 Self-Care for Practitioners

Being a healthcare professional working on the theme of violence can impact our mental health. In this regard, it is crucial to seek for regular exchange (intra, inter, or supervision) to discuss not only challenging cases but also how working with such population affect us on a personal and psychological level. In this context, the use of peer support networks is a valuable resource to cultivate best practices of case management and to share experiences and strategies.

Regardless of the format of care provision (face-to-face or online), such exchange moments are strongly advisable, especially for healthcare professionals primarily engaged in teleconsultation who may have limited physical access to colleagues.

Clinicians using teleconsultations should be aware of the difficulties and the challenges of dealing with violence and abuse and the requirements to do so, continuous education is crucial for staying informed about best practices. For those in teleconsultation, this also means keeping up to date with technological advancements and strategies to enhance the quality of remote care.

24.5 Conclusions

This chapter aimed to highlight the importance, opportunities, and challenges that primary healthcare professionals encounter when managing cases of violence and abuse remotely. Teleconsultation expands access to care for individuals who may face barriers—geographical, economic, or personal—that prevent them from visiting a healthcare center in person. However, conducting online appointments has its specificities, which should be identified in advance to offer the best available care. These specificities include individual competencies (such as preparation, user-friendliness with technological devices, and personal skills to establish rapport online) as well as knowledge of support provision, and legal and ethical considerations.

Teleconsultation offers a new pathway for individuals to disclose experiences of violence and abuse, addressing unmet needs for accessibility, confidentiality, or other personal reasons. However, teleconsultation is not an endpoint in itself. When violence is detected or confirmed, the ultimate goal should be to transition the patient to in-person care at an appropriate facility that can meet their ongoing needs, providing a feasible plan for comprehensive care and follow-up. As primary healthcare professionals, it is our responsibility to recognize that violence may be an underlying, often silent, condition affecting our patients' lives and to ensure that each case is met with the appropriate pathway to support and recovery.

References

1. World Health Organization (WHO. Responding to intimate partner violence and sexual violence against women: WHO clinical and policy guidelines. Geneva: World Health Organization; 2013. http://apps.who.int/iris/bitstream/10665/85240/1/9789241548595_eng.pdf
2. World Health Organization (WHO). Understanding and addressing violence against women. Geneva: World Health Organization; 2012. https://apps.who.int/iris/bitstream/handle/10665/77432/WHO_RHR_12.36_eng.pdf?sequence=1
3. Lohmann, S., Cowlishaw, S., Ney, L. J., & Felmingham, K. (2023). The Trauma and Mental Health Impacts of Coercive Control: A Systematic Review and Meta-Analysis. Trauma, Violence, & Abuse.
4. Coker AL, Smith PH, Bethea L, King MR, McKeown RE. Physical health consequences of physical and psychological intimate partner violence. Arch Fam Med. 2000;9(5):451–7. https://doi.org/10.1001/archfami.9.5.451.
5. Coker AL, Davis KE, Arias I, Desai S, Sanderson M, Brandt HM, Smith PH. Physical and mental health effects of intimate partner violence for men and women. Am J Prev Med. 2002;23(4):260–8. https://doi.org/10.1016/S0749-3797(02)00514-7.
6. World Health Organization (WHO). Preventing intimate partner and sexual violence against women: taking action and generating evidence. Geneva: World Health Organization; 2010. www.who.int/violence_injury_prevention/publications/violence/9789241564007_eng.pdf
7. World Health Organization (WHO). (2014). Global status report on violence prevention 2014. Geneva: World Health Organization. https://www.who.int/publications/i/item/9789241564793
8. European Union Agency for Fundamental Rights (FRA 2014). Violence against women: an EU-wide survey. Main results report Luxembourg: Publications Office of the European Union; 2014. http://fra.europa.eu/en/publication/2014/vaw-survey-main-results
9. Garcia-Moreno C, Jansen HA, Ellsberg M, Heise L, Watts CH. Prevalence of intimate partner violence: findings from the WHO multi-country study on women's health and domestic violence. Lancet. 2006;368:1260–9.
10. Stöckl H, Devries K, Rotstein A, Abrahams N, Campbell J, Watts C, Moreno CG. The global prevalence of intimate partner homicide: a systematic review. Lancet. 2013;382:859–65.
11. World Health Organization (WHO). Global and regional estimates of violence against women: prevalence and health effects of intimate partner violence and nonpartner sexual violence. Geneva: World Health Organization; 2013. https://apps.who.int/iris/bitstream/handle/10665/85239/9789241564625_eng.pdf?sequence=1
12. UNWOMEN (2020): Violence against women and girls: data collection during COVID-19 (17 April 2020). www.unwomen.org/-/media/headquarters/attachments/sections/library/publications/2020/vawg-data-collection-during-covid-19-compressed.pdf?la=en&vs=2339
13. Smith SG, Zhang X, Basile KC, Merrick MT, Wang J, Kresnow M-J, Chen J. The National Intimate Partner and Sexual Violence Survey (NISVS): 2015 data brief – updated release. Atlanta: National Center for Injury Prevention and Control, Centers for Disease Control and Prevention; 2018. www.cdc.gov/violenceprevention/pdf/2015data-brief508.pdf
14. World Health Organization (WHO 2016). Child maltreatment. Key facts (30 September). www.who.int/mediacentre/factsheets/fs150/en/

15. World Health Organization (WHO 2018): Elder abuse. Key facts (15 June). www.who.int/mediacentre/factsheets/fs357/en/
16. Gracia E. Unreported cases of domestic violence against women: towards an epidemiology of social silence, tolerance, and inhibition. J Epidemiol Community Health. 2004;58:536–7.
17. European Commission. Europeans and their views on domestic violence against women. Eurobarometer 51.0. Brussels: European Commission, Directorate General X; 1999.
18. Peterman A, Potts A, O'Donnell M, et al. Pandemics and violence against women and children. Center for Global Development Working Paper 528; 2020.
19. World Health Organization (WHO). COVID-19 and violence against women. What the health sector/system can do. Geneva: World Health Organization; 2020. https://apps.who.int/iris/bitstream/handle/10665/331699/WHO-SRH-20.04-eng.pdf?ua=1
20. World Health Organization (WHO). 2020. Q&A: violence against women during COVID-19. www.who.int/emergencies/diseases/novel-coronavirus-2019/question-and-answers-hub/q-a-detail/violence-against-women-during-covid-19?gclid=CjwKCAjw8J32BRBCEiwApQEKgb6DK86rEZi-I3r5P6qnPOUSZw%2D%2Di1oDNe7kn3ZrQoZ_wrtc9ARufhoCp2EQAvD_BwE
21. Chan G, Cruz-Sánchez M, Bhuptani P, Millman C, Orchowski L. Telehealth and intimate partner violence: a systematic review of telehealth interventions iProc. 2022;8(1):e39326.
22. O'Doherty LJ, Taft A, Hegarty K, Ramsay J, Davidson LL, Feder G. Screening women for intimate partner violence in healthcare settings: abridged Cochrane systematic review and meta-analysis. BMJ. 2014;348:g2913.
23. Gómez Bravo R, Lygidakis C, Feder G, et al. Family Violence Curricula in Europe (FAVICUE): a cross-sectional descriptive study protocol. BMJ Open. 2019;9:e024519.
24. World Health Organization. Health care for women subjected to intimate partner violence or sexual violence. A clinical handbook. 2014; Available from: https://www.who.int/reproductivehealth/publications/violence/vaw-clinical-handbook/en/
25. Rigon S, Dascal-Weichhendler H, Rothschild-Meir S, Gomez BR. Elder abuse and neglect. In: Demurtas J, Veronese N, editors. The role of family physicians in older people care. Practical issues in geriatrics. Cham: Springer; 2022. https://doi.org/10.1007/978-3-030-78923-7_18.

Part IV

Beyond Remote Consultation

Asynchronous Consultations in Primary Care

25

Ulrik Bak Kirk, Luigi Maria Bracchitta, Sara Rigon, and Jacopo Demurtas

25.1 Introduction

Asynchronous consultations in primary care have garnered considerable attention, especially as healthcare delivery models continue to evolve. These consultations enable communication between patients and healthcare providers without the need for real-time interaction. Increasingly recognized for their potential to expand access and improve patient outcomes, asynchronous consultations represent a promising adaptation in healthcare [1]. There was a noted reduction in follow-up appointment rates in secondary and tertiary care settings, indicating that virtual consultations may streamline care pathways [2].

The use of telemedicine, including asynchronous consultations, surged during the COVID-19 pandemic as general practices had to rethink how care was delivered. The need for alternatives to in-person visits led to the adoption of new

U. B. Kirk (✉)
Faculty Fellow, Department of Public Health, Aarhus University, Aarhus, Denmark

Digital Health, Research Unit for General Practice, Aarhus, Denmark
e-mail: ubk@ph.au.dk

L. M. Bracchitta
Primary Care Department, ATS Città Metropolitana di Milano, Milan, Italy

S. Rigon
Casa della Carità, Milan, Italy

J. Demurtas
Clinical and Experimental Medicine PhD Program, University of Modena and Reggio Emilia, Modena, Italy

Family Medicine Department, USL Toscana Sud-Est, Capalbio, Italy

J. Demurtas (ed.), *Remote Consultation in Primary Care*, TELe-Health,
https://doi.org/10.1007/978-3-031-89661-3_25

approaches, such as asynchronous communication, to maintain patient care while minimizing physical interactions [3].

These forms of teleconsultation offer greater flexibility and accessibility by reducing the need for in-person appointments and making more efficient use of healthcare resources. While the concept has existed for some time, its renewed application allows individuals to engage in health communication at their convenience, ushering in a new era of accessible, patient-centered care.

25.1.1 Defining Asynchronous Consultations

Unlike synchronous telemedicine, asynchronous consultations involve communication between a patient and a healthcare professional that takes place at different times. This can be done through various channels such as emails, voicemails, or even faxes. Asynchronous telemedicine typically uses secure messaging platforms like text or online systems and can incorporate decision-making tools. It is used for a range of purposes, including assessing whether patients need further consultation, facilitating communication between patients and healthcare providers, and enabling collaboration among healthcare professionals [4].

A related concept is "store-and-forward" telemedicine, which refers to the process of capturing data (such as paper documents or digital files) and transmitting it later using telecommunications technology to another healthcare provider or party [4].

25.1.2 Added Value of Asynchronous Consultations

A study by Fuster-Casanovas and Vidal-Alaball explored the added value of asynchronous communication between primary care professionals and patients across various countries. This review encompassed 271 articles published since 2010, focusing on the use of asynchronous methods to enhance patient management. Sixteen studies were selected for in-depth analysis, uncovering key themes such as reductions in in-person visits, increased availability of services, characteristics and perceptions of both users and healthcare professionals, as well as facilitators and barriers to implementation [5].

Similarly, literature reviews indicate that asynchronous consultations can lead to increased patient satisfaction, improved health outcomes, and reduced costs, primarily by decreasing the need for in-person appointments [6, 7]. The implementation of virtual consultations was associated with decreased waiting times for appointments, contributing to improved access to care [2].

Research comparing asynchronous (web-based) versus synchronous (in-clinic) screening for depression found that the asynchronous method facilitated timely identification and management of severe depression symptoms. This approach allowed for early intervention, which is crucial in preventing suicide [8].

One of the key advantages of asynchronous consultations is their capacity to support nonurgent communication. For example, Benis et al. discuss "non-queue requests" as a form of asynchronous communication that effectively manages tasks like appointment scheduling or prescription renewals. This approach enhances efficiency by streamlining patient interactions with healthcare systems [9]. Such flexibility is especially valuable in primary care, where the demand for prompt responses can often overwhelm traditional, synchronous communication methods.

Moreover, asynchronous communication has been shown to enhance interdisciplinary collaboration among healthcare professionals. Mardani et al. emphasize that forms of asynchronous communication, such as discharge summaries and referral letters, play a vital role in medication management during transitional care [10].

Similarly, Tran et al. note that electronic consultations foster ongoing discussions between primary care providers and specialists, strengthening collegiality and improving overall care quality [11]. These interactions not only alleviate strain on healthcare systems but also ensure that patients receive timely, coordinated, and appropriate care.

The applicability of asynchronous consultations extends to specialized areas such as telepsychiatry. Balasinorwala et al. demonstrated that asynchronous telepsychiatry is both feasible and effective for managing mental health conditions without the need for real-time interaction [12]. This is especially beneficial in rural or underserved regions where access to mental health services may be limited. Additionally, the use of asynchronous communication in telemedicine has been shown to boost patient satisfaction and reduce unnecessary hospital visits, as highlighted in Jensen's study on digital communication following surgery [13].

Recent experiences have also demonstrated the effectiveness of asynchronous consultations in establishing strong communication between primary care and hepatology, yielding significant results in combating HCV infections through early detection and treatment [14].

A mixed-methods study conducted at Aberdeen Royal Infirmary in Scotland expanded its outpatient asynchronous consultation services, initially implemented in dermatology in May 2020, to gastroenterology and pain management clinics. The study found that asynchronous consultations are not only viable but also acceptable in these areas. The implementation of such services is smoother when they cause minimal disruption to existing administrative processes, though ongoing support is essential [15].

The study offers practical strategies for aiding staff in adopting asynchronous consultations, such as preparing for the nonlinearity of the process and addressing task-related challenges.

Additionally, to ensure digital inclusion, patients require clear explanations, access to technical support, and multiple consultation options.

25.1.3 Pitfalls of Asynchronous Consultations

However, the implementation of asynchronous consultations is not without challenges. For instance, the lack of nonverbal cues in asynchronous communication can lead to misunderstandings, as discussed by Jumreornvong et al. [16].

Additionally, the quality of asynchronous consultations can vary, with studies indicating that not all patients may feel comfortable or adequately supported through these channels [17]. Healthcare professionals could organize training sessions for patients, improving their digital literacy and facilitating the use of asynchronous platforms [18].

Addressing these concerns requires ongoing research and the development of guidelines to ensure that asynchronous consultations meet the needs of diverse patient populations [19]. Some patients may lack access to the necessary technology or the digital literacy required to fully engage in remote interactions [20].

Moreover, ensuring timely responses, protecting patient privacy, maintaining data security, and reducing the risk of miscommunication are essential challenges that must be carefully addressed to enhance the effectiveness and reliability of asynchronous consultations.

There are also concerns regarding the potential for increased workload for healthcare providers, as they need to allocate time to respond to patient messages and inquiries outside of regular appointment hours [21].

To overcome these challenges, healthcare organizations need to invest in a robust technological infrastructure, provide thorough training for both patients and healthcare providers, and establish clear protocols and guidelines for asynchronous communication.

25.2 Examples

25.2.1 Email Consultations in Denmark

In recent years, policymakers worldwide have promoted the implementation of digital patient–clinician interactions, including in Danish general practice, where email consultations became mandatory in 2009 and now account for 21% of all consultations [22].

Using strong structuration theory, a Danish study explored how email consultations were represented at macro, meso, and micro levels, examining the interplay between structures and agents in terms of alignments, tensions, and adjustments [22]. Data were analyzed from policy documents (macro level), clinic websites (meso level), and interviews with 53 GPs and patients (micro level).

The findings indicated that email consultations, as a new health technology, drive changes in consultation practices, professional boundaries, and doctor–patient relationships. Email consultations were thus seen as dynamic components of a socio-technical network, rather than simple tools for health transactions.

The study concluded that future digital communication implementations must consider the multiple influences on telecare practices and recognize patients and clinicians as active agents shaping care based on their opinions, relationships, and values.

Another study explored how patients and general practitioners (GPs) in Denmark perceive the communicative advantages and disadvantages of email consultations through a media-theoretical lens [23].

Using qualitative interview data from general practices in Denmark, gathered from February 2016 to September 2019, the study involved semi-structured interviews with 30 patients and 23 GPs. Three main themes emerged: (a) lower contact thresholds, (b) access to a new interaction space, and (c) access to access.

Patients found email consultations convenient for contacting their GPs, while GPs appreciated the ability to engage with patients they rarely saw, though they expressed concerns about overuse and inappropriate use.

Both patients and GPs recognized email consultations as a medium that invites new types of interactions, including discussions of emotional and sensitive topics. Additionally, email consultations were seen as a way to facilitate easier access to in-person appointments.

From a media perspective, the study highlighted how email consultations create a new communication space with unique possibilities, presenting both opportunities and challenges in adapting traditional GP–patient communication to the written medium.

An additional qualitative study explored GPs' perspectives on the relational potential of email consultations in Denmark [24]. Data were collected through participant observation in four GP clinics and semi-structured interviews with 16 GPs (seven women and nine men, aged 35 to 70). Using inductive thematic analysis, the study found that GPs generally perceive email consultations as unsuitable for relational, socioemotional, and sensitive communication due to interpretational challenges.

However, in established doctor–patient relationships based on mutual knowledge and trust, email consultations were used as a supportive communication channel. Patients could express emotions, and GPs could demonstrate empathy, helping to maintain or even strengthen the relationship.

Thus, while email consultations were context-dependent and most effective alongside face-to-face consultations, they held potential beyond information exchange, contributing to the GP–patient relationship.

Finally, a recent study examined how email consultations in general practice function as a temporal technology, reshaping working conditions and power dynamics between GPs and patients [25].

Drawing on semi-structured interviews with 53 patients, 15 GPs, and two focus group discussions with 17 GPs in Denmark, both patients and GPs were seen as "time workers," adjusting their own schedules and aligning their expectations of each other's time. Email consultations facilitated the recalibration of one person's time to another's, requiring significant effort. This technology not only reshapes the boundaries between GPs and patients but also redefines power relations.

The study highlighted the need for health institutions to critically consider whose time and labor are being "saved" by digital systems like email consultations.

25.2.2 eConsulta Digital Consultation Tool in Catalonia

During the COVID-19 pandemic lockdown, telemedicine became essential for delivering safer patient care, supporting both COVID-19 patients and routine primary care. However, despite the long-standing operation of eConsulta—a teleconsultation service integrated into Catalonia's public health information technology system since late 2015 as a complement to face-to-face consultations—the full integration of telemedicine has yet to be consolidated.

One study aimed to analyze the factors influencing healthcare professionals' intention to use the eConsulta digital consultation tool in a post-COVID-19 context [26]. Using the Technology Acceptance Model as a framework, a model was developed, and a mixed-methods approach was employed, including a questionnaire to gather data.

The analysis revealed that perceived benefits and habitual use of eConsulta were the most significant factors affecting the intention to use the tool. Other influential factors included environmental pressure, technology experience, gender, and the level of eConsulta implementation. In physicians, technology experience and gender were key factors, while in nurses, experience with the tool and the institution where they worked were important.

Overall, the COVID-19 pandemic significantly increased the use of eConsulta, with most healthcare professionals expressing satisfaction and planning to continue using it postpandemic, driven by perceived benefits and environmental pressures.

Another study sought to understand the sociodemographic characteristics of GPs, which are considered crucial for identifying the barriers and facilitators to the adoption of eConsulta [27]. The study aimed to analyze the sociodemographic factors influencing the likelihood of GPs using eConsulta through a retrospective cross-sectional analysis of administrative data and multivariate logistic regression.

The results indicated that GPs more likely to use eConsulta are aged 45–54, rank in the top 20% on the quality-of-care index, have high accessibility, are involved in teaching, and work in high socioeconomic urban areas.

These findings underscored that specific sociodemographic characteristics of GPs influence their use of eConsulta, which should be considered when promoting its broader adoption within the public health system.

An additional study aimed to analyze the profiles of eConsulta users and their reasons for using the service, distinguishing between those who used it before and after the onset of the pandemic [28]. A descriptive, observational study using administrative data was conducted, with the COVID-19 pandemic marked by the state of emergency declared on March 12, 2020, as the key differentiator. The study also categorized users into those who sent messages and those who only received them.

Results showed that during the pandemic, the number of unique eConsulta users nearly tripled, with a peak of 33.10 visits per 1000 inhabitants per month in the first three months. Most users postpandemic were predominantly younger, female, actively employed, and with less complex medical conditions. Health professionals proactively sent more messages, while rural users initiated more conversations compared to higher-income urban users.

The COVID-19 pandemic accelerated the use of telemedicine, helping to sustain contact between citizens and the healthcare system, particularly among younger populations in Catalonia.

Finally, a study aimed to evaluate whether eConsulta could reduce the number of in-person visits to primary care teams [29]. Eighteen GPs from the Central Catalonia Health Region retrospectively classified 2268 eConsulta cases into 13 categories and indicated whether the teleconsultations reduced the need for face-to-face appointments.

The GPs broadly agreed that eConsulta effectively resolved patient queries, avoiding in-person visits in 87.9% of cases. However, increased accessibility also led to higher demand for healthcare support in 27.7% of cases, where patients may not have otherwise initiated contact. Based on these findings, eConsulta could potentially replace 63%–88% of conventional appointments.

The most common uses of the service were for managing test results (35.2%), medical inquiries (16.0%), and repeat prescriptions (12.2%). On average, teleconsultations involved 1.57 messages, with 45.9% of cases requiring only one message.

Overall, 60% of teleconsultations were initiated by the patient. The findings suggested that eConsulta can replace a significant portion of in-person visits, reducing unnecessary clinical interactions in primary care.

25.3 Conclusion

Asynchronous consultations hold the promise of transforming the healthcare landscape, offering a more inclusive, efficient, and patient-centric approach. By harnessing the power of asynchronous communication, healthcare providers can redefine patient care, catalyzing a wave of innovation that amplifies access to care and enhances patient outcomes.

To fully realize this potential, healthcare organizations must address challenges related to technology, workflow integration, and digital equity, while cultivating a culture of digital transformation. Policymakers should incentivize the adoption of digital infrastructures to support the expansion of asynchronous consultations, thereby reducing disparities in access to care [30].

Asynchronous communications represent a valuable solution for improving the efficiency and effectiveness of healthcare systems. They reduce in-person visits, increase user and professional satisfaction, and prove particularly useful during healthcare overloads such as pandemics.

Addressing existing barriers and promoting professional training will be crucial for maximizing the benefits of these technologies. Further research should explore the long-term effects of asynchronous teleconsultations on care quality and health system costs.

References

1. Tushe S, Diwas KC, Ding H, Yeung H. Multichannel healthcare: impact of asynchronous telemedicine adoption on patient flow. Manuf Serv Oper Manag. 2024;27:59. https://doi.org/10.1287/msom.2022.0235.
2. Campbell K, Greenfield G, Li E, et al. The impact of virtual consultations on the quality of primary care: systematic review. J Med Internet Res. 2023;25:e48920. https://doi.org/10.2196/48920.
3. Leighton C, Cooper A, Porter A, Edwards A, Joseph-Williams N. Effectiveness and safety of asynchronous telemedicine consultations in general practice: a systematic review. BJGP Open. 2024;8(1):BJGPO.2023.0177. https://doi.org/10.3399/BJGPO.2023.0177.
4. American Medical Association. Telehealth resource center: definitions 2021. https://www.ama-assn.org/practice-management/digital/telehealth-resource-center-definitions. Accessed 9 Oct 2024.
5. Fuster-Casanovas A, Vidal-Alaball J. Asynchronous remote communication as a tool for care management in primary care: a rapid review of the literature. Int J Integr Care. 2022;22(3):7. https://doi.org/10.5334/ijic.6489.
6. Salsabilla A, Azzahra AB, Syafitri RIP, Supadmi W, Suwantika AA. Cost-effectiveness of telemedicine in Asia: a scoping review. J Multidiscip Healthc. 2021;14:3587–96. https://doi.org/10.2147/JMDH.S332579.
7. Fry MW, Saidi S, Musa A, Kithyoma V, Kumar P. "Even though I am alone, I feel that we are many" – an appreciative inquiry study of asynchronous, provider-to-provider teleconsultations in Turkana, Kenya. PLoS One. 2020;15(9):e0238806. https://doi.org/10.1371/journal.pone.0238806.
8. Sattler A, Dunn J, Albarran M, et al. Asynchronous versus synchronous screening for depression and suicidality in a primary health care system: quality improvement study. JMIR Ment Health. 2024;11:e50192. https://doi.org/10.2196/50192.
9. Benis A, Banker M, Pinkasovich D, Kirin M, Yoshai BE, Benchoam-Ravid R, Ashkenazi S, Seidmann A. Reasons for utilizing telemedicine during and after the COVID-19 pandemic: an internet-based international study. J Clin Med. 2021;10(23):5519. https://doi.org/10.3390/jcm10235519.
10. Mardani A, Griffiths P, Vaismoradi M. The role of the nurse in the management of medicines during transitional care: a systematic review. J Multidiscip Healthc. 2020;13:1347–61. https://doi.org/10.2147/JMDH.S276061.
11. Tran C, Archibald D, Humphrey-Murto S, Liddy C, Keely E. What makes a high-quality electronic consultation (eConsult)? A nominal group study. J Telemed Telecare. 2020;26(4):239–47. https://doi.org/10.1177/1357633X18822885.
12. Balasinorwala VP, Shah NB, Chatterjee SD, Kale VP, Matcheswalla YA. Asynchronous telepsychiatry in maharashtra, India: study of feasibility and referral pattern. Indian J Psychol Med. 2014;36(3):299–301. https://doi.org/10.4103/0253-7176.135384.
13. Høpfner Jensen LW, Kold S, Dinesen B, Husum HC, Skals RG, Eiskjær SP, Elsøe R, Rahbek O. Team-based digital communication reduced patient-initiated phone calls to the hospital and improved patient satisfaction after orthopedic surgery: a randomized controlled trial in 70 patients. Acta Orthop. 2024;95:225–32. https://doi.org/10.2340/17453674.2024.40707.
14. Pérez-Hernández FJ, Morales-Arráez DE, Amaral-González C, González-Méndez Y, Ortega-Sánchez JA, de la Barreda HR, Abreu Alonso I, Ramos López L, Alarcón-Fernández O, Carrillo-Palau M, Hernández-Guerra M. Asynchronous electronic consultation between primary care and specialized care proved effective for continuum of care for viraemic hepatitis C patients. Gastroenterol Hepatol. 2023;46(4):266–73. English, Spanish. https://doi.org/10.1016/j.gastrohep.2022.08.003.

15. Rzewuska Díaz M, Locock L, Keen A, Melvin M, Myhill A, Ramsay C. Implementation of a web-based outpatient asynchronous consultation service: mixed methods study. J Med Internet Res. 2024;26:e48092. https://doi.org/10.2196/48092.
16. Jumreornvong O, Yang E, Race J, Appel J. Telemedicine and medical education in the age of COVID-19. Acad Med. 2020;95(12):1838–43. https://doi.org/10.1097/ACM.0000000000003711.
17. Tuijt R, Rait G, Frost R, Wilcock J, Manthorpe J, Walters K. Remote primary care consultations for people living with dementia during the COVID-19 pandemic: experiences of people living with dementia and their carers. Br J Gen Pract. 2021;71(709):e574–82. https://doi.org/10.3399/BJGP.2020.1094.
18. Jiangliu Y, Kim HT, Lazar M, et al. A medical student-led multipronged initiative to close the digital divide in outpatient primary care. Appl Clin Inform. 2024;15(4):808–16. https://doi.org/10.1055/a-2370-2298.
19. Adams TCE, Lim CT, Huang H. The practice of psychiatric e-consultation: current state and future directions. Harv Rev Psychiatry. 2022;30(3):191–7. https://doi.org/10.1097/HRP.0000000000000338.
20. Rosen R, Wieringa S, Greenhalgh T, Leone C, Rybczynska-Bunt S, Hughes G, Moore L, Shaw SE, Wherton J, Byng R. Clinical risk in remote consultations in general practice: findings from in-COVID-19 pandemic qualitative research. BJGP Open. 2022;6(3):BJGPO.2021.0204. https://doi.org/10.3399/BJGPO.2021.0204.
21. Rosen R, Leone C. Getting the best out of remote consulting in general practice – practical challenges and policy opportunities. Research report. Nuffield Trust; 2022.
22. Assing Hvidt E, Grønning A, Nisbeth Brøgger M, Møller JE, Fage-Butler A. Multilevel structures and human agency in relation to email consultations: a strong structuration theory analysis of the Danish general practice setting. Soc Sci Med. 2021;282:114155. https://doi.org/10.1016/j.socscimed.2021.114155.
23. Grønning A, Assing Hvidt E, Nisbeth Brøgger M, Fage-Butler A. How do patients and general practitioners in Denmark perceive the communicative advantages and disadvantages of access via email consultations? A media-theoretical qualitative study. BMJ Open. 2020;10(10):e039442. https://doi.org/10.1136/bmjopen-2020-039442.
24. Assing Hvidt E, Søndergaard J, Klausen M, Grønning A. Not just an information-delivery tool. An ethnographic study exploring Danish GPs' perspectives on and experiences with the relational potential of email consultation. Scand J Prim Health Care. 2020;38(4):411–20. https://doi.org/10.1080/02813432.2020.1843939.
25. Grønning A, Simonsen LM, Lüchau EC, Hvidt EA, Klausen M. My time, your time, our time. Older patients' and GPs' time sensibilities around email consultations. Health Sociol Rev. 2024;33(1):43–58. https://doi.org/10.1080/14461242.2024.2316742.
26. Saigí-Rubió F, Vidal-Alaball J, Torrent-Sellens J, Jiménez-Zarco A, López Segui F, Carrasco Hernandez M, Alzaga Reig X, Bonet Simó JM, Abizanda González M, Piera-Jimenez J, Solans O. Determinants of Catalan public primary care professionals' intention to use digital clinical consultations (eConsulta) in the post-COVID-19 context: optical illusion or permanent transformation? J Med Internet Res. 2021;23(6):e28944. https://doi.org/10.2196/28944.
27. Fernández OS, Seguí FL, Vidal-Alaball J, Bonet Simo JM, Vian OH, Cabo PR, Hernandez MC, Dominguez CO, Reig XA, Rodríguez YD, Peralta MM, Hermosilla E, León NM, Guimferrer N, González MA, Cuyàs FG, Sust PP. Primary care doctor characteristics that determine the use of teleconsultations in the Catalan public health system: retrospective descriptive cross-sectional study. JMIR Med Inform. 2020;8(1):e16484. https://doi.org/10.2196/16484.
28. Solans O, Vidal-Alaball J, Roig Cabo P, Mora N, Coma E, Bonet Simó JM, Hermosilla Pérez E, Saigí-Rubió F, Olmos Domínguez C, Piera-Jiménez J, Abizanda González M, López SF. Characteristics of citizens and their use of teleconsultations in primary care in the Catalan

public health system before and during the COVID-19 pandemic: retrospective descriptive cross-sectional study. J Med Internet Res. 2021;23(5):e28629. https://doi.org/10.2196/28629.
29. López Seguí F, Vidal-Alaball J, Sagarra Castro M, García-Altés A, García CF. General practitioners' perceptions of whether teleconsultations reduce the number of face-to-face visits in the Catalan public primary care system: retrospective cross-sectional study. J Med Internet Res. 2020;22(3):e14478. https://doi.org/10.2196/14478.
30. Naik N, Hameed BMZ, Sooriyaperakasam N, et al. Transforming healthcare through a digital revolution: a review of digital healthcare technologies and solutions. Front Digit Health. 2022;4:919985. https://doi.org/10.3389/fdgth.2022.919985.

Clinical Decision Support Systems (CDSS) and Symptom Checkers in Primary Healthcare

26

Jacopo Demurtas, Matías Eduardo Díaz Crescitelli, Andreas Meer, Liliana Laranjo, Julius Otieno Oyugi, Ulrik Bak Kirk, and Linda Huibers

26.1 Introduction

Artificial intelligence (AI) is a branch of computer science that aims to develop machine systems capable of behavior comparable to human intelligence. AI programs use data from various interactions to imitate humans and perform tasks, such as learning, planning, knowledge representation, perception, and problem solving. AI focuses on understanding and developing intelligent systems capable of computing effective and safe actions within their environments. This rapidly advancing field is transforming healthcare, particularly by supporting professionals in

---

Jacopo Demurtas and Matías Eduardo Díaz Crescitelli contributed equally with all other contributors.

J. Demurtas
Clinical and Experimental Medicine PhD Program, University of Modena and Reggio Emilia, Modena, Italy

Family Medicine Department, USL Toscana Sud-Est, Capalbio, Italy

M. E. D. Crescitelli
PhD, RN, MSN, Qualitative Researcher, Canary Islands, Spain

A. Meer
CEO In4medicine Ltd., Berne, Switzerland

L. Laranjo
Sydney Medical School, Westmead Applied Research Centre, University of Sydney, Westmead, NSW, Australia
e-mail: liliana.laranjo@sydney.edu.au

J. O. Oyugi
Institute of Tropical and Infectious Diseases (UNITID), University of Nairobi, Nairobi, Kenya

J. Demurtas (ed.), *Remote Consultation in Primary Care*, TELe-Health,
https://doi.org/10.1007/978-3-031-89661-3_26

decision-making processes. The emerging scenario highlights a shift in control of some tasks previously attributable to humans brings up some issues as, for example, the users maintaining decision-making process control, or the need of guarantees in clinical processes [1].

One key area are *clinical decision support systems* (CDSSs), which are evolving to incorporate AI-enabled algorithms, sometimes replacing traditional systems with much more intelligent and adaptable solutions. CDSS functions and advantages described in literature are in patient safety, clinical management, cost containment, administrative functions as well in diagnostic support and patient-facing decision support [2]. CDSSs are software applications designed to assist clinicians in making decisions about patient care. In this scenario, other factors that may influence the processes of everyday clinical life must be considered. AI-enabled CDSSs leverage neural networks, which consist of input layers, output layers, and multiple hidden layers. These hidden layers process the input and guide users toward the appropriate output. However, the inner workings of these hidden layers often remain nontransparent and difficult to interpret.

Using a variety of machine learning and natural language processing techniques, AI-CDSSs are designed as intelligent systems that provide healthcare professionals with decision-making recommendations, either broadly or specific to certain diseases, syndromes, or patterns. It is of importance to integrate this type of entity into daily clinical activities when designing these devices. However, the integration of these systems into primary healthcare needs careful consideration with clinical workflow and compatibility with the existing Electronic Health Records (EHRs). This results in an increased need for interaction for practicing health professionals and training for health students.

In primary healthcare, the integration of CDSSs and symptom checkers represents a relatively new frontier. These innovations have the potential to reduce the workload on clinicians by offering more integrated and efficient systems [3, 4], but also considerable setbacks demonstrated that CDSSs are not without risks [2]. At the same time, the emerging scenario opens the opportunity for ethical as well as social research debates on the implementation of these supporting entities. Additionally, there is need to put in place policies on data sharing and privacy to address security concerns of patients whose data will be used.

This increasing integration of technology into healthcare has introduced CDSSs and symptom checkers as valuable tools in primary care [5]. These tools use machine learning and natural language processing to analyze patient symptoms and offer

U. B. Kirk
Faculty Fellow, Department of Public Health, Aarhus University, Aarhus, Denmark

Digital Health, Research Unit for General Practice, Aarhus, Denmark
e-mail: ubk@ph.au.dk

L. Huibers (✉)
Research Unit for General Practice, Aarhus, Denmark

Department of Public Health, Aarhus University, Aarhus, Denmark
e-mail: huibers@ph.au.dk

personalized diagnostic and treatment recommendations [5, 6]. CDSSs have demonstrated their potential to enhance the quality and consistency of care by providing evidence-based guidance to healthcare professionals at the point of care.

In this chapter, we briefly examine the development and utility of CDSSs in primary healthcare, as well as the role of symptom checkers and self-triage tools.

26.2 Clinical Decision Support Systems (CDSSs)

CDSSs are software applications designed to assist clinicians in making informed decisions about patient care. The definitions outlined below are based on various authors' descriptions from trials and systematic reviews in the field:

- Bates et al. (2003) defines CDSSs as computer-based systems that provide passive or active referential information, reminders, alerts, and guidelines [7].
- Bright et al. (2012) describe CDSSs as electronic systems designed to assist directly in clinical decision-making by using patient-specific characteristics to generate personalized assessments or recommendations for clinicians to consider [8].
- Haynes and colleagues (2010) expand this definition [9], suggesting that CDSSs refer to information systems that support clinical decision-making by linking patient-specific information from electronic health records with evidence-based knowledge. These systems generate case-specific guidance through rule- or algorithm-based software.
- This approach was also adopted in Moja et al.'s review (2014) to determine which studies to include in their analysis [10].

The integration of CDSSs into healthcare is evolving, presenting new opportunities for innovation in diagnosis, therapy, and healthcare management. The COVID-19 pandemic accelerated this evolution. However, despite growing enthusiasm for CDSSs, their adoption is influenced by both human and technological factors:

- Among *human* factors, beliefs, digital literacy, and education play a key role. Professionals, clients, and patients may perceive the use of CDSSs as either a threat or an opportunity, depending on their understanding of the technology's net benefits. A realistic assessment of the human skills required to implement these systems effectively is crucial, especially given the ongoing shortages of professionals and resources across many major healthcare systems. Despite the healthcare systems crisis, both professionals and end-users (patients and caregivers) demand guarantee regarding overall health protection during this time of emerging development of supporting technologies [11].
- The *technological* factors influencing adoption includes transparency, time efficiency, complexity of use, adaptability to clinical environments, respect for knowledge and information delivery, and rigorous scientific evidence processing

[11]. In this context, an emerging range of factors deserving the attention of decision support software producers is emerging from user experience, collected and systematized through qualitative research principal methods.

Despite the apparent advantages of CDSSs, there is still much to explore in the age of AI, particularly regarding the impact on healthcare processes and the patient–doctor relationship, to prevent potential erosion of this dynamic. Addressing these challenges is essential for ensuring that humans and intelligent devices can coexist effectively in healthcare.

Therefore, it is worth considering that AI-CDSSs lack specific human peculiarities, such as emotions, fatigue, stress, as well as sense of inadequacy. The lack of such factors in digital entities seems like an opportunity to increase production in terms of healthcare delivery, from an industrial point of view.

But from another point of view, it brings us face to face up on the fact that missing are those human characteristics (for instance, critical reasoning in detecting a problem or a risk that is not found in the processed data), which often allow us to identify criticalities preserving the different dimensions of the human person. Accordingly, emphasis must be placed on the fact that AI-CDSSs are intelligent to the extent that their users know how to direct processes (inputs) and interpret outputs (user's digital literacy and clinical skills).

Qualitative research experiences with CDSSs are limited and mostly cover the hospital setting. Liberati et al. conducted a Grounded Theory study with the aim of exploring the barriers and facilitators to the adoption of CDSS by hospital professionals [12]. Following the study involving three hospital facilities in Northern Italy, the adoption of CDSS by healthcare professionals is represented as a process consisting of six "placements," depending on the use and perceived mastery of a technology.

Under conditions of low mastery, they perceived the CDSS as threatening, unfamiliar, and difficult to control. On the other hand, participants in conditions of high mastery saw the CDSS as a useful tool, but needing contextual adaptation and integration with the doctors' skills to meet their needs [12]. Thus, whereas in the early placements, the adoption of the CDSS was hindered by representational obstacles, the later placements represented purely technical obstacles to the adoption of the CDSS. Here again, the role of qualitative research emerges. Indeed, the cited study allows hospital administrators the opportunity of looking at a few critical points when implementing these technologies, in order to develop an effective strategy considering their organizational context and staff's technological skills.

In this context, qualitative research serves as a valuable tool for understanding the complexity of human behavior within these environments. It can also guide the development of clinical and design cues and research hypotheses aimed at humanizing these innovative care settings [13, 14].

26.3 Symptom Checkers

As defined by Semigran et al. (2015), symptom checkers are *application or software tools that enable patients to input their symptoms and biodata to produce a set of differential diagnoses and clinical triage advice* [15]. The triage function guides users toward the most appropriate course of action based on the urgency of their symptoms and health status, and the potential diagnosis, which typically includes options such as seeking urgent care, contacting a general practitioner, or managing the issue through self-care.

Digital symptom checkers are becoming an increasingly adopted class of digital health tools, enabling patients to input their symptoms and biodata to generate likely diagnoses and triage advice. However, concerns have been raised regarding the accuracy and safety of these tools:

- In a systematic review from 2022, Wallace et al. evaluated the diagnostic and triage accuracy of symptom checkers. They found that the diagnostic accuracy for the primary diagnosis was consistently low across the included studies, ranging between 19% and 37.9%, despite uniform symptom data input. Triage accuracy, which ranged from 48.8% to 90.1%, was generally higher than diagnostic accuracy. Overall, the accuracy of symptom checkers in both diagnosis and triage was found to be variable and often suboptimal [16].
- Another systematic review by Riboli-Sasco et al. (2023) aimed to summarize the existing peer-reviewed literature on the triage and diagnostic accuracy of online symptom checkers used by laypeople for general health concerns. Their findings echoed those of Wallace et al. (2022), reporting that both diagnostic and triage accuracy varied significantly across different platforms. Diagnostic accuracy was consistently low, often lower than that of healthcare professionals, and most studies demonstrated suboptimal triage accuracy, with only a few exceptions [17].
- A third systematic review by Chambers et al. (2019) focused on digital and online symptom checkers, specifically for urgent health concerns. Their analysis revealed weak evidence regarding patient safety and considerable variation in diagnostic accuracy across systems, which was generally low. Algorithm-based triage was found to be more risk-averse compared to health professionals. Limited evidence was available on patient compliance with online triage advice, though study participants often reported high levels of satisfaction, especially in uncontrolled studies. Younger and more highly educated individuals were more likely to use these services [18].

In conclusion, these reviews found that the accuracy and safety of these tools in general was suboptimal.

26.4 Self-Triage Tools and Chatbots

During the COVID-19 pandemic, numerous apps were launched to help patients assess symptoms potentially related to COVID-19 and provide recommendations on the appropriate level of care and timing for treatment. These apps, often referred to as *self-triage tools,* assist patients in conducting an initial triage. Many of these tools simulate a conversational model using chatbots and may incorporate AI [19]. These tools are closely related to symptom checkers.

Chatbots are software applications that engage in conversational interactions with people using natural language, either through voice or text. In recent years, the deployment of chatbots for healthcare-related purposes has seen a substantial increase, with applications ranging from supporting clinicians in conducting clinical interviews and providing diagnoses to assisting consumers in self-managing chronic conditions [20]. The emergence of highly advanced generative AI chatbots, such as ChatGPT, Bard, or Gemini, powered by large language models (LLMs), has sparked significant mainstream interest due to their potential applications in clinical practice, particularly in healthcare.

A brief overview of recent literature acknowledges the potential but point out concerns also:

- Andrew (2024) consolidates the current literature on LLMs to examine their potential in primary care, concluding that their impact could be vast and transformational. He advocates for a proactive approach to embracing AI, encouraging the healthcare community to educate itself about AI's capabilities and leverage them to enhance healthcare delivery [21].
- In a study by Ayers et al. (2023), the ability of an AI chatbot (ChatGPT) to provide quality and empathetic responses to patient questions was evaluated. This cross-sectional study found that the chatbot generated both high-quality and empathetic responses to patient inquiries posed in an online forum [22].
- Palanica et al. (2019) conducted a study on physicians' perceptions of healthcare chatbots in the United States. The found that physicians recognized both the potential costs and benefits of chatbots, depending on how they are integrated into healthcare. Chatbots may play a positive role in supporting, motivating, and coaching patients, as well as streamlining organizational tasks. However, concerns persist regarding chatbots' ability to fully comprehend human emotions and situations that require expert medical knowledge [23].
- In addition, Laranjo et al. (2018) reviewed the characteristics, applications, and evaluation measures of conversational agents with unconstrained natural language input capabilities used in health-related contexts. They found that the field is still emerging, with the few available studies being quasi-experimental and rarely addressing efficacy or safety. Future research in this area would benefit from more robust experimental designs and standardized reporting methods [24].
- A systematic review by Li et al. (2023) examined the feasibility and effectiveness of conversational agent-based interventions, assessed by randomized controlled trials, in healthcare. They found that conversational agents were feasible, accept-

able, and had positive effects on physical functioning, healthy lifestyles, mental health, and psychosocial outcomes. These agents offer low-barrier access to healthcare services and can act as remote medical assistants, supporting patients' recovery or health promotion before and after treatment. Furthermore, conversational agents can play adjunctive roles in existing healthcare systems, improving service comprehensiveness and allowing healthcare professionals to use their time more efficiently [25].

Understanding and exploring the acceptability, usability, and perceived benefits of using decision-support and self-triage devices by involving different stakeholders (citizens, patients, caregivers, health professionals) becomes essential in this context.

26.5 Safety and Effectiveness of Symptom Checkers and Self-Triage Tools

Recent studies reported suboptimal diagnostic and triage accuracy of symptom checkers, and they have also highlighted an increased rate of overtriage [16–18]. It is crucial that these tools are properly validated and integrated into healthcare systems to enhance, rather than replace, the role of healthcare professionals.

Overtriage in symptom checkers, while often viewed as a drawback, can be somewhat beneficial when these tools are designed for use by patients or caregivers. A certain level of overtriage, provided it is not excessive, may be acceptable in these contexts, as it reflects "safety in case of doubt."

However, overtriage remains a significant concern as it can lead to increased healthcare utilization, longer wait times, and higher costs, which may ultimately reduce the efficiency and accessibility of healthcare systems. Additionally, concerns have been raised regarding the accuracy and reliability of symptom checkers, as they may fail to identify serious conditions correctly or provide appropriate management recommendations in certain cases.

When comparing various studies on symptom checkers, including the work of Semigran et al. [15] and Chambers et al. [18], few studies have focused specifically on emergency or primary care settings. However, a few key studies in these areas are worth noting:

- First, Cotte et al. (2022) analyzed the use of the ADA symptom checker, comparing use of the app with usual hospital triage by the Manchester Triage System [26]. They found that undertriage occurred in 34 out of 378 cases (8.9%), with 59% of these classified as potential avoidable hazardous situations. Overtriage was more common, occurring in 58% of cases. Consequently, the authors reported that a safe assessment was made in 96% of cases. Although the COVID-19 pandemic impacted the study's sample size, the results were notable: 91% of participants were triaged identically or more conservatively by the app compared to usual hospital triage.

- In the study by Meer et al. (2024), the safety and efficacy of the SMASS Pathfinder self-triage tool were assessed with 2,543 patients [27]. None of the patients met the prespecified criteria for potentially hazardous undertriage. Overall, the symptom checker proved to be a safe triage tool in a real-life clinical setting, avoiding hazardous undertriage in emergency consultations without causing significant overtriage.
- In addition, Koskela et al. (2024) evaluated Omaolo, a Finnish symptom checker, in a real-life validation study across multiple primary healthcare centers [28]. The study was conducted using a walk-in primary care model where patients did not need prior contact. Upon arrival, users answered questions from the Emergency Symptom Checker (ESC) and received a triage recommendation, which was then assessed by a nurse. The analysis of 877 patients showed that 97.6% of the assessments were deemed safe. The exact match rate for all symptom assessments was 53.7%, and the rate of exact matches or overly conservative but suitable assessments was 66.6%. For urgent cases requiring treatment, the ESC matched the nurse's conclusion 70.9% of the time, with a sensitivity of 62.6% and a specificity of 69.2%. Importantly, no patient safety concerns were identified during the study.
- Finally, a qualitative study [29] exploring 24 young people's perceptions of the use of symptom checkers for self-triage denoted how symptom checking was perceived as useful for a more personalized assessment than traditional intelligent search engines (Google). Besides, after using a symptom checker, most participants expressed how the platform needed improvements within accuracy, security, and privacy areas, as well as more comprehensible texts (avoiding medical jargon). From this perspective, the qualitative research allows us to broaden the users' position, understanding how to maximize their AI-CDSS user experience.

26.6 Barriers and Facilitators to the Use of CDSSs in Primary Healthcare

Several barriers to the use of CDSSs have been identified, including human and organizational issues, in addition to technological challenges [30]. Moreover, concerns have been raised about the potential for CDSSs to contribute to increased healthcare utilization and costs due to overtriage. However, studies have also identified key facilitators for the adoption of CDSSs, such as improved diagnostic accuracy, enhanced workflow efficiency, and increased patient engagement and self-management. There are also communicational challenges associated with the use of CDSSs, as demonstrated in the ESTEEM trial [31–33].

One notable issue is that the attention required by the tool may impair the communication skills of the clinician or triagist. In some cases, patients being questioned about their symptoms may even change their answers based on the perceived focus on the tool rather than the conversation [33].

The use of AI in decision support also reignited the debate on the impact on the role of healthcare professionals. Questions such as "Can AI replace doctors?" and

"Will doctors who use AI replace those who do not?" are reported in the literature [34]. Thus, an extreme, and at the same time useful view, may be to define them more as "artificial slaves" than as intelligent entities, since they are not comparable to humans in terms of emotional and relational skills but are only capable of performing a large number of specific tasks with high precision in an extremely short time span.

Despite these challenges, the overall evidence suggests that when CDSSs and symptom checkers are properly designed, integrated, and utilized, they can play a valuable role in supporting remote primary care delivery and improving patient outcomes. One way of overcoming these barriers is to consider patients as "fellow workers" and allow them act as cotrainers to prevent doctors falling into some of the traps associated with automated decision support [35]. And in this process, also independent research plays a crucial role, being able to guide and elevate the debate from what producers and principals wish to achieve, to how these entities can be used to support the provision of high-quality healthcare.

26.7 Future Perspectives

The integration of AI and machine learning technologies into telemedicine and CDSSs offers significant promise for the future of primary and emergency care [36]. While challenges such as access, safety, and cost-effectiveness need to be addressed, the potential benefits—including improved diagnostic accuracy, personalized treatment recommendations, and increased patient engagement—are expected to drive further development and adoption within the healthcare sector [4, 10, 37].

Future iterations of self-triage tools may incorporate advanced technologies, such as 3D virtual assistants powered by AI [38]. These tools could leverage mixed or augmented reality environments to enhance the patient experience. Intelligent virtual agents could guide patients through the triage process while continuously learning to handle various healthcare scenarios more effectively [39].

Given that most symptom checker users are relatively young, efforts need to be strengthened in educating users, looking at their culture, age, but above all intercepting the digital and health literacy level of those involved in the process. Integrating these technologies, and especially understanding the processing of LLMs/generative AI tools into the curriculum of health professions students, can enhance the educational experience of these students and better prepare them to adopt high-quality therapeutic strategies involving the use of emerging technologies [30, 40].

Ethical and regulatory considerations regarding the use of digital tools and patient data are an explicit requirement, adding an additional layer of responsibility to the education of future healthcare professionals.

This is the time for aiming at an appropriate design and implementation in healthcare contexts, which scientifically considers the voices of professionals, patients, and caregivers interfacing with these entities [41], and those who will do so in the future. And it is opening the opportunity for a permanent and concrete ethical debate, allowing for a greater level of trust among all users [42].

An ambitious challenge when dealing with these devices is that in the future, qualitative research can inform AI-CDSSs, and that these entities are able to process the findings generated by qualitative research to provide recommendations for users regarding aspects not obtainable through the calculation processes relied upon by these entities. Such skills could increase these technologies' range of action, since they would reach nuances and important suggestions about other aspects of the human sphere not currently achievable using AI-CDSSs.

26.8 Conclusion

As the healthcare landscape continues to evolve, AI and machine learning are becoming indispensable tools in CDSSs, symptom checkers, and self-triage technologies. These innovations hold tremendous potential for transforming primary and emergency care by offering improved diagnostic accuracy, personalized treatment recommendations, and streamlined workflows. However, as these technologies advance, careful attention must be paid to addressing the concerns surrounding their accuracy, safety, and integration into existing healthcare infrastructures.

While symptom checkers and self-triage tools can help alleviate the burden on healthcare systems—particularly in times of professional shortages—issues such as overtriage and the risk of missing serious conditions must be mitigated through rigorous validation and thoughtful design. Ensuring that these tools complement rather than replace the vital role of healthcare professionals will be key to maximizing their benefits.

Barriers to the adoption of CDSSs, such as technical, organizational, and human factors, remain significant. Nonetheless, studies suggest that when these systems are thoughtfully integrated and properly utilized, they can substantially enhance patient outcomes and support the delivery of remote primary care.

Looking forward, future developments in AI-enabled virtual assistants and the use of augmented reality in self-triage tools could further refine and humanize patient care experiences. As AI technology continues to advance, healthcare professionals, patients, and developers must work collaboratively to ensure that these innovations not only improve healthcare delivery but also maintain the essential human elements of care. Through continued research, education, and ethical development, AI-based systems can be a transformative force for the future of healthcare.

References

1. Funer F, Liedtke W, Tinnemeyer S, Klausen AD, Schneider D, Zacharias HU, Langanke M, Salloch S. Responsibility and decision-making authority in using clinical decision support systems: an empirical-ethical exploration of German prospective professionals' preferences and concerns. J Med Ethics. 2023;50(1):6–11. https://doi.org/10.1136/jme-2022-108814.
2. Sutton RT, Pincock D, Baumgart DC, Sadowski DC, Fedorak RN, Kroeker KI. An overview of clinical decision support systems: benefits, risks, and strategies for success. NPJ Digit Med. 2020;3:17. https://doi.org/10.1038/s41746-020-0221-y.

3. Alder H, Michel BA, Marx C, Tamborrini G, Langenegger T, Bruehlmann P, Steurer J, Wildi LM. Computer-based diagnostic expert systems in rheumatology: where do we stand in 2014? Int J Rheumatol. 2014;2014:672714. https://doi.org/10.1155/2014/672714.
4. Golden G, Popescu C, Israel S, Perlman K, Armstrong C, Fratila R, Tanguay-Sela M, Benrimoh D. Applying artificial intelligence to clinical decision support in mental health: what have we learned? Health Policy Technol. 2024;13(2):100844. https://doi.org/10.1016/j.hlpt.2024.100844.
5. Prabhu V, Kannan A, Tso GJ, Katariya N, Chablani M, Sontag D, Amatriain X. Open set medical diagnosis. Cornell University; 2019. https://doi.org/10.48550/arxiv.1910.02830.
6. Kafke SD, Kuhlmey A, Schuster J, Blüher S, Czimmeck C, Zoellick JC, Grosse P. Can clinical decision support systems be an asset in medical education? An experimental approach. BMC Med Educ. 2023;23(1):570. https://doi.org/10.1186/s12909-023-04568-8.
7. Bates DW, Kuperman GJ, Wang S, Gandhi T, Kittler A, Volk L, Spurr C, Khorasani R, Tanasijevic M, Middleton B. Ten commandments for effective clinical decision support: making the practice of evidence-based medicine a reality. J Am Med Inform Assoc. 2003;10(6):523–30. https://doi.org/10.1197/jamia.M1370.
8. Bright TJ, Wong A, Dhurjati R, Bristow E, Bastian L, Coeytaux RR, Samsa G, Hasselblad V, Williams JW, Musty MD, Wing L, Kendrick AS, Sanders GD, Lobach D. Effect of clinical decision-support systems: a systematic review. Ann Intern Med. 2012;157(1):29–43. https://doi.org/10.7326/0003-4819-157-1-201207030-00450.
9. Haynes RB, Wilczynski NL, The Computerized Clinical Decision Support System (CCDSS) Systematic Review Team. Effects of computerized clinical decision support systems on practitioner performance and patient outcomes: methods of a decision-maker-researcher partnership systematic review. Implement Sci. 2010;5(12) https://doi.org/10.1186/1748-5908-5-12.
10. Moja L, Kwag KH, Lytras T, Bertizzolo L, Brandt L, Pecoraro V, Rigon G, Vaona A, Ruggiero F, Mangia M, Iorio A, Kunnamo I, Bonovas S. Effectiveness of computerized decision support systems linked to electronic health records: a systematic review and meta-analysis. Am J Public Health. 2014;104(12):e12–22. https://doi.org/10.2105/AJPH.2014.302164.
11. Olakotan OO, Mohd YM. The appropriateness of clinical decision support systems alerts in supporting clinical workflows: a systematic review. Health Informatics J. 2021;27(2) https://doi.org/10.1177/14604582211007536.
12. Liberati EG, Galuppo L, Gorli M, Maraldi M, Ruggiero F, Capobussi M, et al. Barriere e facilitatori all'implementazione dei sistemi di supporto decisionale computerizzati in ospedale: uno studio "grounded theory". Recenti Prog Med. 2015;106(4):180–91.
13. Challen R, Denny J, Pitt M, Gompels L, Edwards T, Tsaneva-Atanasova K. Artificial intelligence, bias and clinical safety. BMJ Qual Saf. 2019;28(3):231–7. https://doi.org/10.1136/bmjqs-2018-008370.
14. Khalifa M, Albadawy M, Iqbal U. Advancing clinical decision support: the role of artificial intelligence across six domains. Comput Methods Prog Biomed Update. 2024;5:100142. https://doi.org/10.1016/j.cmpbup.2024.100142.
15. Semigran HL, Linder JA, Gidengil C, Mehrotra A. Evaluation of symptom checkers for self diagnosis and triage: audit study. BMJ. 2015;351:h3480. https://doi.org/10.1136/bmj.h3480.
16. Wallace W, Chan C, Chidambaram S, Hanna L, Iqbal FM, Acharya A, Normahani P, Ashrafian H, Markar SR, Sounderajah V, Darzi A. The diagnostic and triage accuracy of digital and online symptom checker tools: a systematic review. NPJ Digit Med. 2022;5(1):118. https://doi.org/10.1038/s41746-022-00667-w.
17. Riboli-Sasco E, El-Osta A, Alaa A, Webber I, Karki M, El Asmar ML, Purohit K, Painter A, Hayhoe B. Triage and diagnostic accuracy of online symptom checkers: systematic review. J Med Internet Res. 2023;25:e43803. https://doi.org/10.2196/43803.
18. Chambers D, Cantrell AJ, Johnson M, Preston L, Baxter SK, Booth A, Turner J. Digital and online symptom checkers and health assessment/triage services for urgent health problems: systematic review. BMJ Open. 2019;9(8):e027743. https://doi.org/10.1136/bmjopen-2018-027743.

19. Demurtas J, Tonelli R, Celotto S, Veronese N, Lagolio E, Rossi F, Clini E, Righi E, Meer A. COVID-Guide: una app per il triage e l'autovalutazione della covid-19 [COVID-Guide: an app for covid-19 triage and self-assessment]. Recenti Prog Med. 2021;112(5):387–91. Italian. https://doi.org/10.1701/3608.35876.
20. Miner AS, Laranjo L, Kocaballi AB. Chatbots in the fight against the COVID-19 pandemic. NPJ Digit Med. 2020;3:65. https://doi.org/10.1038/s41746-020-0280-0.
21. Andrew A. Potential applications and implications of large language models in primary care. Fam Med Commun Health. 2024;12(Suppl 1):e002602. https://doi.org/10.1136/fmch-2023-002602.
22. Ayers JW, Poliak A, Dredze M, Leas EC, Zhu Z, Kelley JB, Faix DJ, Goodman AM, Longhurst CA, Hogarth M, Smith DM. Comparing physician and artificial intelligence chatbot responses to patient questions posted to a public social media forum. JAMA Intern Med. 2023;183(6):589–96. https://doi.org/10.1001/jamainternmed.2023.1838.
23. Palanica A, Flaschner P, Thommandram A, Li M, Fossat Y. Physicians' perceptions of chatbots in health care: cross-sectional web-based survey. J Med Internet Res. 2019;21(4):e12887. https://doi.org/10.2196/12887.
24. Laranjo L, Dunn AG, Tong HL, Kocaballi AB, Chen J, Bashir R, Surian D, Gallego B, Magrabi F, Lau AYS, Coiera E. Conversational agents in healthcare: a systematic review. J Am Med Inform Assoc. 2018;25(9):1248–58. https://doi.org/10.1093/jamia/ocy072.
25. Li Y, Liang S, Zhu B, Liu X, Li J, Chen D, Qin J, Bressington D. Feasibility and effectiveness of artificial intelligence-driven conversational agents in healthcare interventions: a systematic review of randomized controlled trials. Int J Nurs Stud. 2023;143:104494. https://doi.org/10.1016/j.ijnurstu.2023.104494.
26. Cotte F, Mueller T, Gilbert S, Blümke B, Multmeier J, Hirsch MC, Wicks P, Wolanski J, Tutschkow D, Schade Brittinger C, Timmermann L, Jerrentrup A. Safety of triage self-assessment using a symptom assessment app for walk-in patients in the emergency care setting: observational prospective cross-sectional study. JMIR Mhealth Uhealth. 2022;10(3):e32340. https://doi.org/10.2196/32340.
27. Meer A, Rahm P, Schwendinger M, Vock M, Grunder B, Demurtas J, Rutishauser J. A symptom-checker for adult patients visiting an interdisciplinary emergency care center and the safety of patient self-triage: real-life prospective evaluation. J Med Internet Res. 2024;26:e58157. https://doi.org/10.2196/58157.
28. Liu V, Kaila M, Koskela T. Triage accuracy and the safety of user-initiated symptom assessment with an electronic symptom checker in a real-life setting: instrument validation study. JMIR Hum Factors. 2024;11:e55099. https://doi.org/10.2196/55099.
29. Aboueid S, Meyer S, Wallace JR, Mahajan S, Chaurasia A. Young adults' perspectives on the use of symptom checkers for self-triage and self-diagnosis: qualitative study. JMIR Public Health Surveill. 2021;7(1):e22637. https://doi.org/10.2196/22637.
30. Meunier PY, Raynaud C, Guimaraes E, Gueyffier F, Letrilliart L. Barriers and facilitators to the use of clinical decision support systems in primary care: a mixed-methods systematic review. Ann Fam Med. 2023;21(1):57–69. https://doi.org/10.1370/afm.2908.
31. Campbell JL, Fletcher E, Britten N, Green C, Holt TA, Lattimer V, Richards DA, Richards SH, Salisbury C, Calitri R, Bowyer V, Chaplin K, Kandiyali R, Murdoch J, Roscoe J, Varley A, Warren FC, Taylor RS. Telephone triage for management of same-day consultation requests in general practice (the ESTEEM trial): a cluster-randomised controlled trial and cost-consequence analysis. Lancet. 2014;384(9957):1859–68. https://doi.org/10.1016/S0140-6736(14)61058-8. Erratum in: Lancet. 2014;384(9957):1848. Erratum in: Lancet 2024;404(10447):30. doi:10.1016/S0140-6736(24)01354-0
32. Campbell JL, Fletcher E, Britten N, Green C, Holt T, Lattimer V, Richards DA, Richards SH, Salisbury C, Taylor RS, Calitri R, Bowyer V, Chaplin K, Kandiyali R, Murdoch J, Price L, Roscoe J, Varley A, Warren FC. The clinical effectiveness and cost-effectiveness of telephone triage for managing same-day consultation requests in general practice: a cluster randomised controlled trial comparing general practitioner-led and nurse-led management systems with

usual care (the ESTEEM trial). Health Technol Assess. 2015;19(13):1–212., vii–viii. https://doi.org/10.3310/hta19130.

33. Murdoch J, Barnes R, Pooler J, Lattimer V, Fletcher E, Campbell JL. The impact of using computer decision-support software in primary care nurse-led telephone triage: interactional dilemmas and conversational consequences. Soc Sci Med. 2015;126:36–47. https://doi.org/10.1016/j.socscimed.2014.12.013.
34. Sezgin E. Artificial intelligence in healthcare: complementing, not replacing, doctors and healthcare providers. Digit Health. 2023;9:20552076231186520. https://doi.org/10.1177/20552076231186520.
35. Salloch S, Eriksen A. What are humans doing in the loop? Co-reasoning and practical judgment when using machine learning-driven decision aids. Am J Bioeth. 2024;24(9):67–78. https://doi.org/10.1080/15265161.2024.2353800.
36. Pope C, Halford S, Turnbull J, Prichard J. Cyborg practices: call-handlers and computerised decision support systems in urgent and emergency care. Health Informatics J. 2014;20(2):118–26. https://doi.org/10.1177/1460458213486470.
37. Tolmachev I, Kaverina I, Vrazhnov D, Starikov I, Starikova E, Kostuchenko E. Application of artificial intelligence methods depending on the tasks solved during COVID-19 pandemic. COVID. 2022;2(10):1341–78. https://doi.org/10.3390/covid2100098.
38. Adam M, Wessel M, Benlian A. AI-based chatbots in customer service and their effects on user compliance. Electron Markets. Springer/IIM University of St. Gallen. 2021;31(2):427–45.
39. Alowais SA, Alghamdi SS, Alsuhebany N, Alqahtani T, Alshaya AI, Almohareb SN, Aldairem A, Alrashed M, Bin Saleh K, Badreldin HA, Al Yami MS, Al Harbi S, Albekairy AM. Revolutionizing healthcare: the role of artificial intelligence in clinical practice. BMC Med Educ. 2023;23(1):689. https://doi.org/10.1186/s12909-023-04698-z.
40. Thompson C, Mebrahtu T, Skyrme S, Bloor K, Andre D, Keenan AM, Ledward A, Yang H, Randell R. The effects of computerised decision support systems on nursing and allied health professional performance and patient outcomes: a systematic review and user contextualisation. Health Soc Care Deliv Res. 2023:1–85. https://doi.org/10.3310/GRNM5147.
41. Laka M, Carter D, Milazzo A, Merlin T. Challenges and opportunities in implementing clinical decision support systems (CDSS) at scale: interviews with Australian policymakers. Health Policy Technol. 2022;3:100652. https://doi.org/10.1016/j.hlpt.2022.100652.
42. Jones C, Thornton J, Wyatt JC. Enhancing trust in clinical decision support systems: a framework for developers. BMJ Health Care Inform. 2021;28(1):e100247. https://doi.org/10.1136/bmjhci-2020-100247.

Artificial Intelligence, Novel Technologies, and Virtuality

27

Hans A. Eguia and Javier F. Garcia Sanz Donato

27.1 Introduction to Telemedicine and Its Technological Foundations

Telemedicine has risen as an urgent aspect of cutting-edge healthcare, revolutionizing the delivery of medical services by leveraging broadcast communications innovation.

It is growing as a reliable advancement, especially supported by the transformative part played by AI and novel innovations.

Moreover, technological advances that support telemedicine, counting media transmission framework, teleconsultation stages, inaccessible checking gadgets, and electronic health records (EHRs), are helping with this development. Also, new technology resources analyze how AI is being tackled inside telemedicine to drive headways in diagnostics, prescient analytics, and personalized treatment plans, giving telemedicine a key role in healthcare.

H. A. Eguia (✉)
Lægehuset Engdraget, Rudkøbing, Denmark

eHealth – WONCA, Rudkøbing, Denmark

Digital Health Working Group of the Spanish Society of Family Medicine (SEMERGEN), Barcelona, Spain

Danish Society of Primary Care (DSAM), Copenhagen, Denmark

Universitat Oberta de Catalunya, Barcelona, Spain
e-mail: heguia@uoc.edu

J. F. Garcia Sanz Donato
Danish Society of Primary Care (DSAM), Copenhagen, Denmark

Digital Health Working Group of the Spanish Society of Family Medicine (SEMERGEN), Barcelona, Spain

J. Demurtas (ed.), *Remote Consultation in Primary Care*, TELe-Health,
https://doi.org/10.1007/978-3-031-89661-3_27

27.1.1 Overview of Telemedicine

Telemedicine includes a range of healthcare management conveyed remotely, encouraged by broadcast communications innovation (telecommunications technology).

Its roots can be traced back to the early twentieth century when simple shapes of remote restorative meetings were conducted through radio and phone. Over time, telemedicine has advanced in pair with innovative headways, extending its reach and capabilities. Nowadays, telemedicine envelops different modalities, including teleconsultations, telemonitoring, teletherapy, and teleeducation. It serves as an imperative apparatus for overcoming geographical barriers, making advances on healthcare access and upgrading patient monitoring, diagnosis, and treatment.

27.1.2 Foundations of Telemedicine Technologies

The adequacy of telemedicine pivots on an innovative foundation that empowers consistent communication and information trade between patients and healthcare suppliers. Media transmission foundation shapes the cornerstone of telemedicine, giving the fundamental transfer speed and network to reinforce real-time interactions. Teleconsultation platforms, extending from video conferencing programs to portable apps, encourage virtual interviews between patients and professionals, for a remote diagnosis or treatment development. Remote monitoring gadgets, such as wearable sensors and Internet of Things (IoT) gadgets, empower continuous observation of patient vital signs and parameters as well as strengthening adherence to treatment protocols.

Moreover, electronic health records (EHRs) serve as centralized storehouses for patient data, encouraging facilitated care and interoperability in healthcare settings.

The use of these elements has been already tested with positive implications for COVID-19 when they were used as new surveillance strategies showing a new direction as an effective framework for response to future pandemics [1].

27.1.3 Leveraging AI in Telemedicine

Artificial Intelligence (AI) has risen as a game-changer in telemedicine, upgrading its precision, analytics possibilities, and personalized treatment management. AI-enabled instruments in telemedicine use machine learning calculations, picture recognition programs, and Natural Language Processing (NLP) algorithms to analyze patients' situations and medical pictures and distinguish variations from the norm with high accuracy and even increasing productivity.

These systems engage healthcare professionals to create many trained possibilities to speed up the preparation of the consultation and eventually progressing with the presentation of results. Analytics calculation analyzers can manage huge datasets to recognize scales and patterns, empowering proactive mediations and personalized treatment plans custom-made to patients' persistent chronic needs.

By tackling the control of AI, telemedicine is balanced to revolutionize healthcare conveyance, introducing a modern period of exact medication and patient-centered care which will empower them. It is also expected that, in the field of Clinical Information Systems, AI will lead to a more efficient and intelligent patient-oriented health system with an overall improvement in health outcomes [2].

There are some outcomes that could be expected with the use of AI in telemedicine, as early disease detection, better patient accessibility and engagement, more effective screening, and cost implications—savings, reduced unmet needs, and reduced clinical demands [3]. In primary care, work is also being done on NLP, for example with the HOPE project (Health Operation for Personalized Evidence), where AI is used to review EHRs and obtain keywords that are used to search for relevant information in different medical databases such as PubMed, ClinicalTrials, or MedlinePlus [4].

Telemedicine speaks to a worldview move in healthcare development, empowered by progressions in broadcast communications innovation, and driven by the transformative potential of AI and novel advances.

By leveraging media transmission framework, teleconsultation platforms, remote monitoring gadgets, and electronic health records, telemedicine can overcome geographical obstructions, allow progress to care, and eventually improve patient results. In addition, the integration of AI holds a guarantee for advanced upgrading demonstrative exactness, prescient analytics, and personalized treatment arranging inside telemedicine practice.

As telemedicine advances, it is balanced to reshape the scene of healthcare conveyance, introducing a period of available, productive, and patient-centric care.

27.2 Novel Innovations Changing Telemedicine

Telemedicine, as a quickly advancing field, proceeds to be changed by novel innovations that revolutionize the way healthcare is delivered and experienced. Some of the groundbreaking advances that are reshaping telemedicine practice notably include virtual reality (VR), augmented reality (AR), telerobotics, mobile networks improvement, and blockchain, but they are used in different telemedicine stages. Each of these advances offers special capabilities and applications that improve remote healthcare delivery, improve patient outcomes, and drive advancement in telemedicine usage [5].

27.2.1 Virtual Reality (VR) and Augmented Reality (AR) for Enhanced Remote Consultations

VR and AR advances are revolutionizing telemedicine by making immersive, intuitive situations for remote discussions, renewing the preparation/medical training and patient guidance.

VR innovation submerges users in a computer-generated environment, permitting them to associate with virtual objects and scenarios in real time [6].

This empowers healthcare suppliers to conduct remote meetings with patients in a virtual clinic setting, where they can outwardly examine patients, check medical images, and create treatment strategies [7]. AR innovation overlays advanced data onto the patient's see of the genuine world, improving their recognition and understanding of their environment. In telemedicine, AR innovation can be utilized to supply real-time direction and visual aids in surgical strategies, empowering remote surgical assistance, education/training, and preparation [8]. It can also be useful to help the patients' caregivers [9].

Besides, VR and AR innovations encourage virtual patient instruction and rehabilitation programs, permitting patients to lock into an immersive encounter that would promote health education, self-management (patient empowerment), and treatment adherence.

There are several fields where VR with telepresence has already being used, such as in telerehabilitation [10], with good results not only in mobilization but also in cognitive rehabilitation [11].

Its use in training different procedures—as surgical protocols or examination of patients—is also well known [12].

The use of VR/AR has also been shown to be effective in the field of ophthalmology, helping to improve access to specialized medicine, and reducing diagnostic error and underdiagnosis [3]. The potential use of these tools has been recently enhanced with the appearance of the Metaverse program from the company Meta, with possibilities more accessible to health professionals in pain management use [13].

Metaverse may prove itself an exceptional educational tool, offering the possibility of interactive digital lessons, allowing to dissect and to study an anatomical apparatus in detail, to navigate within it, not only to study but also to see the evolution of the pathological processes, and to simulate in advance surgical or medical procedures on virtual patients [14].

27.2.2 Tele-Robotics and Remote Surgical Assistance

Tele-robotics is transforming surgery by empowering out-of-reach surgical procedures and interventions through mechanical frameworks controlled by healthcare professionals. These mechanical frameworks consist of specialized surgical instruments and cameras mounted on automated (robotic) arms, which are controlled by specialists from a remote area utilizing teleoperation innovation technology. This permits specialists to perform minimally invasive strategies, such as laparoscopic surgery and robotic-assisted surgery, with exactness and accuracy from a distance. Tele-robotics also empowers unapproachable surgical help, where experienced specialists can give direction and supervision to less experienced specialists performing methods in inaccessible or underserved areas [8]. Moreover, telerobotics assists telesurgery, where specialists can perform complex strategies on patients found thousands of miles away, leveraging progressed mechanical autonomy and media transmission innovations to overcome topographical boundaries and access to better surgical care.

It is also expected that robotic systems will have tremendous potential in the future implementation of different fields such as cerebrovascular procedures where there are many professionals with little clinical experience, helping with procedures such as thrombectomies for acute stroke [15].

Robotic systems may play a significant role also in the field of Ambient Assisted Living (AAL) with Internet of Things-based monitoring systems.

AAL encompasses several different products and services which may enable people to live independently in their environment, providing also an improvement of their quality of life, notably relevant for older people and patients [16–18].

Robots have been developed to help chronic and/or older patients with their mobility (wheelchairs, exoskeletons, walking aids); provide equipment to help people with personal care such as eating and drinking; robots may help with home maintenance such as cleaning and cooking; some robots were conceived to play as companion—many of which use telepresence systems and can have access to telemedicine systems; other robotic systems help with cognitive training (known as emotional enhancers) [19].

These technologies can be used, blended, and combined in the future provision of primary care. The use of sensors proposed has shown positive clinical effects both in laboratory tests and in outpatient tests in different scenarios [20].

27.2.3 Future Mobile Connectivity: Enabling High-Speed Data Transmission and Low-Latency Communication

The appearance of the 5G network is empowering high-speed information transmission and low-latency communication between patients and healthcare suppliers. 5G systems offer quicker information speeds and lower latency compared to previous generations of mobile innovation, making it perfect for applications that require real-time interaction and high-bandwidth information exchange, such as telemedicine.

With a 5G network, healthcare suppliers can conduct high-definition video discussions, transmit large medical images, and stream real-time physiological information with almost no delay, upgrading the quality and proficiency of distant healthcare delivery.

In addition, the 5G network empowers the multiplication of associated medical gadgets and IoT sensors, allowing constant observation of vital signs and monitoring of the patient at all times without the need for physical consultations, and all in real time.

The use of mobile networks with 5G allows to interact with applications that almost everyone uses, such as WhatsApp, not only for instant communication but also as a form of geolocation in cases of emergencies in areas that are unknown to us (for instance, tourists in other countries), helping to reach emergency teams up to 5 min apart from nonuse [21].

27.2.4 Blockchain in Telemedicine: Securing Patient Data and Streamlining Transactions

Blockchain innovation holds a guarantee for changing telemedicine by giving secure, straightforward, and tamper-proof capacity and exchange of patients' information as well as therapeutic/medical records.

Blockchain may be a record innovation that empowers decentralized capacity and confirmation of exchanges over a network of computers, guaranteeing information judgment and security through cryptographic calculations and agreement mechanisms.

In telemedicine, blockchain can be utilized to form unchanging records of understanding data, EHRs, and treatment plans, which are open to authorized healthcare professionals and patients while protecting patients' data security and privacy [22].

In addition, blockchain can streamline regulatory forms (administrative process), such as insurance/malpractice claims handling and charging, by mechanizing confirmation and approval of exchanges, reducing administrative steps, and increasing proficiency in telemedicine operations [23, 24].

The integration of blockchain technology with AI can generate a significant difference in health by promoting the implementation of analytical technology that is integrated into better risk management and patient care, which will lead to medical systems improving their efficiency, reducing costs, and aiming toward a more democratized health [25–27].

All this is because blockchain allows the storage of EHRs information in a cryptographic way that can be better understood by AI, improving the global use of this data [28].

27.2.5 Integrated Telemedicine Platforms and Ecosystems

Integrated telemedicine programs and ecosystems are reshaping the scene of inaccessible healthcare delivery by giving comprehensive arrangements for educating in healthcare [5], supplier collaboration, and administrative management. These platforms bring together a wide extent of telemedicine administrations and functionalities, which encompass teleconsultations, remote monitoring, EHRs, and appointment scheduling.

Integrated telemedicine platforms offer consistent integration with existing healthcare frameworks and workflows, empowering healthcare suppliers to convey high-quality care remotely while streamlining regulatory administration tasks and diminishing operational costs [29]. Besides, these platforms cultivate collaboration and communication between multidisciplinary care groups, empowering facilitated care and continuity of treatment for patients over distinctive specialities and settings.

Integrated telemedicine platforms and environments streamline healthcare access by giving comprehensive solutions for patient care, healthcare-provider collaboration, and administration management [30]. As these advances proceed, they hold the potential to revolutionize the telemedicine practice, making healthcare more available, proficient, and patient-centered within the computerized age.

27.3 Virtuality in Telemedicine Practice

Virtual clinics and telehealth platforms serve as computerized center points (digital hubs) for remote discussions, empowering patients to get to healthcare services from the security of their homes or even from very remote areas. These platforms give secure, user-friendly interfacing for planning consultations, conducting virtual visits, and communicating with healthcare suppliers through video conferencing, messaging, or normal telephone communication [31].

Virtual clinics offer a wide extent of services, including primary care, hospital specialist consultations, mental well-being counselling, and follow-up visits, permitting patients to get care without the requirement for in-person visits.

In addition, telehealth platforms integrated consistently with EHR and other healthcare frameworks are empowering healthcare providers to get access to patient information, report experiences, and facilitate care over distinctive specialities and settings [32, 33].

27.3.1 Telepresence and Telecollaboration Tools for Multidisciplinary Care

Telepresence and telecollaboration instruments encourage real-time communication and collaboration between multidisciplinary care groups, empowering facilitated care and treatment arranging for complex medical conditions.

Telecollaboration instruments empower multidisciplinary care groups to work together over diverse areas and specialities, encouraging case discussions, treatment arranging, and decision-making in real time. Additionally, telepresence and telecollaboration instruments empower interest in medical conferences and surgical methods, permitting specialists to share information, counsel on cases, and give mentorship to less experienced colleagues.

It also improves persistent engagement and fulfilment by including patients in their care choices and treatment plans, cultivating a sense of strengthening and possession over their well-being.

Virtual patient instruction and remote rehabilitation programs use immersive innovations to teach patients about their medical conditions, treatment alternatives, and self-management encounters with procedures. Out-of-reach recovery programs (e.g., for drug/alcohol users) as remote rehabilitation programs utilize VR-based works, virtual reality gamification, and movement-following sensors to deliver personalized rehabilitation for patients recouping from surgery, injuries, or chronic conditions. Gamification has shown also potentially effective features in mHealth apps for medication adherence [34]. These programs empower patients to take an interest in treatment sessions from their own homes, diminishing barriers to getting to the rehabilitation programs, making strides in adherence to treatment plans, and advancing prompt recuperation and autonomy.

Virtual treatment is used to empower patients to get to mental well-being back from the consolation and protection of their homes. These protocols utilize VR situations, telepresence platforms, and digital communication devices to encourage psychotherapy, counselling, and even support groups for patients with mental health conditions, such as depression, anxiety, PTSD, and substance abuse disorders [35]. Virtual treatment sessions permit patients to participate in evidence-based interventions, such as cognitive behavioral treatment (CBT), mindfulness-based treatment, and exposure treatment, delivered by authorized advisors and counsellors prepared in virtual care treatments [36]. In addition, virtual treatment platforms offer highlights such as secure informing, video conferencing, and virtual reality situations, improving patient engagement, confidentiality, and therapeutic support.

27.4 Conclusions: Future Directions and Challenges

As telemedicine continues to evolve, it presents both exciting opportunities and notable challenges in shaping the future of healthcare delivery. Therefore, it is crucial to understand the segment that examines the potential future use of telemedicine and the key challenges that must be addressed to fully realize its potential.

One of the most promising future directions in telemedicine is the integration and advancement of artificial intelligence and machine learning technologies. AI-powered tools such as diagnostic systems, predictive analytics, and personalized treatment algorithms are expected to become increasingly sophisticated and precise, enabling healthcare professionals to deliver more efficient, accurate, and tailored care to patients globally. Furthermore, AI and ML advancements have the potential to automate scheduling, streamline administrative processes, and enhance clinical decision-making, freeing up healthcare professionals to focus on more complex and high-value aspects of patient care.

An additional prospective direction in telemedicine is the expansion of remote consultations, monitoring, and telehealth services to encompass a wider range of medical conditions and patient populations.

While the future of telemedicine holds great promise, there are several challenges and considerations that must be addressed to realize its full potential and overcome barriers to adoption. One key challenge is ensuring access to telemedicine services, especially for underserved and vulnerable populations who may lack access to technology or reliable Internet connectivity. To address this, stakeholders must invest in digital infrastructure, expand broadband availability, and provide specialized support not only to patients but also to healthcare professionals to ensure the proper and equitable use of these tools, regardless of socioeconomic status or geographic location.

References

1. Kostkova P, Saigí-Rubió F, Eguia H, Borbolla D, Verschuuren M, Hamilton C, et al. Data and digital solutions to support surveillance strategies in the context of the COVID-19 pandemic. Front Digit Heal. 2021;0:89.
2. Hackl WO, Neururer SB, Pfeifer B. Transforming clinical information systems: empowering healthcare through telemedicine, data science, and artificial intelligence applications. Yearb Med Inform [Internet]. 2023;32(01):127–37. Available from: http://www.thieme-connect.de/DOI/DOI?10.1055/s-0043-1768756
3. Ramessur R, Raja L, Kilduff CLS, Kang S, Li JPO, Thomas PBM, et al. Impact and challenges of integrating artificial intelligence and telemedicine into clinical ophthalmology. Asia-Pacific J Ophthalmol [Internet]. 2021;10(3):317–27. Available from: https://linkinghub.elsevier.com/retrieve/pii/S2162098923001056
4. Eguia H, Sanchez-bocanegra C, Fernandez-Llatas C, Saigí-Rubió F. Using natural language and health ontologies in hope recommender system: evaluation of use in primary care. Preprint [Internet]. 2024; Available from: https://www.researchgate.net/publication/379723502_Using_Natural_Language_and_Health_Ontologies_in_Hope_Recommender_System_Evaluation_of_Use_in_Primary_Care
5. Ezeamii VC, Okobi OE, Wambai-Sani H, Perera GS, Zaynieva S, Okonkwo CC, et al. Revolutionizing healthcare: how telemedicine is improving patient outcomes and expanding access to care. Cureus [Internet]. 2024;16(7) Available from: https://pubmed.ncbi.nlm.nih.gov/39099901/
6. Rhee T, Thompson S, Medeiros D, dos Anjos R, Chalmers A. Augmented virtual teleportation for high-fidelity telecollaboration. IEEE Trans Vis Comput Graph [Internet]. 2020;26(5):1923–33. Available from: https://ieeexplore.ieee.org/document/8998353/
7. Talevski J, Semciw AI, Boyd JH, Jessup RL, Miller SM, Hutton J, et al. From concept to reality: a comprehensive exploration into the development and evolution of a virtual emergency department. J Am Coll Emerg Physicians Open [Internet]. 2024;5(4) Available from: /pmc/articles/PMC11269764/
8. Ammendola M, Vescio F, Al Ansari M, Hila J, Rizzo L, Romano R, et al. Metaverse and telementoring: from surgery to workshop. Surg Innov [Internet]. 2024;31(2):212–9. Available from: https://pubmed.ncbi.nlm.nih.gov/38378041/
9. Albright L, Ko W, Buvanesh M, Haraldsson H, Polubriaginof F, Kuperman GJ, et al. Opportunities and challenges for augmented reality in family caregiving: qualitative video elicitation study. JMIR Form Res [Internet]. 2024;8:e56916. Available from: https://formative.jmir.org/2024/1/e56916
10. Sarpourian F, Sharifian R, Poursadeghfard M, Khayami SR, Erfannia L. Comparison of the clinical effectiveness of telerehabilitation with traditional rehabilitation methods in multiple sclerosis patients: a systematic review. Telemed e-Health [Internet]. 2024; Available from: https://www.liebertpub.com/doi/10.1089/tmj.2023.0412
11. Mantovani E, Zucchella C, Bottiroli S, Federico A, Giugno R, Sandrini G, et al. Telemedicine and virtual reality for cognitive rehabilitation: a roadmap for the COVID-19 pandemic. Front Neurol [Internet]. 2020:11. Available from: https://www.frontiersin.org/article/10.3389/fneur.2020.00926/full
12. Morsy H, Scott C, Jairath R, Ghetti C, Chu C, Sutcliffe S, et al. Telemedicine: the new "virtual reality" of female pelvic medicine and reconstructive surgery? Female Pelvic Med Reconstr Surg [Internet]. 2022;28(3):e80–7. Available from: https://journals.lww.com/10.1097/SPV.0000000000001149
13. Cerda IH, Therond A, Moreau S, Studer K, Donjow AR, Crowther JE, et al. Telehealth and virtual reality technologies in chronic pain management: a narrative review. Curr Pain Headache Rep [Internet]. 2024;28(3):83–94. Available from: https://link.springer.com/10.1007/s11916-023-01205-3

14. Massetti M, Chiariello GA. The metaverse in medicine. Eur Hear J Suppl [Internet]. 2023;25(Supplement_B):B104–7. Available from: https://academic.oup.com/eurheartjsupp/article/25/Supplement_B/B104/7135792
15. Rabinovich EP, Capek S, Kumar JS, Park MS. Tele-robotics and artificial-intelligence in stroke care. J Clin Neurosci [Internet]. 2020;79:129–32. Available from: https://linkinghub.elsevier.com/retrieve/pii/S0967586820313527
16. Demurtas J, Veronese N. The role of family physicians in older people care. 2022.; Available from: https://www.amazon.com/Family-Physicians-People-Practical-Geriatrics/dp/3030789225
17. Memon M, Wagner SR, Pedersen CF, Aysha Beevi FH, Hansen FO. Ambient assisted living healthcare frameworks, platforms, standards, and quality attributes. Sensors (Basel) [Internet]. 2014;14(3):4312. Available from: /pmc/articles/PMC4003945/
18. Mangini L, Wick JY. Wandering: unearthing new tracking devices. Consult Pharm. 2017;32(6):324–35.
19. Payr S, Werner F, Werner K. AAL robotics: state of the field and challenges. Stud Health Technol Inform [Internet]. 2015;212:117–24. Available from: http://www.ncbi.nlm.nih.gov/pubmed/26063266
20. Bleda AL, Melgarejo-Meseguer FM, Gimeno-Blanes FJ, García-Alberola A, Rojo-Álvarez JL, Corral J, et al. Enabling heart self-monitoring for all and for AAL – portable device within a complete telemedicine system. Sensors [Internet]. 2019;19(18):3969. Available from: https://www.mdpi.com/1424-8220/19/18/3969
21. Eguia H, Vinciarelli F, Curioso WH, Sanz FJ, Sotelo CO, Sanchez C, et al. Use of the geographical information system integrated in smartphone to reduce transportation time for general medical care in Ibiza, Spain. Acad J Heal Sci Med Balear ISSN-e 2255-0560. 2022;37(1):86–90. [Internet]. 2022;37(1):86–90. Available from: https://dialnet.unirioja.es/servlet/articulo?codigo=8254787&info=resumen&idioma=SPA
22. Ghadi YY, Mazhar T, Shahzad T, Amir Khan M, Abd-Alrazaq A, Ahmed A, et al. The role of blockchain to secure internet of medical things. Sci Rep. [Internet] 2024. 2024;14(1):1–31. Available from: https://www.nature.com/articles/s41598-024-68529-x
23. Sahu H, Choudhari S, Chakole S, Sahu H, Choudhari SG, Chakole S. The use of blockchain technology in public health: lessons learned. Cureus [Internet]. 2024;16(6) Available from: https://www.cureus.com/articles/255674-the-use-of-blockchain-technology-in-public-health-lessons-learned
24. Mahdi SS, Ullah Z, Battineni G, Babar MG, Daood U. The telehealth chain: a framework for secure and transparent telemedicine transactions on the blockchain. Ir J Med Sci [Internet]. 2024:1–9. Available from: https://link.springer.com/article/10.1007/s11845-024-03728-z
25. Tagde P, Tagde S, Bhattacharya T, Tagde P, Chopra H, Akter R, et al. Blockchain and artificial intelligence technology in e-health. Environ Sci Pollut Res [Internet]. 2021;28(38):52810–31. Available from: https://link.springer.com/10.1007/s11356-021-16223-0
26. Omidian H. Synergizing blockchain and artificial intelligence to enhance healthcare. Drug Discov Today [Internet]. 2024;29(9):104111. Available from: https://linkinghub.elsevier.com/retrieve/pii/S1359644624002368
27. Lacson R, Yu Y, Kuo TT, Ohno-Machado L. Biomedical blockchain with practical implementations and quantitative evaluations: a systematic review. J Am Med Informatics Assoc [Internet]. 2024;31(6):1423–35. https://doi.org/10.1093/jamia/ocae084.
28. Hiwale M, Walambe R, Potdar V, Kotecha K. A systematic review of privacy-preserving methods deployed with blockchain and federated learning for the telemedicine. Healthc Anal. 2023;3:100192.
29. Anawade PA, Sharma D, Gahane S. A comprehensive review on exploring the impact of telemedicine on healthcare accessibility. Cureus [Internet]. 2024;16(3) Available from: https://pubmed.ncbi.nlm.nih.gov/38618307/
30. Jain S, Jain PK. 5G technology for healthcare and its health effects: wonders, dangers, and diligence. J Fam Med Prim Care [Internet]. 2022;11(11):6683–6. Available from: https://journals.lww.com/jfmpc/fulltext/2022/11000/5g_technology_for_healthcare_and_its_health.12.aspx

31. Anis S, Zelinsky M, Shuaib U, Hartwig E, Simpson M, Fernandez HH, et al. Introducing virtual shared medical appointments as a novel treatment platform for functional movement disorders. Tremor Other Hyperkinetic Mov. 2024;14(1)
32. Annunziata CM, Dahut WL, Willman CL, Winn RA, Knudsen KE. Reflections on the state of telehealth and cancer care research and future directions. JNCI Monogr [Internet]. 2024;2024(64):100–3. https://doi.org/10.1093/jncimonographs/lgae008.
33. Dai Z. Telehealth in long-term care facilities during the Covid-19 pandemic – lessons learned from patients, physicians, nurses and healthcare workers. BMC Digit Heal [Internet]. 2023;1(1) Available from: /pmc/articles/PMC9872077/
34. Tran S, Smith L, Carter S. Understanding patient perspectives on the use of gamification and incentives in mHealth apps to improve medication adherence: qualitative study. JMIR mHealth uHealth [Internet]. 2024;12:e50851. Available from: https://mhealth.jmir.org/2024/1/e50851
35. Bogdanski E. The effects of virtual reality telemedicine with pediatric patients diagnosed with posttraumatic stress disorder: exploratory research method case report. JMIR Form Res [Internet]. 2023;7:e34346. Available from: https://formative.jmir.org/2023/1/e34346
36. Jingili N, Oyelere SS, Ojwang F, Agbo FJ, Nyström MBT. Virtual reality for addressing depression and anxiety: a bibliometric analysis. Int J Environ Res Public Health [Internet]. 2023;20(9):5621. Available from: https://www.mdpi.com/1660-4601/20/9/5621

Remote Consultations in Primary Care: Investigations in the Age of Telemedicine

28

Jacopo Demurtas, Keith Thompson, Brian Geller, and William Cherniak

28.1 Investigations in the Age of Telemedicine

The definition of telemedicine has been established for many years. As defined by the WHO:

> Telemedicine is defined as the delivery of health-care services where distance is a critical factor, by all health-care professionals using information and communication technologies for the exchange of valid information for diagnosis, treatment and prevention of disease and injuries all in the interests of advancing the health of individuals and their communities (1).

J. Demurtas
Clinical and Experimental Medicine PhD Program, University of Modena and Reggio Emilia, Modena, Italy

Family Medicine Department, USL Toscana Sud-Est, Capalbio, Italy

K. Thompson (✉)
Department of Family Medicine, Schulich School of Denistry and Medicine, Western University, London, ON, Canada
e-mail: kthomps@uwo.ca

B. Geller
Department of Family Medicine, Schulich School of Denistry and Medicine, Western University, London, ON, Canada

Department of Family Medicine, University of Saskatchewan, Saskatoon, Canada

W. Cherniak
Department of Family Medicine, Schulich School of Denistry and Medicine, Western University, London, ON, Canada

Department of Family and Community Medicine, Division of Emergency Medicine, University of Toronto, Toronto, Canada

J. Demurtas (ed.), *Remote Consultation in Primary Care*, TELe-Health,
https://doi.org/10.1007/978-3-031-89661-3_28

While we may have good understanding and definitions of the terminology of telemedicine and its various aspects of care, we still have not seen robust studies that would bring validation of all aspects of telemedicine within the domains of patient health outcomes, provider adoptions, and healthcare system economic outcomes. The future of investigations in this "age of telemedicine" will no doubt focus, not solely on the advancement of the technological aspects of devices and systems created, but on better understanding of how such technologies incorporated into the clinical care workflows impact healthcare systems. There will also be a need to address the "digital divide" that the technologies of telemedicine create. One-half of the globe has great challenges achieving equivalent levels of healthcare equity enjoyed by wealthier nations (2), and our technological advancements may be biased to those individuals with proper connectivity and resources that provide access to the required devices for telemedicine visits, thus only worsening healthcare disparities around the globe. The pressure upon primary care providers currently is to service larger volumes of patients within the context of diminishing resource supports and develop or participate in models of care that are high-volume, low physician touch programs.

How might telemedicine investigations address these needs for family doctors around the world?

How might the investigations promote reconciliation of the foundational "mission statements" of primary care (as suggested by Dr. Ian McWhinney in his "Textbook of Family Medicine" (3)) within the evolving telemedicine age?

What might be the appropriate platform for codesigning systems that lessen the administrative burden for family physicians yet are intuitive and user friendly for the patients they serve?

This chapter will outline some of the global research work being done/planned and provide framework for primary care to develop/collaborate on their own investigational research and further validation of telemedicine adoption within clinical practice to address these population health needs. The research would also ideally promote trust and ease of adoption of the information and communication technology (ICT) needed to serve patients within the context of longitudinal care—a founding principle for family medicine (3).

We will start by outlining some of the basic concepts around study design in the context for telemedicine investigations.

28.2 Methodological Approaches to Telemedicine Investigations

Methodological approaches to investigational studies in telemedicine may be quite varied and dependent upon the research question asked. In-depth review of this topic will be beyond the scope of this chapter, but an excellent source of further reading and systematic review can be found in: *The Handbook of eHealth Evaluation—An Evidence-based Approach* (4)

> In the mid-1990s, the National Library of Medicine (NLM) requested that the Institute of Medicine (IOM) develop a broad framework for telemedicine evaluation. In 1996, based on the deliberations of a 15-member expert committee, the IOM released its report, *Telemedicine: A Guide to Assessing Telecommunications in Health Care*. The report presented a framework built upon five main evaluation elements: (1) quality of care and health outcomes, (2) access to care, (3) health care costs and cost-effectiveness, (4) patient perceptions, and (5) clinician perceptions (IOM 1996) (5).

The Office of the Assistant Secretary of Planning and Evaluation released a publication in November 2020 the "Assessment of approaches to the evaluation of telemedicine." This publication built upon the prior work from the 1996 IOM expert committee and is another excellent resource for outlining key ingredients and focus for telemedicine investigations.

The most reliable study design to determine outcomes for telemedicine programs would be the randomized clinical trial or RCT. When designing a telemedicine RCT, it is essential to consider the specific objectives and outcomes needed to measure. Telemedicine interventions are not fully standardizable, so evidence from RCTs should be combined with "real-world" data—routinely collected patient-level data—to capture the effects of these interventions (6).

These randomized clinical trials should ideally be pragmatic and decentralized to best capture outcomes given the heterogenous make-up of primary care practices (7).

The need for DCTs has become more urgent due to the COVID-19 pandemic, which demonstrated the potential for digital technologies to support the continuation of clinical trials under restrictive conditions.

It is also important to consider patient populations when designing the study. The statement "nothing about me without me" is a colloquial reference but important mode of operation for successful and meaningful studies to be completed (8).

Some common outcomes for telemedicine studies include patient satisfaction, clinical effectiveness, cost-effectiveness, and access to care.

Study design should define its primary and secondary outcomes, the target population, inclusion and exclusion criteria, and the trial's duration. The methodology most applied to gather evidence-based medical data is PICO (9).

This method helps researchers and healthcare professionals to develop focused and answerable research questions that can guide systematic reviews, literature searches, and the design of clinical studies. When applied to telemedicine investigations, the PICO method can help in comparing the effectiveness, feasibility, and outcomes of various telemedicine interventions as outlined in Table 28.1 (9).

These are just a few examples of possible primary and secondary outcomes for telemedicine RCT. The specific outcomes will depend on the objectives of the trial, the disease or condition being studied, and the telemedicine intervention being tested.

Table 28.1 Primary and secondary outcomes for telemedicine research

Primary outcomes:
Clinical effectiveness: Improvement in specific health outcomes, such as reduction in blood pressure, HbA1c levels (for diabetic patients), or symptom scores (e.g., depression or pain scores). The choice of the specific outcome will depend on the disease or condition being studied
Hospitalization rates: Reduction in the number of hospitalizations or emergency department visits for the target population, indicating better management of chronic conditions or improved access to care through telemedicine
Treatment adherence: Improvement in adherence to medication, lifestyle changes, or other prescribed treatments, as telemedicine may enable better monitoring and support for patients
Patient satisfaction: Assessing patients' satisfaction with the telemedicine intervention compared to standard care, using validated satisfaction questionnaires or surveys
Secondary outcomes:
Cost-effectiveness: Evaluating the cost-effectiveness of the telemedicine intervention compared to standard care, considering direct and indirect costs, such as cost savings due to reduced hospitalizations, transportation costs, and time savings
Access to care: Measuring the impact of telemedicine on access to care, such as the number of patients receiving timely care, reduced waiting times for appointments, or increased access to any care in remote or underserved areas
Quality of care: Assessing the quality of care provided through telemedicine compared to standard care, using established quality indicators or measures relevant to the specific intervention
Provider satisfaction: Evaluating healthcare providers' satisfaction with the telemedicine intervention, considering factors such as workload, ease of use, communication quality, and perceived impact on patient care
Patient engagement and self-management: Assessing whether telemedicine intervention leads to increased patient engagement in their care or improved self-management of their condition

Modified from Ref. (9)

28.3 Different Dimensions and Domains of Telemedicine Investigations

There are several domains/subdomains that will be the focus of future telemedicine investigations. The modalities of remote patient consults and the infrastructures needed to support these virtual encounters are quite extensive, but the main areas of focus may include:

1. Virtual Reality (VR) and Augmented Reality (AR): VR and AR can transform telemedicine by enabling immersive, lifelike consultations and medical training. Research in this area will focus on improving the quality of virtual experiences, developing realistic simulations, and creating tools for remote collaboration between healthcare professionals.
2. 5G and Beyond Connectivity: Telemedicine, particularly involving real-time video visits, relies on stable, high-speed Internet connections for effective communication and data transfer. Research in 5G and beyond connectivity will be

crucial for providing the necessary infrastructure for seamless, real-time video-enabled telemedicine services, especially in rural and underserved areas. The challenges of Internet access and digital divides are created by adoption of digital health systems. The needs for developing nations and remote rural will no doubt include technologies supported by lower bandwidth solutions. Research into the use of low bandwidth solutions which could be rapidly deployed and are less reliant on complicated networks to maintain. Research into these solutions will be essential in order to keep telehealth access equitable.

3. Data Privacy and Security: Telemedicine generates large amounts of sensitive patient data, necessitating robust data privacy and security measures. Research in this area should focus on developing advanced encryption techniques, secure data storage, and privacy-preserving technologies to ensure the protection of patient information. *Data "infostructure"*—global examples of mature data lakes and interoperability—supports innovation in this area with programs such as Novartis Foundation Health Hub tech Africa.
4. Wearable and IoT Devices: Wearable devices and the Internet of Things (IoT) can enhance telemedicine by providing continuous health monitoring and real-time data collection. Research should be conducted to develop more advanced, user-friendly devices with longer battery life, better data accuracy, and seamless integration with telemedicine platforms.
5. User Experience (UX) and Accessibility—Telemedicine platforms should be easy to use and accessible to a wide range of patients, including those with disabilities and limited technical skills. Research in UX and accessibility will help develop intuitive interfaces, voice-controlled systems, and assistive technologies that ensure telemedicine is inclusive and user-friendly. Systems user interface—to accommodate cultural, linguistic appropriate services, and patients with limitations due to disabilities.
6. Health Equity and Policy—UN-SDG#3—how this might apply to primary care and telemedicine programs, how is the research focusing on outcomes and measures of maturity and success in digital health systems, HHR building capacity within weakened HC systems, current challenges and research focus to improve allied and specially trained community health workers to support population health needs. Telemedicine can help address health disparities by increasing access to care in underserved populations. Research should be conducted to understand the barriers to telemedicine adoption and to develop policies and strategies to promote health equity and accessibility.
7. Clinical Outcomes and Cost-Effectiveness—Predictive Analytics—in relation to disease management, hospital to home, and public health needs within a geographic region. Research should be conducted to assess the clinical outcomes and cost-effectiveness of telemedicine interventions compared to traditional care. This evidence will be crucial in supporting the widespread adoption of telemedicine by healthcare systems, insurers, and policymakers.

By focusing on these areas of research, telemedicine has the potential to become more effective, accessible, and efficient, ultimately improving healthcare for millions of people around the world.

We will explore the specific use case of hypertension as it relates to telemedicine programs around the world looking at these examples and their relevance to family medicine.

28.4 The Case Study of Hypertension: The Global Epidemic Needing High Patient Volume–Low Physician Touch Solutions

The WHO defines primary care as the point of contact and entry to healthcare systems (10). McWhinney outlines several foundational principles for family medicine or primary care. One of those principles is:

> A Family Physician views his/her practice as a population at risk (3).

Certainly for patients under the umbrella of a primary care provider, the current digital health technologies may support population health programs to improve outcomes among patients with various noncommunicable diseases (NCDs) like diabetes or hypertension. Primary care providers may run EMR reports to determine the performance of their population programs, getting patients to target for various treatment guidelines.

How does this look on a global scale, however, and where might future research focus to improve healthcare outcomes in underserved regions or low middle income countries (LMICs)?

The current reality from World Bank and WHO statistics are that half the global population lacks access to proper healthcare … (11). The result is health inequity for diagnosing and treating conditions like hypertension for much of the global population.

Currently in the world, there are "More than 700 million people with untreated hypertension" (12).

The ability to treat this condition globally already falls short, especially in LMIC. There is added demand for healthcare workers to supply growing medical needs in most nations, and current shortfalls for the health human resource supplies are expected to grow. There is a predicted global shortage of healthcare staff by 2030 of 15 million, with the greatest burden upon LMIC (13).

The disparity of information communication technologies may not be as severe as the disparity for healthcare. In fact, the World Bank stats suggest nearly 70% of the poorest, 20% in developing countries have access to cellular technology (14), and 59% of the globe has Internet access such that 92% of that access is by mobile technology (15).

There are also challenges in defining and tracking the funding of primary healthcare given the disparity of definitions.

The Primary Care Spend model, shown in Fig. 28.1, is one proposal that tries to unify tracking health care expenditures agnostic of definitions of terms for primary care (16).

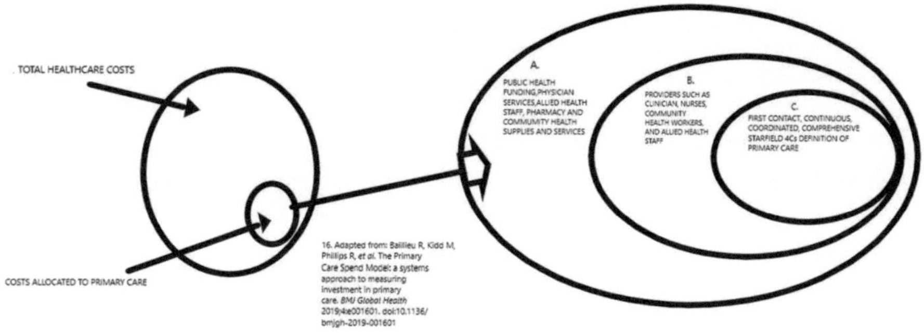

Fig. 28.1 The primary care spend model. (Adapted from Ref. Bailieu et al.)

The Primary Care Spend model, thus applied to the context of managing a disease such as hypertension, can highlight the challenges of managing this condition purely in the context of primary care providers being readily accessible and continuous contact within the patient journey, especially in regions of low provider to patient ratios. Regions of sub-Saharan Africa are below 1.2/10,000 population (17) and WHO guidelines suggest a minimum of 2.6/1000 (18).

Thus, it is easy to see the near impossible task to supply human health resources to manage NCD such as hypertension in these regions.

It is conceivable within a carefully structured program leveraging community health worker, or specially trained community workers armed with technology supports, one could provide the essential elements to treat the leading NCD of hypertension with minimal input from a primary care physician.

While regulatory requirements across the globe may allow only physicians to prescribe medications for the treatment of hypertension, decanting the initial screening and assessment to specially trained and technology supported community workers will improve the efficiency of primary care patient workflows and allow physicians to manage high-volume, low-touch patient populations, and essential need in regions with tens of thousands of patients per provider.

Cellular mobile technology is an ideal platform to partner with newer medical devices to measure blood pressure and screen for hypertension. Given over 1 billion people worldwide suffer from hypertension, it would be impossible to dispense cuff-based blood pressure measurement devices to everyone; however, it is much more conceivable to reach an exceptionally large portion of the hypertensive population in the globe using programs such as validated cloud-based software able to capture blood pressure readings using the ubiquitous technology of smart phones or any Internet connected device with a camera for Reflected Photoplethysmography systems currently being validated and tested for this model of population health. The democratization of web-based technologies like this would improve screening and monitoring of hypertension worldwide. Given 46% of patients are unaware they have the disease (19), we would expect improved outcomes in global management for this condition with improved access to the devices needed to monitor blood pressure measurements.

The other advantage to programs as cloud-based technology is the ability to capture large volumes of population health data. That data can be assessed anonymously and meet the regulatory requirements of each region for privacy and security and provide "snap shots" of population health within a given region. Health authorities could plan public health needs relevant to NCDs based upon dashboards created from the residents in the community scanning with software as medical device or wearables, thus providing real-time analysis of the population prevalence of NCDs like hypertension.

Social innovation is also a critical ingredient to successful population health, especially for LMIC. While in developed nations, patients have come to expect physicians to be the primary contact or entry point for any healthcare, clearly this is not the case in all regions of the world. It is not feasible for a single physician to provide adequate care to thousands of patients without access to allied health or collaborative care approaches. Nurses and pharmacists are key providers of healthcare in LMIC such as Africa. Organizations like Project Hope (20) and Path (21) have formalized stakeholder and partner business model funding with access to technology and social innovation such as training of community workers to improve healthcare equity in LMICs.

Programs such as "Digisahayam" under PHFI (22) have successfully demonstrated supporting remote telemedicine access into remote and underserviced regions of India. The Digisahayam platform provides not only telemedicine access but also arms community healthcare workers with AI-based decision support tools bring skill and expertise normally provided in the context of a physician encounter. The program is being scaled to other provinces and regions within India and globally.

While these models of primary care may well serve LMIC and marginalized populations, it does raise the question of task shifting and ultimately how decanting clinical tasks and workflows to other allied health professionals will impact family practice as a profession (23):

> Task shifting is an approach to help address the shortage of healthcare workers through reallocating human resources. Task shift from physicians to allied healthcare professionals in primary care appears to increase service provision and cost-effectiveness. Services shifted include the provision of care and coordination of patients with chronic diseases as well as independent prescribing.

We have learned from the pandemic that virtual care and its associated technologies are key ingredients to serving patient care needs outside of the normal face-to-face primary care workflows. The next obvious step is to address the healthcare inequity that results from the digital divides we are creating. We will need to improve access to care using mobile platforms, but partner those new digital workflows with socially innovative methods that allow for high-volume, low physician touch servicing of large populations.

The application of mobile technology to managing hypertension may also benefit developed nations. The ability to engage patients at home, point-of-care programs, may improve outcomes for conditions like hypertension and lower overall healthcare costs. A program called "Hello Heart" recruited patients with hypertension. "In this cohort study of 28 189 US adults with elevated blood pressure or hypertension participating in a hypertension self-management program with a blood pressure monitor and connected smartphone application with clinically based digital coaching, most participants achieved and maintained lower blood pressure during a follow-up period that lasted as long as 3 years" (24). The cost savings for this program over 3 years of follow-up were verified by a third-party program from the validation institute. The outcomes captured included reductions in BP, weight, and cholesterol profiles. The most significant findings, however, were the savings of 1865 USD per patient per year due to reduced cardiovascular events and a reduction in hospitalizations of 3 days per patient per year during the study duration.

While this study is not specific to family medicine, it is foundational research suggesting that digital health interventions for chronic disease management can have a significant impact on patient outcomes, both reducing disease complications as well as healthcare cost reductions.

This type of program should be replicated for other NCD programs within primary care. Facilitated by allied health professionals in the community, engaging patients where they live and work, moving primary care from the constraints of the office-based encounter will be the coming focus of further research and validation of both mobile health interventions and software as medical device technology applied to telemedicine programs.

This type of program is an example of reconciling one of the foundational principles of family medicine within the evolving digital ecosystem.

28.5 The Evolution of Homecare

Another foundational principle for family physicians defined by McWhinney is:

> The family physician sees patients in their homes (3).

Visiting patients via telemedicine during the pandemic became the defining moment for primary care around the globe. Unfortunately, there was little if any time for family physicians to prepare for the rapid shift to telemedicine. Similarly, there was little if any guidelines for appropriate use of telemedicine in the context of the types of medical visits performed by family physicians in their offices.

28.6 Conclusions

In this rapidly evolving era of telemedicine, as we stand on the precipice of technological advancement and global health paradigm shifts, it is imperative that we anchor our investigations in the core principles of primary care.

The journey through the landscape of telemedicine, from its theoretical underpinnings to the practical applications in managing noncommunicable diseases like hypertension, underscores the critical need for innovative research, equitable access, and adaptive healthcare models.

Our exploration has not only highlighted the promise of digital health technologies in enhancing patient outcomes and system efficiencies but also illuminated the significant challenges of the digital divide and healthcare equity.

As we chart the course forward, the synergy between technological innovation and primary care principles must guide our approach to telemedicine research. Embracing the potential of virtual and augmented realities, advanced connectivity, and wearable technologies, we must also remain steadfast in our commitment to patient-centered care, accessibility, and health equity. The examples of hypertension management through telemedicine offer a blueprint for addressing global health challenges, showcasing the potential to transcend geographical barriers and resource limitations. However, the success of these endeavors hinges on our ability to conduct robust, evidence-based investigations that not only validate telemedicine interventions but also ensure they are integrated seamlessly into the fabric of primary care.

In conclusion, the future of telemedicine in primary care is replete with opportunities and challenges alike. As we strive to harness the power of digital health, let us do so with a clear vision of improving healthcare delivery and outcomes for all, guided by the enduring values of equity, accessibility, and compassionate care. The journey ahead is not without its hurdles, but with collaborative efforts, innovative research, and a commitment to bridging the digital divide, we can unlock the full potential of telemedicine to revolutionize primary care for the betterment of populations worldwide.

References

1. World Health Organization, International Telecommunication Union. National eHealth strategy toolkit. Geneva: World Health Organization; 2012. https://apps.who.int/iris/handle/10665/75211. Last accessed 5 Feb 2023
2. Tracking universal health coverage: 2017 global monitoring report. World Health Organization and International Bank for Reconstruction and Development/The World Bank; 2017. Licence: CC BY-NC-SA 3.0 IGO.
3. Freeman T, McWhinney IR. McWhinney's textbook of family medicine. 4th ed. New York: Oxford University Press; 2016. p. 5–6–17–19. https://doi.org/10.1093/med/9780199370689.001.0001. Thomas R. Freeman
4. Lau F, Kuziemsky C, editors. Handbook of eHealth evaluation: an evidence-based approach [internet]. Victoria: University of Victoria; 2017. Available from: https://www.ncbi.nlm.nih.gov/books/NBK481590/
5. Office of the Assistant secretary for planning and evaluation; Assessment of approaches to the evaluation of Telemedicine. Available from: https://aspe.hhs.gov/reports/assessment-approaches-evaluating-telemedicine. Last accessed 25 Mar 2023.
6. Oliveira Hashiguchi T. Bringing health care to the patient: an overview of the use of telemedicine in OECD countries, OECD Health Working Papers, No. 116. Paris: OECD Publishing; 2020. https://doi.org/10.1787/8e56ede7-en.
7. Gussoni G, Manfellotto D, editors. Implementing decentralized clinical trials in Italy: why and how? Multistakeholder expert opinion on priorities for methodology, regulatory affairs, ethics and training. Verona: Fondazione Smith Kline; 2022. Tendenze Nuove – Special Issue 2/2022

8. Wise J. Shared decision making must move from rhetoric to reality, says king's fund. BMJ. 2011;343:d4734. https://doi.org/10.1136/bmj.d4734.
9. Brown D. A review of the PubMed PICO tool: using evidence-based practice in health education. Health Promot Pract. 2020;21(4):496–8. https://doi.org/10.1177/1524839919893361.
10. WHO online publications, Primary Care definition. Available from https://www.who.int/teams/integrated-health-services/clinical-services-and-systems/primary-care. Last accessed 8 Apr 2023.
11. WHO News release. Available from https://www.who.int/news/item/13-12-2017-world-bank-and-who-half-the-world-lacks-access-to-essential-health-services-100-million-still-pushed-into-extreme-poverty-because-of-health-expenses. Last accessed 8 Apr 2023.
12. World Health Organization. More than 700 million people with untreated hypertension [Internet]. 2021. Available from: https://www.who.int/news/item/25-08-2021-more-than-700-million-people-with-untreated-hypertension. Last accessed 9 Apr 2023.
13. Project HOPE. The global health worker shortage: 10 numbers to note [internet]. 2022. Available from: https://www.projecthope.org/the-global-health-worker-shortage-10-numbers-to-note/04/2022/. Last accessed 9 Apr 2023.
14. World Development Report 2016: Digital Dividends. Overview booklet. Washington, DC: World Bank. License: Creative Commons Attribution CC BY 3.0 IGO.
15. Internet users in the world 2021|Statista. Available from: https://www.statista.com/statistics/617136/digital-population-worldwide/. Last accessed 8 Apr 2023.
16. Baillieu R, Kidd M, Phillips R, et al. The primary care spend model: a systems approach to measuring investment in primary care. BMJ Glob Health. 2019;4:e001601. Available: http://www.euro.who.int/en/health-topics/Health-systems/primary-health-care/main-terminology. Last accessed 8 Apr 2023
17. WHO Global Health Observatory Data. Available from https://www.who.int/data/gho/data/indicators/indicator-details/GHO/medical-doctors-(per-10-000-population. Last accessed 8 Apr 2023.
18. WHO Publications – The World Health Report, October 2006. Available from https://www.who.int/publications/i/item/the-world-health-report%2D%2D-2006%2D%2D-working-together-for-health. Last accessed 8 Apr 2023.
19. WHO fact sheets- hypertension. Available from https://www.who.int/news-room/fact-sheets/detail/hypertension. Last accessed 8 Apr 2023.
20. Project Hope. Available from https://www.projecthope.org/. Last accessed 8 Apr 2023.
21. Path – Better Lives. Available from https://www.path.org/. Last accessed 8 Apr 2023.
22. Digisahayam: An assisted telemedicine solution [Internet]. Public Health Foundation of India and Centre for Chronic Disease Control; 2023. Available from: https://www.digisahayam.org/. Last accessed 5 May 2023.
23. Leong SL, Teoh SL, Fun WH, Lee SWH. Task shifting in primary care to tackle healthcare worker shortages: an umbrella review. Selangor: Faculty of Pharmacy, Cyberjaya University College of Medical Sciences; School of Pharmacy, Monash University Malaysia; Institute for Health Systems Research, National Institutes of Health; Asian Centre for Evidence Synthesis in Population, Implementation and Clinical Outcomes (PICO), Health and Well-being Cluster, Global Asia in the 21st Century (GA21) platform, Monash University; Faculty of Health & Medical Sciences, School of Pharmacy, Taylor's University; [date of publication].
24. Gazit T, Gutman M, Beatty AL. Assessment of hypertension control among adults participating in a mobile technology blood pressure self-management program. JAMA Netw Open. 2021;4(10):e2127008. https://doi.org/10.1001/jamanetworkopen.2021.27008.

MIX
Papier aus verantwortungsvollen Quellen
Paper from responsible sources
FSC® C105338

If you have any concerns about our products,
you can contact us on
ProductSafety@springernature.com

In case Publisher is established outside the EU,
the EU authorized representative is:
Springer Nature Customer Service Center GmbH
Europaplatz 3, 69115 Heidelberg, Germany

Printed by Libri Plureos GmbH
in Hamburg, Germany